Borders of Care

Borders of Care

Immigrants, Migrants, and the Fight for Health Care in the United States

BEATRIX HOFFMAN

The University of Chicago Press
Chicago and London

The University of Chicago Press, Chicago 60637
The University of Chicago Press, Ltd., London
© 2025 by The University of Chicago
Published 2025
Printed in the United States of America

34 33 32 31 30 29 28 27 26 25   1 2 3 4 5

ISBN-13: 978-0-226-82084-2 (cloth)
ISBN-13: 978-0-226-82086-6 (paper)
ISBN-13: 978-0-226-82085-9 (e-book)
DOI: https://doi.org/10.7208/chicago/9780226820859.001.0001

Library of Congress Cataloging-in-Publication Data

Names: Hoffman, Beatrix Rebecca, author.
Title: Borders of care : immigrants, migrants, and the fight for health care in the
    United States / Beatrix Hoffman.
Other titles: Immigrants, migrants, and the fight for health care in the United States
Description: Chicago ; London : The University of Chicago Press, 2025. | Includes
    bibliographical references and index.
Identifiers: LCCN 2024020845 | ISBN 9780226820842 (cloth) | ISBN 9780226820866
    (paperback) | ISBN 9780226820859 (ebook)
Subjects: LCSH: Immigrants—Medical care—United States—History. | Latin
    Americans—Medical care—United States—History. | Health services
    accessibility—United States—History. | United States—Emigration and
    immigration—Government policy.
Classification: LCC RA448.5.I44 H64 2025 | DDC 362.1086/9120973—dc23/
    eng/20240605
LC record available at https://lccn.loc.gov/2024020845

♾ This paper meets the requirements of ANSI/NISO Z39.48-1992
(Permanence of Paper).

For my students

Contents

Two Broken Systems

On September 9, 2009, President Barack Obama stood in front of the US Congress and made a promise. His new health care program, Obama announced, "would not apply to those who are here illegally." From the Republican side of the chamber came a shout: "You lie!" But it turned out that excluding undocumented immigrants was just about the only thing that the two parties could agree on when it came to health care reform. The final version of the law specified that undocumented people would not be allowed to obtain any coverage under the Affordable Care Act (Obamacare), even if they paid for it with no help from the government.

The exclusion of undocumented immigrants from health programs was nothing new. The approximately ten million undocumented people living in the United States are banned from Medicare and Medicaid, the two largest federally financed health insurance systems. Even *legal* immigrants are excluded from these programs for their first five years in the country. Some states offer limited coverage for undocumented children and pregnant women, but mostly undocumented people must rely on hospital emergency rooms or medical clinics that do not inquire about citizenship status. Because of the country's harsh system of immigration enforcement, immigrants and their families are often fearful of trying to access even the services they are legally entitled to. As a result, many receive no care at all. Both undocumented and legal immigrants have very low rates of insurance coverage, and they use less medical care than any other group in the country.[1]

Since undocumented immigrants make up a significant portion of the US population, and entire sectors of the economy are dependent on their labor, keeping them uninsured does not make sense from a public health perspective. Their exclusion from health care is an immigration policy, not a health policy. And attacking immigrants as a burden on medical resources, as many politicians do, deflects attention from our most pressing problem, which is that both the health care system and the immigration system are fundamentally broken.

Despite the coverage expansions of the Affordable Care Act, the US remains the only high-income nation that does not ensure that all of its citizens have access to health care. In 2020, twenty-eight million Americans under age sixty-five (8.6 percent) were uninsured.[2] Millions who *do* have insurance face high out-of-pocket costs and a shortage of primary care. Americans experience more medical debt and medical bankruptcies than anyone else in the world. The health care system is primarily run by private, profit-driven insurance, hospital, and pharmaceutical industries that use their political power to block meaningful reforms. Health care in the US is also embedded in the nation's long history of racial injustice, resulting in severe inequalities in access to care and higher rates of sickness and death for poor people and people of color.[3] Even before the COVID-19 pandemic, economic inequality and the lack of investment in public health were conspiring to bring down the average life expectancy in the US.[4]

If measured in dysfunction and human suffering, the immigration system is also a calamity. Although the US is known as a nation of immigrants, it should also be described as a nation of immigration control and restriction. Exemplified by the Chinese Exclusion Act of 1882 and the discriminatory national origins quotas of 1924, laws and practices for admitting and rejecting immigrants have been heavily based on race. Avenues for legal immigration are severely restricted, with waiting lists for applicants from certain countries measured in years and even decades, leading millions to attempt unauthorized border crossings.[5]

At the same time, the US has continually relied on immigrants as a low-paid workforce. Undocumented migrants make up a significant portion of workers in agriculture, construction, cleaning and maintenance, home health services, hotels, and restaurants. Essential sectors of the economy, especially food production and processing, would collapse without immigrant workers.[6] Intensified border controls, immigration policing, and a vastly expanded system of detention have not been able to stop the continual flow of undocumented or asylum-seeking arrivals, who come because of poverty, violence, and repression in their countries and the continuing demand for their labor in this country.

The immigration and health systems are also intertwined, in what might be called the immigration/health nexus. Most familiarly, immigrants have been associated with infectious diseases. The idea that foreigners will bring disease has been behind numerous immigration policies and practices, such as excluding people who are sick or disabled from entering the country, medical inspection and detention of migrants at borders, immigrant quarantines, and scapegoating immigrant groups as health threats. This nexus was starkly visible in the Title 42 policy, implemented under Trump and temporarily continued by Biden, that expelled millions of migrants in the name of preventing the importation of COVID. Yet public health research and history show that blaming immigrants for epidemics is scientifically incorrect and is not an effective public health strategy,[7] and also that the most significant threat to migrants' health comes *after* they have entered the US.[8] Policies like Title 42 pose as health laws but act as immigration restriction laws. Similarly, restrictive immigration laws have serious health consequences, as this book will show.

As a historian of the US health system, I began thinking about the immigration/health nexus while working on my previous book, *Health Care for Some*. As the title implies, in that book I argued that health care in the US is organized around exclusions. Instead of providing access for all, the country has rationed care and coverage based on factors like employment, income, race, location, and age. As well as letting many people fall through the cracks, the American way of rationing continually reinforces the idea that not everyone is deserving of inclusion or of good health. Immigration status provides another category for rationing. Just as I was finishing that earlier book, the exclusion of the undocumented from Obamacare was announced, and I knew that questions about the place of immigrants in the US health system would drive the research that has become *Borders of Care*.

The title of this book intends to capture the reality of rationing. People who cross national borders to enter the US face another border when they are in need of medical help: the many ways that care is fenced off. While this country hungrily ingests the labor power of immigrants to build and manufacture and serve in the lowest-paying and often most dangerous jobs, it refuses to accept responsibility for addressing the injuries, chronic conditions, and other health burdens resulting from that employment and the poverty that often accompanies it. The result is another border between people and the health care they need.

The US is not the only nation that benefits from the labor of immigrants while excluding them from most access to care. Countries with universal health systems also do so. Including all citizens in care can still mean the exclusion of noncitizens.[9] Even so, there is something distinctive about the US care/immigration nexus. The borders of care apply to people entering the country and to those already here. In the US, citizens as well as newcomers experience health care exclusion. For both citizens and immigrants, hospital emergency rooms are the only places where they are legally guaranteed access to care (and only within limits).[10] Both the health and immigration systems are preoccupied with drawing boundaries of deservingness. The suffering caused by health care denial and cost burdens is something that many citizens and noncitizens share. Understanding how immigrants in particular have experienced and responded to the rationing of care can help expose and undermine the broader premise of exclusion that warps the US health system.

This book narrates a national story across a broad sweep of time, from 1848 to the present, but with a focus on local examples that show how historical developments were shaped and experienced on the ground. Finding the sources to piece together this history was an adventure. There is no single archive on immigrant health care in the US. I delved into collections on immigration history to find references to health care, and health care history records to find references to immigrants. Most fruitful were the records of organizations and individuals who directly confronted the immigration/health nexus, ranging from activist physicians and nurses to the United Farm Workers of America. *Borders of Care* synthesizes this new primary source research with the work of many other historians and interdisciplinary scholars who have, over the past few decades, built the vibrant fields of migration studies, Latino and borderlands history, public health history, and the history of social movements.

In order to tell the story of the immigration/health care nexus and the borders that affect us all, this book highlights the themes of exclusion, inclusion, and activism. While the chapters proceed chronologically, these three themes (which often overlap) appear throughout.

Starting in the mid-nineteenth century, *exclusion* of immigrant populations from health care was accomplished through methods such as residency requirements; racial, ethnic, and language discrimination; bars on using public health programs; and the threat of deportation. Immigrants were forced into dangerous workplaces and overcrowded housing, and then blamed and stigmatized when they got sick. They were segregated into barrios, tenements, and Chinatowns that suffered from lack of services and government neglect. Mexican Americans and Mexican immigrants seeking medical care were targeted in the mass deportations of the 1930s and 1950s, and deportation was used as punishment for braceros (guest workers) who attempted to use their modest health insurance benefits. Immigrants with HIV were excluded from the country, prohibited from obtaining legal residency, and even placed in detention. State laws such as California's Proposition

187 attempted to ban health services for undocumented people, and federal Medicare, Medicaid, and Affordable Care Act rules excluded them. Governments, hospitals, and clinics used immigration enforcement as a weapon to prevent people from obtaining care. The immigration detention system has a long history of medical neglect and the denial of care.

Yet immigrants and migrants have also, at particular times and places, been *included* in health care. Religious orders and settlement houses cared for immigrant communities. Church groups and public health nurses provided services to migrant farmworkers, and the FDR and Kennedy administrations established federal programs for migrant health. Local governments looked the other way as public hospitals and clinics kept their doors open to undocumented patients. Federal community health centers and hospital emergency rooms became the only medical facilities required to treat people regardless of citizenship status. Some states made exceptions to Medicaid bans and created programs to cover undocumented children and pregnant women.

These avenues for access were always limited and inadequate, and too often they focused on protecting immigrants' and migrants' health only because it benefited employers or protected the public against alleged disease threats. Immigrants and migrants have rejected this instrumental definition of care and engaged in *activism* on behalf of both their own access to health, and the right to health for all. In the face of exclusion, they organized mutual aid societies and ethnic hospitals to provide their communities with medical care and benefits. They went on strike and organized unions to fight back against workplace conditions that were dangerous to their health. They fought to enter medical and nursing schools and become health care providers, and demanded rights to multilingual practitioners and interpreter services. They opened clinics that not only provided care to the underserved, but also included community members in health education and democratic governance.

In addition to the themes of exclusion, inclusion, and activism, this book shows how US health care and immigration policies have intersected and influenced each other. Health care policies often serve as proxies for immigration policies; the banning of undocumented immigrants from the Affordable Care Act is a clear example, because it supports an anti-immigrant agenda rather than a public health goal. And immigration policies aim to shape the health care system: the five-year waiting period imposed on legal immigrants' access to Medicaid, for example, was ostensibly intended to reduce health cost burdens on the federal budget. The immigration policies of deportation and repatriation have also been used as ways for hospitals and local health services to supposedly save money, by deterring or removing people who need expensive medical care.

Immigrants have been continually scapegoated as burdens on the health system. Yet the history uncovered in *Borders of Care* shows that the opposite is true. Exclusion, poverty, deportation fears, and racial discrimination prevented immigrants from getting care and kept their health care utilization rates low. At the same time, immigrants benefit and improve US health care. They provide a major financial contribution to the health system as well as to the economy, because they pay more in taxes than they use in services. Immigrant doctors and nurses fill critical shortages and provide care to underserved communities.[11] And immigrants' activism has, again and again, improved the overall health system for both citizens and noncitizens. For example, as this book will show, lawsuits brought by immigrants and migrants ended up establishing new rights to informed consent, local public health services, and emergency room access for everyone in the US.

Immigrants' roles in strengthening health and the economy have long been ignored or made invisible. For a short time, it seemed that the COVID-19 pandemic would finally bring their contributions to light. Immigrants made up a significant percentage of workers in industries that were defined as essential, including food processing, agriculture, and health care. As a result of their exposure on the job, noncitizen workers were disproportionately vulnerable to sickness and death from COVID. Immigrant workers got sick and died so that Americans could continue to have meat, fruits and vegetables, and medical services. Yet the sudden visibility of their sacrifices did not lead to easing immigration enforcement or expanding access to health care. Instead, both the Trump and Biden administrations doubled down on labor exploitation in the workplace and harsh controls on the border. Working people—citizen and noncitizen—were made even more vulnerable when pandemic safety protections and temporary sick leave and other workplace benefits ended. Due to continued gridlock in Congress, undocumented workers have not been rewarded with a path to citizenship or inclusion in health coverage. Until May of 2023, Title 42 continued to be used to expel migrants legally attempting to seek asylum at the border. Yet the US needs immigrant workers more than ever to address labor shortages and for its economy to function.[12]

This book seeks to use history to understand why and how the US continually requires the exploitation of immigrant and migrant workers, while also punishing them by putting their health at risk and refusing them care. And it tells a parallel story of how immigrants and migrants fought back, demanding and expanding rights to health, care, and dignity for all.

✲

The terminology and categories used in *Borders of Care* require some explanation. This book traces the history of groups that have been defined as immigrants, migrants, and/or noncitizens. In the word's most narrow definition, "immigrant" refers to people who come to the United States with the intention to settle permanently. "Migrants" are people who move around inside the country for work and also who come from other countries for work but intend to return home. Recently, the term "migrant" has been used even more expansively to include refugees and asylum seekers. While I try to be specific in describing people as immigrants, migrants, refugees, and so on, precision in terminology is not always possible, especially since an individual's or group's status can change depending on policy transformations and historical contexts.

The same is true of the categories "legal," "illegal," and "undocumented." Such categories are created and changed by laws and policies, and also by people's circumstances. For example, Chinese workers could enter the US as "legal" immigrants until 1882, when the Chinese Exclusion Act made many categories of Chinese arrivals "illegal." A Mexican bracero (guest worker) in the 1950s who labored "legally" on a US ranch could become an "illegal alien" if he remained in the country after his contract expired. (Although the word "undocumented," which is preferable to the derogatory designation of "illegal," was not widely used until the 1980s, I use that term rather than "illegal immigrant" or "illegal alien," except in direct quotes from primary sources, throughout the book.)

Borders of Care has "migrants" as well as "immigrants" in the book's subtitle to include not just refugees and asylum seekers, but also people who are US citizens but still migrate for work. Mexican Americans, Asian Americans, and Black Americans, as well as white Americans, have been important to the migratory agricultural workforce, at times toiling alongside workers from other countries. Puerto Ricans are US citizens, but they also migrate when moving from the island to the mainland.

Additionally, Mexican American populations who have lived in portions of the present-day United States for centuries are an important part of the story told in *Borders of Care*. Many Mexican people in the Southwest never migrated or immigrated; instead, when the US took over the region following its invasion of Mexico, "the border crossed them." Mexicans who became US citizens after the Treaty of Guadalupe Hidalgo in 1848 were not immigrants or migrants, but they started to be treated as foreigners or second-class citizens in their own land.[13] The fate of Mexican Americans has also been inextricably tied to that of Mexican immigrants and migrants. For this reason, Mexican Americans are included alongside immigrants and migrants as the subjects of this book. When making broad or conclusive statements, and in chapter titles, I sometimes use the term "immigrants" to encompass all these groups.

Borders of Care begins in the Southwest, where the border would violently change. Although long-term Mexican residents might not move physically after their land was taken by the United States, the creation and maintenance of borders still deeply affected them—and their health care.

1

Immigrant Health Threats, Immigrant Health Action

Borders Crossing People

In the centuries following the Spanish invasion and conquest of Mexico in 1521, the places now called California, Texas, New Mexico, Utah, Nevada, most of Colorado and Arizona, and parts of Wyoming, Kansas, and Oklahoma, all came under Spanish control. Mexico City was the populous and vibrant center of Spanish North America, while Texas and California were its remote frontiers.

Starting in the eighteenth century, Spanish priests and soldiers were sent north from Mexico to set up missions and military garrisons. Their brutal quest to extend Spain's reach included killing or capturing the Indigenous people of these regions, as well as compelling them to labor and to convert to Catholicism. Disease played a major role in the conquest, as some native populations were decimated by epidemics brought by the newcomers. To fully exploit the resources of the frontier, the Spanish forced Indigenous people to labor in construction, farming, and mining. In California, the mission system, which lasted until 1823, served as involuntary labor camps. Because of the missions' severe overcrowding, bad sanitation, and harsh labor conditions, the native people imprisoned there suffered shockingly high mortality rates.[1]

Health and medicine played additional roles in the conquest. Native Californians in the missions who tried to use their own healing techniques were punished. But, at the same time that they tried to suppress traditional medicine, the Spanish invaders adopted Indigenous practices that helped them survive the new climate and diseases they encountered in the frontier regions. Franciscan priests in California utilized Indians' knowledge of local plants to provide medical care in the missions. In the Texas region, Spanish newcomers learned from the Indigenous people that a tincture from the *chaparro amargosa* plant was effective against dysentery and that the *cenizo* flower (also known as Texas sage) could cure jaundice.[2]

On this frontier, "all but the largest towns and military posts lacked doctors and hospitals."[3] But in some surprising ways, the "North of Mexico" was also a region of medical progress and innovation, at least for its European population. Continuing epidemics of smallpox led the Spanish Crown to impose public health laws and practices, even in its most remote colonies. It had long been known that inoculation with fluid or scabs from infected people helped protect against that dread disease. In 1796 the Scottish physician Edward Jenner proved that the safer cowpox would have the same protective effect, and a few years later Spanish king Charles IV launched "the world's first immunization campaign," sending orphaned children vaccinated with cowpox (as conveyances for their lymphatic fluid) to all areas of the Spanish empire. The new vaccines arrived in Texas in 1805. They were administered in fort hospitals by military physicians and made available to the poor free of charge. There was some resistance to the vaccines in the frontier territories, but the campaign was highly effective in Bexar (San Antonio), the government center of Spanish Texas.[4]

A Spanish royal order also led to the opening of a frontier hospital in San Antonio in 1805. Apart from the rudimentary hospitals housed in military forts, this was the very first such institution in the present-day US west of the Mississippi. The hospital was set up in the Mission San Antonio de Valero, which would later be known as the Alamo. It was a military hospital for Spanish soldiers, but it also treated civilian residents of this town of around five thousand people.[5] By 1807, the San Antonio hospital had thirty beds and a pharmacy. Early residents of Texas were also protected by "certain wise sanitary regulations," including requirements for the removal and burial of dead animals.[6]

But war and invasion threatened health care for the settlers of Spanish Texas. The medical historian P. I. Nixon believes that the San Antonio hospital did not survive past 1812, because keeping it open was too expensive and also "Spain's hold on Texas was becoming less secure."[7] We do know that San Antonio was attacked by a joint US-Mexico paramilitary expedition in early 1813, a precursor of the events that would lead to Mexican independence from Spain in 1821 and, later, to the US takeover of the Southwest.

After 1821, the government of independent Mexico still emphasized public health. In the 1830s Mexico began requiring that all its soldiers, including those on the frontier, be supplied with mosquito nets. (Although this was long before mosquitos were understood as the vectors of malaria and yellow fever, the government wanted to protect its troops from annoying bites by the insects, with the unintended benefit of avoiding infection.) Frontier officials in San Antonio imposed rules for medical training and licensing. Mexico City sent updates to frontier governments on the continuing campaign against smallpox and ordered local officials to keep lists of vaccines administered.[8]

Mexico initially welcomed Anglo (white US) immigrants from the East to its northern territories, but it soon became evident that many of the newcomers were not interested in becoming Mexican; instead, they intended to purchase or take Mexican lands and expand slavery to the region. Most US colonizers (many of whom could be termed "illegal immigrants" under Mexican law) brought white supremacist beliefs and looked down on their Mexican hosts as racially inferior. Ignoring the region's attention to public health, they used the scarcity of formal medical care in Mexican Texas as part of their justification for racist views and practices.

In their accounts of life in Mexican Texas, Anglo migrants described a lack of doctors, hospitals, and pharmacies, and noted locals' reliance on traditional and self-help medicine.[9] Rather than seeing this as resourcefulness, they took it as evidence of backwardness. A "significant number" of migrants also exploited medical shortages by pretending to be doctors. Although few of them actually had medical training, "people in the region welcomed these presumed Anglo-American physicians," according to historian Jorge A. Hernández, because of their desire for more doctors.[10]

In one horrific example, two white colonists committed fraud and brutally exploited Mexican Texans' need for medical care. Anglo tobacco smuggler John Webber arrived in San Antonio in 1827 and, seeing that the town had "no regular physicians," pretended to be a doctor. He began seeing large numbers of patients and prescribing them "liberal" doses of tartar emetic, a chemical compound that led to violent vomiting. Another white migrant/colonizer, Noah Smithwick, accompanied Webber on his visits. Smithwick's description of the "doctor's" practice is grotesquely racist and reveals that Webber's intent was not just to deceive, but also to torture:

> I looked on the Mexicans as scarce more than apes and could with difficulty restrain my enjoyment at the situation when the medicine got in its work, seemingly turning the poor devils inside out, they meanwhile swearing and praying alternately. And I felt no twinge of remorse for the monstrous imposition we were practicing upon them when they finally emerged from the doctor's heroic treatment looking as dry and shrunken as so many pods of *chili colorado* (their favorite article of diet), and loaded him with thanks for his ministrations.[11]

Smithwick took the patients' thanks as evidence of their ignorance, but "he-roic" treatments like tartar emetic were also widely—if more judiciously—used by European and US physicians during this time period. The violent effects of purgatives and emetics were seen as proof of their effectiveness.[12] If residents of San Antonio sought "Doctor" Webber's treatments despite their awful effects, this was likely because they thought they were getting access to genuine medical care. We don't know how many patients sickened, died, or recovered following Webber's ministrations, but the story stands as testimony to the region's continuing demand for doctors and the colonizers' willingness to exploit it for profit. It is also a painful example of how medical "treatment" could be used for abuse rather than healing.

The United States relied on notions of Mexican inferiority as part of its justification for annexing Texas in 1845, invading Mexico in 1846, and taking control of all Mexican territories north of the Rio Grande in 1848. As histo-rian Mark Alan Goldberg argues, ideas about health and sanitation shaped how Mexican Americans in the Southwest were treated, and continued to be treated, after "the border crossed them." The region's poverty and lack of formal medical institutions provided ammunition for US settlers to portray Mexican residents as backward when it came to health. They attributed poor housing and lack of clean water to Mexican people's "dirtiness" and "indo-lence." US settlers and visitors to the Southwest noted how locals relied on medicinal plants, self-treatment, and religious practices to maintain health and attributed these practices to Mexicans being "superstitious" rather than to their efficacy or the lack of other medical options. At the same time, US arriv-als eagerly appropriated many Mexican traditional cures and local knowledge for their own medical care.[13]

Racist stereotypes solidified even in the face of Mexican Americans' con-tinued efforts to obtain access to better care. No formal medical training was available to them, but local residents welcomed the arrival of German immi-grant physicians to practice in Texas in the 1850s.[14] San Antonio still lacked a hospital, and in 1855, the Spanish-language newspaper *El Bejareño* pleaded for a remedy. Cholera was ravaging the Ohio and Mississippi valleys and had even arrived in New Orleans, the paper noted, and for San Antonio, "the dan-ger is imminent. . . . To us it seems that no institution is more vital than a hospital." The newspaper called for "all the classes of society to unite their strength to reach this important goal."[15]

San Antonio did establish a Board of Health in 1858. It's notable that this first Board of Health listed one member with a Spanish name, but by 1866 there were no longer any Spanish-surnamed members.[16] According to histo-rian David Montejano, by the mid-1850s "San Antonio had been half-deserted by its Mexican population," primarily due to the loss of their land (by both co-ercion and violence) and to relentless racial harassment.[17] Whatever window of opportunity had existed for a Mexican American resident to join the Board of Health swiftly closed. No permanent hospital would open in San Antonio until 1869.[18] By then, people of Mexican origin had become a minority in the city that had once been theirs.

For centuries, the Southwest and California have been home to Spanish-speaking people. Anglos immigrated there, and then, like the Spanish before them, invaded and took those lands for the United States. Mexican citizens in the region became US citizens, as stipulated in the 1848 Treaty of Guadalupe Hidalgo. Yet from that day forward, they were treated as "foreigners in their own land."[19]

Ideas about health and medicine played an important role in this transfor-mation of longtime residents into foreigners. The Anglo colonizers focused on how Mexicans and then Mexican Americans were medically different, whether due to their medical practices, shortages of hospitals and medical services, or their poverty and sanitary conditions. They ignored how wars and conquest had contributed to the region's medical scarcity and how Mexican governments and people had participated in vaccination campaigns, estab-lished and followed public health laws, and voiced demands for more hos-pitals and doctors. As historians have powerfully shown, their supposed medical difference also imprinted people of Mexican origin as racially distinct and inferior.[20]

This racial stigmatization had material—and medical—consequences for Mexican Americans. As the white populations of the Southwest and Cali-fornia grew, Mexicans were segregated into neighborhoods called *barrios* or *colonias*. *Barrios* were not only separated, but also suffered medical neglect and a lack of public health services.

In Santa Barbara, California, the Pueblo Viejo barrio was considered by city governments as "unworthy of municipal concern and taxpayer dollars," according to historian Albert Camarillo. When a diphtheria epidemic broke out in 1876, children of the neighborhood were not provided with medical care. In the 1890s, years after fire protection became a standard part of mu-nicipal services, the barrio still had no fire hydrants.[21] Historian Mario T. García describes how, in the early twentieth century, residents of the El Paso, Texas, barrio of Chihuahuita had to bathe in the river because they lacked an adequate supply of municipal water. Residents repeatedly petitioned the city for improvements, but the Anglo part of town got paved streets and side-walks several years before Chihuahuita did. The El Paso barrio also had no hospital.[22]

The few medical services that were available to people of Mexican origin were segregated and poorly funded. Starting in 1919, Los Angeles County established a system of municipal health centers. They did open some facilities in barrios, which became known as "Mexican clinics." In the Los Angeles neighborhood of Belvedere, historian Natalia Molina writes, a separate Mexican clinic was established so that the "white public would not have to attend the same clinic as the area's Mexican residents." Molina demonstrates that Los Angeles's Mexican clinics were clearly separate and unequal; they were given far less funding and resources than the clinics designated "for Americans only."[23]

As the El Paso barrio residents' demands show, people sometimes pushed back against segregation and neglect. A health rights movement would grow especially in California, a state with a long history of racial segregation and medical mistreatment of immigrants.

Chinese Immigration and Medical Discrimination

Starting with the Gold Rush in 1848, thousands of Chinese immigrants began coming to California. They filled crucial jobs in agriculture, mining, and building the railroads. Some worked as storekeepers and merchants. Chinese segregation was even more starkly drawn than that of Mexicans. In San Francisco, Los Angeles, and gold mining towns throughout the state, Chinese workers (most of whom were men) lived separately in "Chinatowns."

Even as Chinatowns became densely populated, their residents were denied basic health services. In San Francisco, Chinese people were barred from all hospitals and clinics, even though on arrival they were required to pay a "head tax" that funded the county hospital. In 1854, Presbyterian missionary William Speer, a champion of San Francisco's Chinese community, "pleaded with authorities" to spend some of the immigrants' head tax money on a permanent hospital for Chinatown, but his request was denied.[24]

Three decades later, a Chinese immigrant, Chun Chung, tried to challenge hospital discrimination. Chun was "poor and friendless" and required long-term hospital care for his phthisis (tuberculosis), but in 1881 authorities refused him admission at San Francisco's County Hospital due to his race. Apparently some of the doctors who witnessed his plight complained to the city government, and the mayor called a special meeting of the Board of Health to discuss the public hospital's practice of excluding Chinese patients.[25]

Even though one forward-thinking physician announced that he "thought a Chinaman had an equal right as anybody else to demand admission to the hospital," the San Francisco Board of Health ended up endorsing the hospital's policy of discrimination. They agreed with the views of another doctor at the hearing, who "deemed it an outrage to commingle Chinamen, suffering from sundry filthy and incurable diseases, with civilized citizens." The city would not leave such sufferers to die in the streets; instead it would send them to a separate outbuilding of the smallpox hospital, where a few Chinese patients and "an African" had already been placed. This building "could accommodate about 20 more," the Board of Health estimated. They did not mention the condition of the facility, whether adequate care was provided there, or whether it was wise to cram so many tubercular patients into the segregated space.[26]

Racial discrimination fueled a vicious cycle in which segregated Chinese communities increasingly suffered from overcrowding, poor sanitation, and lack of medical services. In turn, whites condemned all Chinese as "filthy," "uncivilized," and a threat to public health. These stereotypes were then used as justification for denying care and resources to Chinese residents. The movement for excluding Chinese from the country altogether was mostly driven by fears of labor competition, but stigmatizing Chinese people as disease carriers added to the racial hostility behind the exclusion drives.

The Chinese Exclusion Act, passed in 1882, banned Chinese laborers from immigrating to the US (there were exceptions for merchants and a few other occupational categories) and made all Chinese people ineligible for US citizenship, regardless of how long they had been in the country. In the words of historian Erika Lee, "The Exclusion Act marks the first time in American history that the United States barred a group of immigrants because of its race and class."[27]

Under the new exclusion regime, Chinese people who were already US residents needed special permission to return if they left the country. Along with new arrivals applying for entry under the law's exemptions, returning Chinese residents were subject to an arduous medical inspection and could be held indefinitely in detention barracks while their cases were scrutinized by officials. A negative decision meant deportation, no matter how long the applicant had lived in the US.

Arriving Chinese people could be excluded from entry if a medical examiner suspected them of carrying a parasitic or contagious disease, but the detention process itself often made healthy people sick. The building where immigrants and returning residents were confined after their arrival in San Francisco was notoriously overcrowded and unsanitary. Erika Lee tells the story of US resident Wong Fong, who returned from a visit to China in 1895. He was denied reentry and held in the barracks for several weeks. He then became extremely ill. Wong hired a lawyer to challenge his detention and

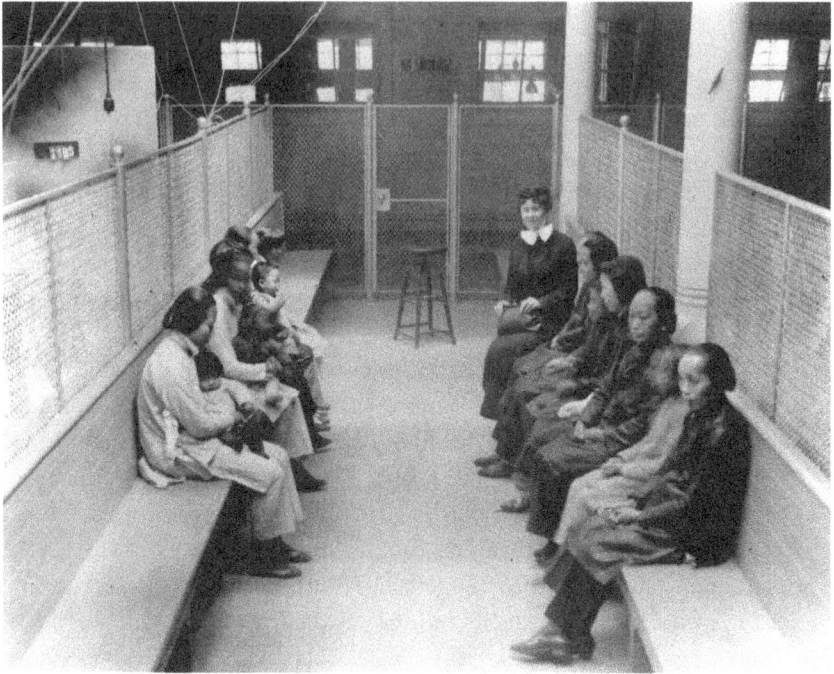

FIGURE 1.1. Angel Island Immigration Station, California, early twentieth century. A social worker meets with women and children held in a detention pen. US National Library of Medicine.

complained that authorities had refused his requests for Chinese herbs and medicines to alleviate his sickness. He lost his case, and the official who deported him mocked his illness and his dietary preferences.[28]

Chinese detainees were also denied medical care. In 1899, Ho Mun, a Chinese merchant arriving in San Francisco for the first time, was denied entry and "kept in the detention shed" where "he became seriously ill," but authorities "refused medical care for him for over two months," Lee recounts. "Ho's lawyers finally succeeded in moving him to the county jail, but he died a few days later." According to inspection reports, Ho's was not the only death caused by the unsanitary conditions in the San Francisco detention shed. Detainees continued to file complaints about overcrowding, sickness, and fire hazards until the facility—also known as the "Chinese jail"—closed in 1909.[29]

But inspections and detention of Chinese arrivals continued at Angel Island, the immigration facility in San Francisco Bay that operated from 1910 to 1940. Angel Island was the port of entry for all immigrants arriving on the West Coast, but Chinese people were detained much longer than other groups—two to three weeks that at times could "stretch into months." In 1924, the San Francisco–based Chinese Benevolent Association "bitterly complained to President Calvin Coolidge and Secretary of Labor J. J. Davis about the unhealthy conditions on the island which had allegedly caused several detainees to sicken and die." To fight for improvements, detainees formed their own advocacy group, the Angel Island Liberty Association. H. M. Lai writes, "As late as 1932, the Angel Island Liberty Association was forced to negotiate with the authorities to provide soap and toilet tissue for the detainees."[30]

These examples show not just how medical stigmatization was connected to medical abuse and neglect, but also that the Chinese community has a long history of protesting against this treatment. A notable number of detainees had legal representation. This was due to a strong infrastructure, based in Chinatown, of mutual aid and self-help organizations (mutual aid will be discussed later in this chapter).

European Immigration: Disease Threats and Public Charges

Between 1845 and 1849, a blight destroyed Ireland's potato crop. Nearly one million Irish people died of starvation or disease, and tens of thousands of poor tenant farmers were evicted and became homeless. This disaster led to a great wave of emigration. An estimated two million Irish left their country, including 1.5 million who came to the United States, joining an already significant Irish population in many US cities.[31] With the new wave of immigration, the Irish overtook the English and Germans to become the largest European immigrant group in the eastern US.

Many of the Irish newcomers arrived sick. They were already weakened by famine, and the crowded and perilous ocean voyage subjected them to outbreaks of contagious disease aboard ship. Although the vast majority survived their journeys, the vessels crammed with poor immigrants became known as "Coffin Ships" because of their association with disease and death.[32]

Like Mexicans in the Southwest and Chinese in California, Irish immigrants were stigmatized as carriers of disease. Their sickness was blamed on their behavior or inherent racial tendencies, not the conditions of poverty, famine, or overcrowding that they suffered. When large numbers of Irish New Yorkers died during the cholera epidemic of 1832, the Board of Health attributed their vulnerability to their "intemperance and lack of cleanliness." That terrible epidemic led many Americans to associate cholera with the Irish, a population already under suspicion for their Catholicism.[33]

To address fears that Irish immigrants would bring cholera and other diseases into the country, New York and Boston strengthened the quarantine facilities at their ports of entry. Quarantining of ships (holding them in port for a number of days before allowing cargo or people to leave) was a significant public health activity of local governments in the nineteenth century. Espe-cially following the yellow fever epidemic of 1793, which originated in Phila-delphia's busy port, officials focused on foreign ships as the source of deadly diseases. The influx of large numbers of poor Irish people shifted their con-cern from cargo to humans. In New York, immigrants were inspected upon arrival, and if they showed signs of sickness, they were sent to one of New York's quarantine hospitals.

Due to fears of contagion, quarantine hospitals were located in remote parts of town, including Ward's Island (in the East River) and Staten Island. Sick immigrants became virtual prisoners there. It is notable, however, that these facilities were called "hospitals." Unlike the detention sheds of San Fran-cisco, it seems that quarantine hospitals did actually provide some medical and nursing attention to their inmates.[34] Still, the facilities were primarily cus-todial; rather than treating disease, their primary purpose was to segregate immigrants from the local population.

Quarantine hospitals were sites of mistreatment as well as care and con-finement. In 1856, according to historian Hidetaka Hirota, Irish American newspapers published exposés of abuse and neglect of immigrants at the Ward's Island quarantine hospital, including a report that an Irish patient suffered an assault by two hospital staff. The *New York Citizen* newspaper informed readers that quarantined immigrants at Ward's Island, "including women with infant children[,] were 'left destitute of food for days' and 'sick passengers are very grossly maltreated.'"[35]

Local residents were aware that quarantine hospitals contained sick immi-grants, and they feared and resented having such facilities in their midst. Staten Island citizens even rioted and burned down their famous quarantine hospital in 1858.[36] The existence of immigrant quarantine hospitals further added to the stigmatization of groups like the Irish as inherently diseased and unwelcome in American society.

As Irish neighborhoods grew due to the famine migration, they contin-ued to suffer epidemics of sickness, including cholera and typhus. The actual causes of these diseases—contaminated drinking water and body lice—were not known at the time, but it was obvious that outbreaks were concentrated among poor people who were crowded together, whether in a ship's hold or in a tenement building. Some immigrants who passed their initial inspec-tion may actually have had undetected contagious diseases on arrival, but many Irish were also sickened by the conditions in their new neighborhoods, homes, and workplaces. As one contemporary described it, New York City's huge and growing immigrant population lived in "filth, overcrowding, excre-ment, putrid exhalations, and disease."[37]

When immigrants became sick, many could no longer work or care for their families, and ended up in the city's hospitals and almshouses (poorhouses). Hospitals were still primarily places for the sick poor, where they could be removed from the community and also serve as "teaching material" for physicians and medical students. By the 1850s, the vast majority of hospital patients in New York, Philadelphia, and Boston were Irish immigrants.[38]

Immigrants' high rates of hospitalization led to another type of stigma. People who became dependent on charity or government assistance, including public hospitals, were defined as paupers or "public charges." During the great wave of Irish immigration, as Hirota has shown, local governments increasingly used public charge accusations to deport significant numbers of immigrants. In Massachusetts, state immigration officials would raid hospitals and poorhouses, bodily remove sick and disabled immigrants, and put them on ships heading back across the Atlantic.[39]

State deportations of pauper or public charge immigrants influenced the federal Immigration Act of 1882, which was passed by Congress the same year as the Chinese Exclusion Act. These laws marked the beginning of full federal control over immigration. The 1882 act stated that an immigrant "unable to take care of himself or herself without becoming a public charge" should be excluded from entering the US. A few years later, the Immigration Act of 1891 provided funds for deporting public charge immigrants already in the country. Although public charge designations would not be extensively used for deportations or repatriation until the 1930s, thousands of would-be immigrants were excluded for this reason every year.[40]

In 1892, the Ellis Island Immigration Station opened in New York harbor, with an expanded system of medical inspection. This coincided with a great wave of new immigrants from southern and eastern Europe. Like the Irish before them, Russian Jews and Italian Catholics were feared as potential importers of disease. Immigrants dreaded the infamous inspections, but only a small percentage of people arriving at Ellis Island were completely excluded for medical reasons.[41]

Southern and eastern European immigrants were not yet restricted from entry solely because of their race or country of origin, but their experiences at Ellis Island in some ways reflected those of Chinese immigrants on the West Coast. They were more subject to detention and quarantine than their wealthier or northern European counterparts. Poor passengers in steerage (third class) were treated differently than first- and second-class arrivals. For example, during a cholera epidemic in 1892, Russian Jewish passengers who arrived in steerage were forced into a heavily overcrowded quarantine facility, where the conditions ended up giving many of them the disease, and forty-four of them died. First-class passengers from the same ship were only briefly quarantined in a luxury hotel.[42] Restrictive measures intended to prevent epidemics could end up making previously healthy immigrants sick or even killing them.

And, like the Chinese organizations and the Irish American press, newer immigrant groups spoke out against discrimination. In 1892, New York's Yiddish-language newspapers protested the treatment of Russian Jews during the cholera scare, complaining that the quarantined were exposed to disease and subject to "murderous injustice and inequalities."[43] Another way that immigrant communities tried to push back against pervasive medical discrimination was by creating their own health care institutions.

Origins of Access: Immigrant and Ethnic Hospitals

The first hospitals in the American colonies were opened in the eighteenth century by Protestant denominations in cooperation with local governments. Both the more prestigious hospitals like Pennsylvania Hospital in Philadelphia and huge free urban hospitals like Bellevue in New York were founded and run by local elites. These hospitals might care for immigrants, but that was not their explicit purpose.

This began to change in the 1830s with the appearance of Catholic hospitals. Catholic nuns had provided medical and nursing care since colonial times, but the growth of US Catholic communities due to immigration led religious orders to begin creating their own freestanding medical institutions. Mullanphy Hospital in Saint Louis, Missouri, opened in 1832, was the first private Catholic hospital in the US; by 1885, the country had 154 of them.[44]

The opening of Philadelphia's first Catholic hospital was a direct response to the rise in Irish immigration. In the 1840s, sick and poor immigrants overflowed the city's two existing hospitals. Philadelphia's Irish community came under attack when anti-Catholic riots broke out in 1844. The city's Catholics came together to provide support for refugees from the Irish famine and also to organize against the riots and discrimination. Their work culminated in the incorporation of Saint Joseph's Hospital in 1849. Philadelphia's *Catholic Herald* newspaper explained why a hospital was an important institution for new immigrants: "Many arrive . . . in the most destitute condition—debilitated by disease incident to a long voyage, in a crowded vessel." A Catholic hospital would provide "the best medical aid," away from "the contagious atmosphere of the crowded rooms in which [immigrants] are so often obliged to congregate."[45]

Hospitals for Jewish communities in the US were also founded as a response to immigration and discrimination. As historians Alan and Deborah Kraut write, "Jewish hospitals have a venerable history arising from the twin traditions of community self-help and resistance to anti-Semitism." Anti-Semitism prevented many Jewish physicians from obtaining hospital appointments, so Jewish hospitals were intended to provide professional opportunities as well as patient care. The first Jewish hospital in the United States opened in Cincinnati, Ohio, in 1850, following a cholera epidemic. New York's famed Mount Sinai Hospital was founded in 1852, and Chicago's Michael Reese Hospital in 1872. The largest wave of Jewish hospital building came during the 1890s with the new immigration of Jews from Russia and other parts of eastern Europe. By the early twentieth century, there were 113 Jewish hospitals in the US.[46]

These hospitals intended to combat discrimination and also to protect cultural traditions that were under threat. Jewish leaders argued that members of their communities should not be subject to the nonkosher diets and Christian proselytizing that they experienced in Protestant- and Catholic-run hospitals. Patients would benefit from being treated by doctors and nurses who spoke their own language, whether German, Russian, or Yiddish. In Jewish hospitals, patients who died would also be protected from autopsy and burial practices that violated their religion.[47]

Ethnic and religious hospitals maintained immigrant difference but could also open a path to immigrant assimilation or acculturation (blending in with the dominant US society and culture). Hospitals were prestigious institutions that signaled a community had "arrived." Campaigns to build and maintain hospitals demonstrated immigrants' desire for acceptance into mainstream American life. For example, in 1923 Boston's Italian-language newspaper praised the community members who had contributed to a hospital fund. An Italian American hospital, the newspaper assured donors, would not only provide medical care but "will have a tendency to help our race in this country."[48] In this way, immigrant hospitals were similar to the hospitals founded by Black Americans at the end of the nineteenth century in response to Jim Crow and as part of explicit campaigns of "racial uplift."[49]

Hospital building campaigns also created and strengthened an immigrant elite, including physicians, philanthropists, and hospital administrators. These leaders tended to be longer-settled assimilated or first-generation immigrants who felt they had a duty to uplift the less fortunate newer immigrants. Ethnic and religious hospitals were not established or controlled by the patients they intended to serve: the poor, workers, and new arrivals. And most of these hospitals moved away from their initial focus on the poor and ended up providing only a limited amount of care to those most in need. Hospitals were expensive to build and maintain, and by the end of the nineteenth century, formerly "charity" hospitals were admitting greater numbers of patients who could pay. Increasingly, poor immigrants had to rely on public hospitals and clinics, rather than the hospital named for their church or homeland.[50]

Attempts by immigrants to establish hospitals were sometimes met with resistance. This was especially the case when the immigrant group was stigmatized as racially distinct, excludable, and a threat to public health. For the Chinese in San Francisco, their campaign to build a hospital was inseparable from their fight against racial discrimination and immigrant exclusion.

As mentioned earlier, Chinese immigrants arriving in San Francisco had to pay a tax for a city hospital that they were not allowed to use, and hospitals and tuberculosis sanatoriums refused to admit Chinese patients. In 1875, the Chinese community tried to organize its own hospital in Chinatown, but the city denied permission. A second attempt in 1888 to build a Chinese hospital on the outskirts of the city was also turned down, as was a hospital building effort by Protestant missionaries and the Chinese consulate in 1899.[51]

Chinatown was already home to flourishing Chinese apothecaries (pharmacies) and practitioners of traditional medicine. By 1856, there were fifteen drug stores and five Chinese doctors in the neighborhood. Although the American Medical Association labeled Chinese practitioners as "irregular" and "quacks," many white residents of San Francisco visited the area to utilize their services, which were less invasive and more affordable than Western doctors'.[52]

In February of 1900, neighborhood leaders succeeded in opening a free clinic in Chinatown called the Tung Wah Dispensary. Tung Wah provided both traditional Chinese medicines and Western treatments, and it was staffed by both Chinese and white practitioners. The dispensary also employed a full-time interpreter to help with communication between the English-speaking doctors and Chinese patients. Although both Chinese and Euro-American donors funded the hospital, its board of directors was entirely Chinese.[53]

The clinic's opening coincided with the announcement that a Chinese worker in the city had died of bubonic plague. Believing that Chinatown was the origin of the disease, San Francisco authorities quarantined the neighborhood and ordered Tung Wah physicians to report all suspicious cases and to release any dead patients for autopsy. But clinic staff pushed back against the city's attempts to associate the disease with their community. They insisted that there was no plague in Chinatown, and they fought to keep control of death certificates and to protect residents from autopsies, which the community viewed as a desecration of bodies. Although a handful of plague cases did

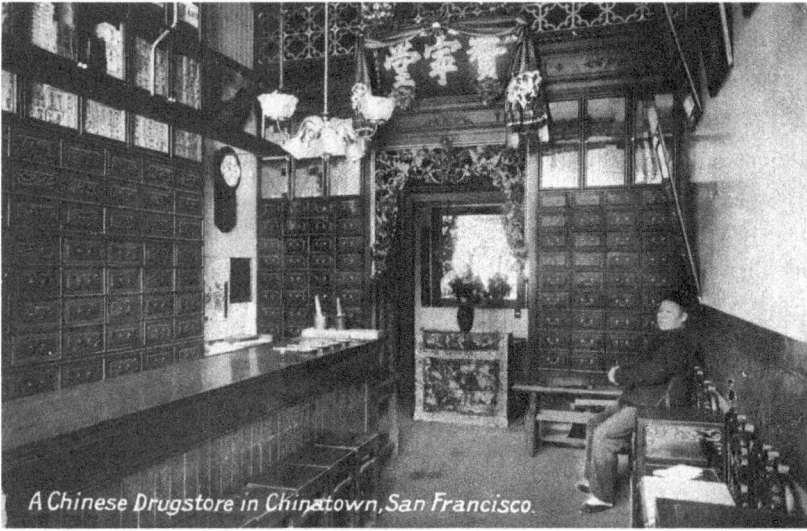

A Chinese Drugstore in Chinatown, San Francisco.

FIGURE 1.2. A Chinese drugstore in Chinatown, San Francisco, 1800s. US National Library of Medicine.

appear at the clinic in subsequent years (the disease was present in California until 1905), by resisting the city's most draconian measures Tung Wah had demonstrated its new role in the medical leadership of Chinatown.[54]

Chinese community leaders continued to raise funds to expand the Tung Wah clinic into a "modern hospital." In 1925, they finally succeeded with the opening of a five-story, fifty-five-bed Chinese Hospital in the heart of Chinatown. Like Tung Wah, the Chinese Hospital was staffed by both Chinese American and white physicians. To accommodate a continuing suspicion of Western medicine among Chinatown residents, the hospital also supported a free clinic run by traditional practitioners. The Chinese Hospital flourished and continues to exist in San Francisco today.[55]

Like the Chinese, Jews, and African Americans, Mexican residents and immigrants suffered severe medical neglect and segregation. However, they were less successful in establishing hospitals as part of their efforts against discrimination. Primarily, this was due to their status as a colonized people. After the US takeover in 1848, California's Mexican population experienced a devastating loss of land and power. A small elite remained, particularly in fast-growing Los Angeles. In 1856, a group of nuns from the Maryland-based Daughters of Charity of Saint Vincent DePaul arrived in Los Angeles. The city fathers, who included both Anglos and Californios, the longtime Spanish-speaking residents, "pledged money and support in raising a countywide subscription" for a hospital. The sisters opened an orphanage, and then a charity hospital in 1859.[56]

Yet, by the end of the century, this first city hospital (called variously the Los Angeles Infirmary, the Sisters Hospital, and Saint Vincent's) ended up serving only a small number of Mexican American patients. The dilution and disempowerment of Spanish-speaking elites due to the colonial takeover after 1848 helps explain why Los Angeles's Catholic hospital did not have a Mexican identity.[57] In the 1920s, as the city's Mexican population blossomed, Mexican American civic leaders again called for a hospital for their own community but were not able to raise sufficient funds.[58] Mexican residents and immigrants would turn their focus to building mutual aid institutions to partly address the lack of medical services in their communities.

Where they existed, ethnic hospitals were limited in their ability to address immigrants' health needs and push back against medical discrimination. Often, they reinforced class hierarchies and adopted the moneymaking ethos required to survive in the US hospital system. Yet in some ways, ethnic and religious hospitals founded by and for immigrants contributed to the expansion of health care access for all. Early Catholic hospitals, writes Gail Farr Casterline, "made a genuine contribution to civic welfare in areas where few municipal services existed." Historian Charles Rosenberg notes that "the new ethnic hospitals would expand the categories of those treated: many, for example, made a point of admitting chronic, and often aged, patients, a group generally excluded by the older private hospitals." Ethnic hospitals also opened their wards to cancer, contagious, and tuberculosis (TB) patients. Tung Wah clinic in San Francisco treated many patients with TB. When Jewish organizations in Denver, Colorado, began fundraising to open a tuberculosis hospital in 1889, "no institution in Denver would admit penniless consumptives, and many poor victims of the disease lived and died on the city's streets." While breaking down ethnic barriers and building communities, hospitals founded by and for immigrants also sought to erode discrimination based on health conditions.[59]

Care in the Community: The Henry Street Settlement and Public Health Nursing

In 1893, two recent graduates of the New York School of Nursing moved to the city's Lower East Side. Lillian Wald and Mary Brewster intended to open a settlement house, where nurses and social workers would live among and serve the immigrant residents of the neighborhood. Settlement houses began as a social reform movement in England in the 1880s, and Jane Addams had founded the most famous American settlement, Hull House, in Chicago in 1889. Wald and Brewster were inspired by these models, and as nurses they made health care the centerpiece of their Henry Street Settlement.

Wald was from an affluent German-Jewish family that had been in the US since 1848. German-Jewish immigrant financier Jacob Schiff supported Wald's goals and helped her purchase the building that would become the Henry Street Settlement. At the height of southern and eastern European immigration, the Lower East Side of New York City was the largest immigrant neighborhood in the world. German immigrants first settled there in the 1850s due to the growing number of jobs in garment factories. By the 1890s, the neighborhood was home to hundreds of thousands of Jews, Italians, and Irish, living in densely packed tenement apartment buildings.

The Lower East Side was viewed as a ghetto where immigrants lived in squalor and posed a threat to the general public's health. During infectious disease outbreaks, New York health authorities targeted the neighborhood's Jews and Italians for quarantine and detention in contagious disease hospitals.[60] Lillian Wald brought a different vision to the problem of poor health on the Lower East Side. Like other Progressive reformers, she argued that poverty and illness stemmed from social conditions, not from individual morality or racial characteristics, and that these conditions should be addressed by both philanthropic work and government action. The activity she named "public health nursing"—nurses visiting the poor in their homes—would, she believed, both save lives and lead to social change.[61]

Henry Street nurses climbed steep tenement stairs and traversed the roofs of apartment buildings to reach as many families as possible. In 1913, they made two hundred thousand visits to 22,168 patients—more than were served by the Lower East Side's hospitals. Their nursing care was so effective in reducing mortality rates that the Metropolitan Life Insurance Company contracted with Henry Street to provide nurse visits to their low-income policyholders as a way of saving money for the company. Henry Street ran its own tuberculosis surveillance and control program before the city of New York did. Henry Street nurses also conducted inspections of factories and other workplaces and examined workers for health problems.[62]

A 1921 Henry Street survey of a new block under its jurisdiction described the conditions their nurses encountered. The block was home to over 1,200 people in 344 families, mainly Irish and Italian (mostly Sicilian). The survey found unemployment to be "acute" in thirty families; in some households "they seem to be living on credit from the neighboring stores." In the apartments, few rooms had windows; there were no bathtubs, and hallway toilets were shared among families. Only three houses had electric lights, and only one had hot water.[63]

In a single month, the Henry Street nurse assigned to this block provided bedside care for a myriad of medical conditions: "one with diagnosis of bronchial asthma and two with mal-nutrition and gastritis," one patient with acute bronchitis, one with scarlet fever, and one case of osteomyelitis. "Three deaths have occurred on the block last month, one an adult with diphtheria, one a child with chronic cardiac valvular disease and acute rheumatic fever, and one a baby of five months with pneumonia."[64] Virtually all of these health problems were preventable and could have been alleviated by less crowding, better ventilation and sanitation, adequate food, and regular medical care. A subsequent editorial in *Henry Street Nurse* stated, "Having to grapple each winter with a pneumonia epidemic largely due to overcrowding," nurses know "that a large proportion of diseases can be laid at the door of poor living conditions. . . . As public health nurses . . . we plead on the grounds of health for better tenements."[65]

Visiting nurses also encountered families who needed help navigating the immigration system, especially its targeting of poor people via public charge accusations. One Italian woman, who had been in the country for only six months, ended up without her husband when he was "sent to Ward's Island as incurable insane." She was pregnant and already had two little girls. Her case was reported to the Department of Public Charities, and since her husband had become a public charge, the family "required immediate deportation." But advocacy by Henry Street succeeded in getting the deportation order withdrawn. To avoid further public charge accusations against the family, Henry Street nurses made sure to deliver the woman's baby at home, rather than sending her to a taxpayer-supported hospital.[66]

Lillian Wald's vision proved transformative. From providing one-on-one care to patients at their bedsides, Henry Street's activities grew to form the basis of significant municipal and labor reforms. Looking back on the settlement house's achievements in 1934, a nursing journal noted that "milk stations, first aid rooms, the Bellevue School of Midwifery, school nurses, tuberculosis oversight in the home, tenement house inspection, social services at city hospitals—all grew out of private demonstrations by Henry Street nurses which were later taken over as city functions."[67]

But, like ethnic hospitals, settlement houses were provided *for* immigrants, not primarily *by* them. Wald and many donors were assimilated Jews, and Henry Street's nurses were almost entirely native-born white middle-class women. Few, if any, spoke Yiddish, Italian, or the other languages needed to

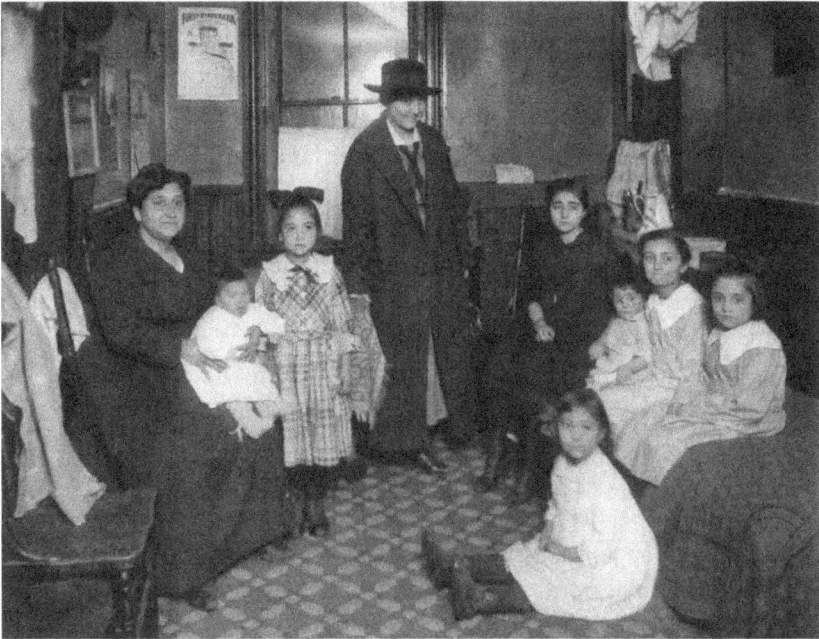

FIGURE 1.3. A public health nurse and the Italian family she cared for during the influenza pandemic, Boston, 1918. The father had died of the flu. James V. Donnaruma Papers, Box 2, Folder 11, Immigration History Research Center Archives, University of Minnesota.

communicate with their charges. In their newsletters, Henry Street nurses even poked fun at immigrants' accents and their charming malapropisms. (One nurse reported a conversation with an Italian patient's friend in this way: "She no spik English . . . I spika good English. I talka for her. She wanta know what's the temper-fever?")[68] At the same time that they pushed for housing and workplace reforms, visiting nurses also tried to change their immigrant patients' behaviors and to combat their "ignorance." Nurses and social workers came from outside to live in the neighborhoods they served; settlement houses were not started or run by members of their own communities. But there was another type of organization that did prioritize immigrant empowerment: the mutual aid society.

Immigrant Self-Help: Mutual Aid

Mutual aid is a form of self-help in which people with something in common—a craft, trade, religion, ethnicity, neighborhood, and so on—combine resources to provide support and assistance to each other. The practice can be traced back to diverse origins, including medieval guilds in Europe and cooperative savings societies in West Africa.[69] Unlike philanthropy or welfare, mutual aid is not dependent on donations from the wealthy or help from the government.

The earliest mutual aid societies in what is now the United States were founded in New Mexico "almost immediately after the Spanish arrived," in 1598. These societies, according to historian José Amaro Hernández, were called *cofriadas* or *confraternidades* (lay brotherhoods) and were primarily religious, but they also assisted their members with some "basic needs," including care "for the sick and needy."[70] We don't know what this care consisted of, since early societies left very few records.

Two centuries later, in 1794, Spanish settlers founded Los Penitentes (Confraternity of Brothers of Our Father Jesus of Nazareth) in Santa Fe, New Mexico. It swiftly spread to become the largest mutual aid society in the region. Hernández estimates that membership may have been as high as two-thirds of the entire Spanish population of what are now New Mexico and Colorado. Although it was still mostly for religious activities, Los Penitentes also pooled its members' resources to provide funeral benefits. (The fear of death without a decent burial was one of the strongest motivations for mutual aid in poor communities). Like many mutual aid societies, Los Penitentes was all male, but it did have women's auxiliaries, known as *auxiliadora de la morada* (auxiliary of the lodge). The women's activities included "nursing the sick," but again, records don't give details on the care they provided.[71]

After 1848, mutual aid societies provided both continuing protection and ethnic solidarity for Mexican Americans, and essential support for new immigrants from Mexico. Starting in the 1890s, Mexican immigrants founded hundreds of local societies in Texas and Arizona. These were based not on religious orders but on Mexican *mutualistas*, which were organizations of workers, and some even functioned as trade unions.[72] As Mexican immigrants increasingly settled in the Midwest to take industrial jobs, they brought the *mutualista* idea with them. In 1925, the researcher Paul Taylor counted thirty-five Mexican mutual aid societies in Chicago, Illinois, and Gary, Indiana, alone.[73]

Like ethnic hospitals, many *mutualistas* were formed as a community response to discrimination. As xenophobia and attacks on Mexican Americans intensified in the late nineteenth century, the mutual aid society became an instrument of protection against violations of immigrants' civil rights. For example, after Arizona in 1914 passed legislation limiting the number of Spanish-speaking workers that businesses could hire, the Liga Protectora Latina mutual aid society was flooded with new members. In Texas, a wave of violence and lynching against Tejanos in the 1910s spurred the organizing of several new *mutualistas*.[74]

The *mutualistas'* ethnic and political solidarity function has overshadowed their role as medical providers, but it appears that most of them offered some sort of health care benefits. Death benefits (life insurance) were extremely important to members, but so were sick benefits—a small payment if the member couldn't work due to illness. Societies employed doctors to examine members who claimed sick benefits. The Alianza Hispano Americana, an Arizona *mutualista* founded in 1894, offered "money to pay for doctor's fees and medicine," as well as unemployment and disability benefits.[75] Medical discrimination played a role in the *mutualistas'* popularity; for example, commercial insurance companies refused to sell life insurance to Mexican Americans "because it was believed that they all had tuberculosis."[76] Also, it seems that *mutualistas* did not discriminate based on citizenship; the Alianza Hispano Americana enrolled both US- and Mexican-born members.[77]

Another important mutual aid society, the Cruz Azul Mexicana (Mexican Blue Cross), expanded throughout the Southwest during the 1920s. The Cruz Azul was founded by Mexican women in San Antonio, Texas, to assist the poor of the community. It was distinct from other *mutualistas* not just because it was founded and controlled by women, but also because it received direct support from the government of Mexico via the Mexican Consulate. In 1924, the Cruz Azul in San Antonio raised enough funds to open a free medical clinic. However, an attempt in Los Angeles to open a clinic based on the San Antonio model foundered when organizers weren't able to get enough support from local physicians.[78]

Mutual aid also became a fixture of life for European immigrants in the Northeast. The region had a long tradition of self-help organization, starting with free Black people in Philadelphia, who founded the Free African Society in 1784. German Jews had banded together since at least the 1840s to provide medical care to their less fortunate compatriots. In 1843, the German Society in New York City recruited German-speaking physicians who "agreed to treat the poor gratis upon presentation of a certificate of need" issued by the society. In the early twentieth century, the Hebrew Sheltering and Immigrant Aid Society provided newly arriving Jews with "excellent baths" and a "physician and a nurse," all at no cost.[79]

During the new immigration of the 1890s, mutual aid among eastern European arrivals boomed. By the early twentieth century, thousands of *Landsmanshaftn*—associations of immigrants from the same hometown— "enrolled a quarter of New York Jews."[80] A major reason for the popularity of the *Landsmanshaftn* was that, in addition to providing life insurance and sick benefits, they developed systems of prepaid medical care for their members. In what the medical profession called (and often derided as) "contract practice," each society hired its own doctors. So, "for the cost of just one or two visits ($2–3) from a private physician, a working-class family secured the services of a society doctor for the entire year," writes historian Daniel Soyer. These physicians had to work hard: as Soyer describes it, "In addition to office hours . . . the societies required their doctors to make house calls." Like the Henry Street nurses, *Landsmanshaftn* MDs found themselves "forced to climb up and down tenement stairs in the Lower East Side, Harlem, and Brooklyn." Some *Landsmanshaftn* also provided members with sanatorium treatment for tuberculosis, and a few even opened their own hospitals.[81]

Mutual aid also emerged among immigrant workers in Florida. The first Cuban mutual aid society formed in Key West in 1871, but the most remarkable flowering of association activity occurred in Ybor City (part of Tampa), the center of Florida's cigar-making industry. Cigar factories were dangerous places for workers; windows were kept closed to keep the tobacco from drying out, and the workers suffered high rates of tuberculosis and other respiratory diseases. A yellow fever epidemic in 1887 led to a flurry of organizing among cigar workers, and by the early twentieth century, Ybor City was home to five mutual aid societies organized by Spanish, Italian, and Cuban immigrants.[82]

The cigar workers' mutual aid societies built a remarkable system of medical care. Both of Ybor City's Spanish clubs opened modern hospitals, called *sanitarios*, in 1905 and 1906. El Centro Asturiana's medical complex "included a pharmacy, X-ray lab, a modern operating room, beds for sixty patients and a pavilion." Membership in the society was only $1.50 a month for full benefits. The Italian and Cuban mutual aid societies contracted with the two Spanish hospitals for services for their members. For Ybor City's immigrant women, historian Nancy Hewitt notes, "the medical care provided by the clubs—including midwifery, emergency medical care, and prescriptions—was the single most important benefit of club membership." The clubs also provided jobs for women as nurses and midwives.[83] Thanks to the mutual aid hospitals, two other historians write, "Ybor City's cigarmakers and their families could expect better health services than almost anyone in Tampa."[84]

But it was a different story for Afro-Cuban cigar makers. At first, Cuban mutual aid societies in Ybor City were open to both Black and white members, but by 1900 both Jim Crow restrictions and Cuban racial hierarchies were forcing Afro-Cubans to create their own clubs. La Unión Martí-Maceo formed out of two Black mutual aid societies in 1904. This club "provided complete medical care for members and benefits for sickness and death, in

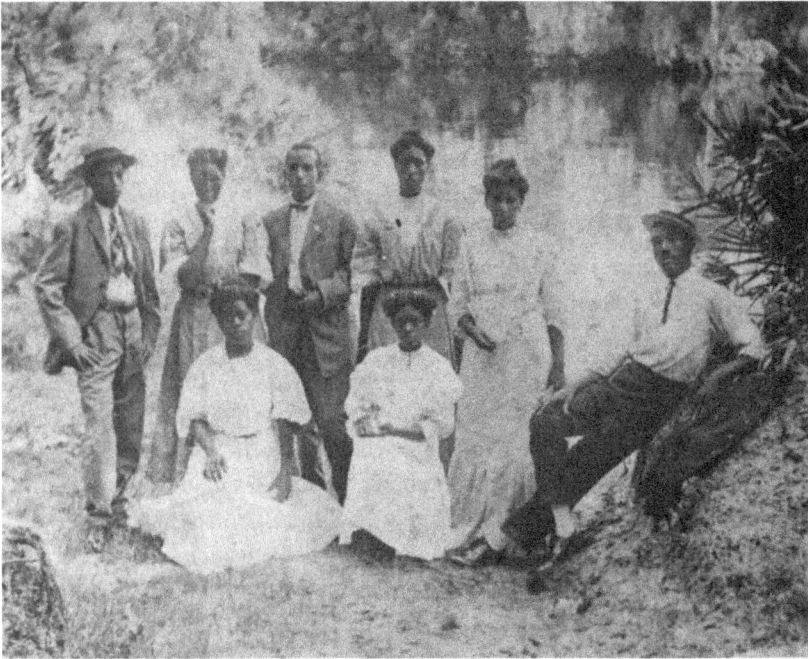

FIGURE 1.4. Mutual aid organizations provided sociability as well as medical care and other benefits. These members of Sociedad La Union Martí-Maceo, an Afro-Cuban mutual aid society in Florida, were photographed at a picnic around 1900. New York Public Library.

addition to a variety of social and cultural activities."[85] However, the Afro-Cuban society did not have the resources to open a hospital. Black Cubans were excluded from Florida hospitals under Jim Crow, so Ybor City's mutual aid societies utilized a unique and expensive method of obtaining care for their Black members: they provided funds for travel back to Cuba for hospital treatment.[86] Although Florida's Cuban cigar makers achieved notable success in organizing mutual aid based on national, language, and workplace solidarity, race still divided them. Racial exclusion was also practiced by some Mexican mutual aid societies; as late as the 1940s, lodges of the Alianza Hispano Americana refused to accept "members of the Negro or Mongolian races." (But by 1955, Alianza would embrace civil rights and work with groups like the NAACP in school segregation battles.)[87]

Immigrant mutual aid societies may have been founded partly in response to discrimination, but their role as civil rights advocates was limited. Clubs of European, Asian, and Latino immigrants, writes Hernández, "placed a high value on local freedom and autonomy often conflicting with other goals; for example, unity."[88] This is evident in the racial separation of the Cuban cigar

workers' societies. *Landsmanshaftn* could promote a Jewish American identity but also encouraged continuing identification with immigrants' home
villages. The organizations of San Francisco's Chinatown were probably the
best example of how mutual aid could provide powerful institutional support
for immigrant civil rights activism, but the societies also reinforced a form
of class elitism and, unlike the Cuban and Jewish clubs, were not worker led.
By definition, due to its very specific membership requirements, immigrant
mutual aid practiced exclusion and the rationing of care.

But in other ways, mutual aid expanded notions of health democracy and
rights. The organizations were managed and directed by the members themselves. By opening their own hospitals and hiring their own doctors, immigrants were able to demand "medical care on their own terms."[89] Their own
terms included prepayment, affordability, democratic governance, coverage of
conditions excluded elsewhere like tuberculosis, and benefits for dependents.
A study of Florida mutual aid concludes that "immigrant associations antici-
pated socialized medicine. Indeed, Ybor City residents took care of their own
in ways still not duplicated by American standards."[90]

These immensely popular organizations gave members care in their own
languages and nurtured immigrant medical talent. They helped new arrivals
survive and thrive in the difficult adjustment to life in the United States. By
offering both benefits and participation in governance, mutual aid advanced
their members' sense of belonging and perhaps of citizenship, without requiring that they abandon their immigrant identities.

Workplace Hazards and Workplace Action

For immigrants (as for all workers), health and livelihood were inseparable.
Dangerous and exploitative working conditions could lead to disease, injury,
and even death, and medical discrimination against immigrants was rampant
in workplace settings. Mutual aid and labor organizing could be mechanisms
for demanding better conditions and creating new types of health provision
for workers.

Railroad hospitals were among the earliest forms of health care available
to immigrant workers. The railroad industry depended heavily on Irish, Italian, Chinese, and Mexican labor. Dangerous work and high rates of injury
led railroad companies to develop limited medical programs, decades before
workers' compensation existed. Beginning in the 1860s, railroad hospital associations in the US West required workers to contribute a sum from their
paychecks to support company hospitals and doctors. In some communities, such as Fort Worth, Texas, the railroad hospital was the only hospital.[91]

For employer-provided health care, the goal was not primarily to enhance immigrant health, but to keep workers on the job. Bosses governed the plans, and benefits did not cover workers' families. And many, perhaps all, railroad benefits entirely excluded Chinese workers.[92]

Mining was another immigrant-heavy industry that was extremely dangerous for laborers. Injuries, diseases, and deaths fell disproportionately on certain immigrant groups. Underground miners at California's New Almadén mercury mines suffered injury and death from cave-ins, errant blasting, and breathing in the cinnabar ore dust. Above ground, mercury poisoning plagued workers at the reduction furnaces, where they sorted and roasted the cinnabar ore and inhaled quicksilver fumes. Historian Stephen Pitti writes that in the 1890s, a government report showed that "Mexicans had a much higher rate of fatalities in the mine—nearly four times greater—than did 'Anglo Americans' . . . while only 8.5 whites per one thousand died at New Almadén, Mexicans suffered from a death rate of 30.5 per thousand." In addition to direct exposure at the mine site, the debilitation and death caused by mercury poisoning also afflicted Mexican workers and their families disproportionately. The company town was segregated, with Mexican and other Spanish-speaking families forced to live in a settlement directly downwind from the mine's furnace. The employer had provided medical care since the 1860s, but Mexican workers protested that the care was inadequate and that they were denied treatment by company doctors. Rather than taking steps to make the workplace safer, the company doctors blamed Mexican workers for their own illnesses.[93]

In Arizona's copper mines, where both resident and migratory Spanish-speaking workers were paid a lower "Mexican wage," immigrant miners suffered high rates of tuberculosis and other respiratory diseases, as well as work accidents. The fatality rates were so high that the Mexican consul in Phoenix received constant requests "to help families of dead miners return to Mexico."[94] Their continual endangerment led to protests by Mexican miners, many of whom were members of mutual aid societies. During the Clifton-Morenci copper strike of 1903, Alianza lodges pushed for better health conditions, including locker rooms so workers could change out of their wet clothes before walking home, and "demanded free hospitalization and life insurance."[95] In an era when most labor unions discriminated against Mexican workers, mutual aid amplified their voices; as a local newspaper observed, "The Mexicans belong to numerous societies and through them they can exert some form of organization to stand together."[96]

European immigrant miners who were not subject to exclusion by unions were able to organize their own health care institutions. In hard-rock mining, they objected to employer-run medical care that could actually hurt immigrants; for example, one Colorado Fuel and Iron Company physician stated that his job was "to help keep the Greek and Italian people down," and some miners had to pay a "hospital fee" where no hospital existed. Historian Alan Derickson describes how multiethnic white workers organized the Western Federation of Miners in 1893 and began building their own medical institutions; by 1925, there were twenty-five miners' hospitals in the mountain states. These "small to very small" hospitals, which focused on surgery, were entirely worker owned and run: "democratic decision-making and rank-and-file participation, customary in the miners' movement, guided the founding of these institutions," Derickson notes. Like the mutual aid societies, miners' hospitals valued immigrant empowerment as well as health care provision.[97]

Migrant farmworkers faced major hazards on the job, including heat, dust, backbreaking labor, and a complete lack of sanitary facilities. Labor camps where workers and their families lived were so crowded and filthy that outbreaks of contagious disease, including dysentery and typhoid, were a regular occurrence.[98] There is evidence of labor organizing among Chinese and Japanese farmworkers in California in the 1880s and 1890s and of a brief alliance between Japanese and Mexican farmworkers in the sugar beet fields in 1903.[99] The first farmworkers' collective action to gain much publicity was the Wheatland hop workers' strike in Stockton, California, in 1913, organized by the Industrial Workers of the World ("Wobblies"). The strike exposed the "filth and sanitary neglect" on hop ranches, where laborers caught dysentery from overflowing toilets and were forced to work in the scorching heat without any drinking water.[100] Strike meetings were held in multiple languages, including Arabic, German, Greek, Italian, and Spanish. The hop workers' strike ended when armed gunmen organized by the rancher provoked a riot, three people were killed, and strike leaders (including a Swedish immigrant) and dozens of workers were arrested and beaten. Nevertheless, the strike led to the first state investigations of farm labor sanitary conditions in California.[101]

In the factories of the nation's cities, immigrant workers faced a variety of hazards. In the 1910s, the pioneering medical researcher Alice Hamilton found hundreds of cases of lead poisoning among industrial workers, and "They were almost always foreigners." She reported that immigrants, especially those who did not speak English, were deliberately given the most dangerous jobs and could not understand what little safety information was provided.[102]

The Triangle Factory fire in New York City in 1911, which took the lives of 146 garment workers, mainly young Jewish immigrant women, drew national attention to the problem of crowded, hazardous "sweatshops." The sweatshops were also breeding grounds for contagious disease, particularly tuberculosis. In 1913, the International Ladies' Garment Workers' Union (ILGWU) opened the Union Health Center in New York's garment district, where union members could receive free medical treatment and tuberculosis care. "The Center cannot be run as an impersonal institution dispensing charity," an observer noted, "because the worker has himself built and paid for the clinic."[103]

In addition to organizing unions and building institutions, immigrant workers participated in the Progressive movement for workplace health and safety legislation. Pauline Newman, the founder of the ILGWU Union Health Center, was a Lithuanian-born garment worker who became the most prominent Jewish immigrant spokesperson for the campaign for compulsory worker health insurance from 1915 to 1920. Russian Jewish immigrant Isaac Rubinow, who like Newman was a socialist, was also among the health insurance movement's leaders.

The compulsory insurance proposals, which would have been the first step toward creating a national health insurance program in the US, were defeated at the height of the antiradical Red Scare in 1919. Socialist and labor activists and the legislation they supported came under attack by antisocialist politicians, and immigrant "agitators" faced deportation for their political views. Opponents of health insurance legislation also took advantage of the ultrapatriotic atmosphere of World War I to condemn the proposals as inherently "un-American." Xenophobia, particularly the idea that immigrants were undeserving of health care due to their racial habits, also played a role in the defeat of the legislation. A factory worker who signed a petition against the health insurance proposal explained, "I didn't want to support some dago's wife every time she had a baby."[104] ("Dago" was a racial slur against Italians.)

Among the supporters of the doomed health insurance bills were numerous labor unions whose immigrant members suffered high rates of workplace disease, including the garment workers, the United Mine Workers, the International Brotherhood of Foundry Employees, the Tunnel and Subway Constructors' Union, and unions of steam engineers, textile workers, and paper mill workers. The president of the Granite Cutters Union stated in 1919, "To wage earners health insurance is next in importance to compensation for industrial accidents."[105]

Granite workers in particular suffered grievous losses in the "Spanish flu" pandemic of 1918–19. Already-high rates of tuberculosis in industries like granite cutting, in which workers inhaled large amounts of rock dust or silica, obscured how much influenza was an occupational disease for immigrant workers during that pandemic. In the Barre, Vermont, granite industry, more than one hundred laborers, mostly Italian immigrants, perished of influenza in just three weeks in the fall of 1918.[106]

Apart from this example, we know little about how the influenza pandemic affected immigrants compared with the general population. Most historical and contemporary accounts posit that sickness rates were similar among various racial and ethnic groups. But it seems notable that the US city that did the best job in curbing influenza, Saint Louis, Missouri, distributed public health information not just in English, but also in Polish, Russian, Yiddish, Hungarian, Italian, Bohemian, and Spanish.[107]

What is clear is that medical neglect and discrimination against immigrant communities led to some dire consequences during the 1918 pandemic. In the El Paso, Texas, barrio, thirty-seven people died of influenza in a twenty-four-hour period—even as there were *zero* deaths in the Anglo part of town. According to Mario T. García, "22 sick people were discovered in one room. Although the Associated Charities of the city sent some volunteers . . . the lack of doctors and nurses who could speak Spanish hampered its efforts." There was no hospital in the barrio, and the coroner reported that "many Mexicans who died had not been treated by a physician." The "devastation" of the epidemic, writes García, "exposed the deplorable scarcity of health services for Mexicans." In Los Angeles, the public health department blamed Mexican residents for the influenza epidemic, and even sent guards to quarantine Mexican neighborhoods.[108]

Between 1848 and 1924, immigrants and their advocates developed a wide range of institutions that provided medical care. The institutions varied in their accessibility and exclusivity. Some were only open to members of particular groups, or to patients who could pay. They also differed in the extent to which they offered paternalism or empowerment to immigrants. But they all reflected immigrants' desire for health and health care, and their definition of medical access as an aspect of survival, dignity, and belonging.

This time period encompasses many examples of immigrant activism for health. Immigrants raised funds for hospitals, created and joined mutual aid societies, went on strike, organized unions, objected to abuses by the immigration system, protested unsafe working conditions, petitioned for municipal services, and advocated for health care legislation. Many of these efforts were, again, on behalf of discrete groups, but sometimes immigrant health actions and institutions pointed toward greater access to care for all. This included hospitals that welcomed patients with tuberculosis and were open to the whole community, mutual aid and union health programs that imposed fewer exclusions for preexisting conditions, and groups that organized on behalf of safe workplaces and for worker health insurance.

But immigrant health institutions and activism could not stem the tide of repression and lawmaking that sought to keep immigrants as second-class citizens, and to end further immigration altogether. The US excluded people who were suspected of being sick or unhealthy, and sometimes deported those who got sick after arrival. The immigration inspection regime continued to send the message that newcomers—especially those of certain races—were inherently diseased and a threat to public health. All immigrants remained subject to deportation on public charge grounds, and Asians were almost entirely excluded. The efforts of immigrant workers to improve their conditions through organizing and strikes were suppressed, often brutally. And in the 1920s, a new era of restriction began that would not only drastically reduce immigration from Europe, but would also reinforce prejudice against those groups already in the US. At the same time, the new national origin quotas did not limit immigration from Western Hemisphere countries, which meant that workers from Mexico and the Caribbean could continue to serve as an exploitable labor force. Exploitable, and also deportable.

2

Health Care in the Era of Restriction and Expulsion

The famous phrase "a nation of immigrants" obscures how the US has restricted immigration and citizenship since its beginnings, and how restriction has been based on racial discrimination. The 1790 Naturalization Act specified that only immigrants who were "free white persons" were eligible for citizenship. Political movements demanding federal immigration restriction grew in the 1850s with the formation of the anti-Catholic, anti-Irish American (Know Nothing) Party. Starting in the 1880s, the Chinese Exclusion Act and subsequent laws barred most Asian immigrants from the US and made all Asians ineligible for citizenship. These laws were based on ideas that Chinese people were racially inferior and that they competed unfairly with American workers for jobs. In the 1890s, nativists or restrictionists began arguing for reducing or stopping immigration altogether. They were influenced by "scientific" racism, which classified the large numbers of southern and eastern Europeans entering the country as biologically undesirable and a threat to American racial purity.[1] Congress responded in 1897 by passing a bill requiring a literacy test for immigration, but it was vetoed by President Grover Cleveland.

World War I and the Russian Revolution intensified a fear of foreigners, and in 1917 Congress passed "the first widely restrictive immigration act." The Immigration Act of 1917 imposed a literacy test, barred almost all immigrants from a broad "Asiatic Zone" beyond China, and specified a large number of conditions for refusing admission, including tuberculosis, other "loathsome or contagious disease," mental or physical defects, and "likely to become a public charge."[2]

Restrictionists next demanded a quota system to reduce the immigration of undesirable groups. The Immigration Acts of 1921 and 1924 placed numerical limits on immigration for the first time in US history, capping entries at

355,000. These laws also instituted quotas based on nationality that favored immigrant groups who had been in the country before 1890. This led to the near elimination of immigration from southern and eastern Europe. Under the Immigration Acts, all nationalities ineligible for citizenship were barred entirely, so Asians were almost completely excluded. The Fourteenth Amendment to the Constitution (1868) had made Black people born in the country citizens, but Congress still discriminated against Black immigrants by providing African countries with only a tiny number of quota slots.[3]

The national origins quotas addressed the demands of the eugenics movement to protect the native white stock of the United States from pollution by foreign bloodlines. While disease and disability had always been categories for exclusion, eugenicists argued that certain "races" were constitutionally weak and unfit for American life. Not only were they more prone to disease, they also had an inherent racial tendency to fall into poverty and become public charges. But the 1924 immigration restriction was only a partial victory for eugenicists and scientific racists. Countries in the Western Hemisphere were exempt from the entry quotas. This was due mainly to the power of agricultural and railroad interests in the Southwest and California, who insisted on a continued supply of cheap labor from Mexico.

Health and the Debate over Restricting Mexicans

For several years after 1924, Congress debated whether Mexico and other Western Hemisphere countries should be added to the quota system. Although the Treaty of Guadalupe Hidalgo after the US-Mexico War had conferred US citizenship on Mexicans in the acquired territories and so implied that Mexicans were a "white" race, restrictionists argued that Mexicans were actually Indigenous and therefore nonwhite, making them even more racially undesirable than southern and eastern Europeans.[4]

During debates in Congress, both supporters and opponents of Mexican restriction used racial arguments about health to support their cause. (All the speakers were white/Anglo; no Mexican immigrants or Mexican Americans were invited to provide testimony.) Restrictionists insisted that Mexicans had racial tendencies to be diseased and to become public charges. G. B. Ocheltree, who headed the California Immigration Study Commission, presented testimony that Mexicans were a race of dependent peasants who drove down wages for American workers. They knew "nothing about sanitation," and their high fertility rates meant that they would produce generations of children "of a type that does not hesitate to beg for charity." Ocheltree argued that the Mexican worker would not return home but instead go "into permanent quarters in the cities, where he becomes a public charge, and the farmer must draw a fresh supply from Mexico."[5]

But representatives of agricultural and mining regions argued against restricting Mexicans. Entire industries relied on a low-paid and flexible labor supply from Mexico. Restriction would mean "economic disaster" for his district, argued Rep. John Gardner of Texas. Anti-restrictionists agreed that Mexicans were racially different, but in ways that actually made their continued admission to the US desirable. Mexicans' bodies rendered them fit for labor that other groups would refuse. Gardner said that only Mexican workers would undertake the backbreaking work of digging up trees and underbrush to create farmland. In addition, "These people live on less than American labor lives on." Mexican workers would not populate American cities; they always went back over the border to their home villages when the harvest season was over, Gardner insisted.[6]

The employers of migrant labor won the day, and Western Hemisphere countries continued to be exempt from immigration quotas. This did not mean that movement across the border was unrestricted. Visa requirements, medical inspections, and the brand-new Border Patrol would do little to slow the flow of workers from Mexico but did a lot to redefine many migrants as "illegal" and thus subject to deportation.[7]

Immigration control at the US-Mexico border had a medical component. After an outbreak of the lice-borne disease typhus in 1916, the US government quarantined the border city of El Paso, Texas. In order to enter the US from Ciudad Juárez, Mexicans were required to submit to a delousing process that included being stripped, bathed, and sprayed with a combination of soap and kerosene. Many people from Juárez worked daily in El Paso, and apart from being humiliating, the typhus baths added additional time and difficulty to their commute.

Shortly after the new requirements began, a remarkable protest erupted. A rumor spread that naked bathers were being secretly photographed. A group of Mexican domestic workers heading to work to El Paso, led by a seventeen-year-old woman named Carmelita Torres, refused the baths and began attacking the streetcars and other vehicles that crossed the bridge between the two cities. The two days of protests, which became known as the "Bath Riots," failed; the US would continue to require Mexican commuter workers to be bathed and disinfected. The quarantine regime in El Paso persisted until the 1930s, even though no threat of typhus from Mexico existed, and forced disinfection would become part of border entry requirements for Mexican "guest workers" in the 1940s and 1950s.[8]

Despite the resistance of people like Carmelita Torres, stereotypes of

Mexicans as diseased and unhealthy continued to be used to argue for restriction and also justified discrimination against Mexicans in the US. Chicago physician Benjamin Goldberg warned that "in importing Mexican laborers," employers were "also importing a race sizzling with susceptibilities" to disease. Stricter immigration laws would "in some measure offer a health protection to the American citizen." An economics professor at the University of Wisconsin called for reducing Mexican immigration because, among other reasons, "their infant mortality and general morbidity rates are very high."[9]

In the 1920s, it did become evident that the rapidly growing Mexican immigrant communities were suffering severe health problems, including high rates of tuberculosis and infant mortality. Restrictionists argued that Mexicans brought their diseases with them and that they had an inherent racial susceptibility to poor health. They ignored or downplayed evidence that immigrants' health problems were due to their exploitative work and living conditions and to discrimination and neglect.

Tuberculosis, a contagious disease that usually affected the lungs, was incurable before the age of antibiotics, and often fatal. From the nineteenth to the early twentieth century, tuberculosis, also called consumption, was the leading cause of death in the US. It was also a long-term chronic condition that could lead to years of disability. The disease was especially devastating for Black and immigrant populations. Since the turn of the twentieth century, tuberculosis had been declining for all groups in the United States, but Black mortality from the disease continued to be disproportionately high.[10]

There were few statistics comparing Mexicans to other groups, but the existing studies were alarming. A 1927 survey in Chicago concluded that tuberculosis morbidity in Mexicans was *ten times* higher than in the general population, reported the physician Goldberg, who was the head of Chicago's Municipal Tuberculosis Sanatorium. He argued that unrestricted immigration could only lead to higher disease rates: "Who will solve this problem when the Mexican population in Chicago amounts, as it eventually may because of the drift eastward of this race, to two or three hundred thousand?"[11]

Goldberg did talk about some of the workplace and home conditions that exacerbated the spread of consumption among Mexican immigrants. He noted that among the tuberculosis patients at Cook County Hospital, "practically all the Mexicans were unskilled laborers." The Mexican men who made up the low-wage workforce at Chicago's railroad, stockyard, and steel industries, and their families, lived in "box cars and colonies [that] make it difficult to escape infection. Box cars have no light, ventilation, running water, or toilets." Enforcing housing regulations against overcrowding would help, Goldberg said. At the same time, he undercut his own statements by insisting that it was Mexicans' racial difference that made them susceptible to infection. "The Mexican is below medium stature, of inferior muscular development and under excessive labor demands will rapidly break," he wrote. Even though he had just acknowledged that Mexicans were acquiring tuberculosis in Chicago due to their housing and work environments, he referred to health problems as something that the Mexican "brings with him."[12]

Evidence that Mexican immigrants did not bring sicknesses, but rather acquired them in the United States, was plentiful. Historian Zaragosa Vargas writes that "exposure to diseases was a sacrifice Mexicans made for the good money they were able to earn in the North." For new arrivals in Detroit, "Unhealthy living conditions and improper nutrition coupled with cold weather produced a high incidence of tuberculosis, measles, and rickets."[13] In Los Angeles, where TB was ravaging the Mexican community, studies showed that most immigrants acquired the disease after arrival; in 1926, four-fifths of Mexican heads of households with tuberculosis had been in the US for more than five years.[14] Yet, like Goldberg in Chicago, Los Angeles authorities continued to depict Mexicans as "agents of disease rather than its victims," as the historian Emily Abel puts it.[15]

Infant Mortality and Immigrant Midwives

High rates of infant mortality also marked Mexican immigrants as racially different. In Arizona in the 1920s, for example, the death rate among Mexican American infants was 205 per one thousand, while for Anglos it was 77.8 per one thousand. Health authorities and restrictionists pointed to Mexicans' "racial" tendencies—large families and allegedly poor hygiene practices—as the cause. Yet infant mortality, like tuberculosis, was highest among low-wage workers, especially migrant workers in the Southwest, who lived in conditions of poverty. A study by the US Children's Bureau showed that poor nutrition and overwork among new mothers made breast-feeding difficult, and that "feeding infants with sanitary bottles was nearly impossible for migrant women who lacked clean water and adequate kitchen equipment."[16]

Like tuberculosis, infant mortality was a nationwide problem that disproportionately affected poor and working-class communities. In 1921, following the victory of women's suffrage, Congress passed the Sheppard-Towner Act (Maternity and Infancy Protection Act), which provided matching grants to states for hiring public health nurses and educators to implement programs to reduce infant and maternal mortality. The government campaign to "save mothers and babies" included "Americanization": teaching immigrant mothers about US diets, medical care, and child-rearing. Immigrant women overwhelmingly relied on midwives from their own communities to assist in childbirth. One of the goals of the Sheppard-Towner programs was to impose registration requirements on midwives and to train them in hygienic childbirth methods; another was to force older and uncooperative midwives out of practice.[17]

Government-funded nurses and health educators who visited rural communities portrayed immigrant midwives as another example of health backwardness. A Texas report described Mexican midwives as "illiterate, usually dirty and in rags, gesticulating, oftentimes not able to talk or understand the English language."[18] Rather than seeing midwives' Spanish fluency as an advantage for communicating with patients, some Sheppard-Towner workers took it as evidence of ignorance. (At least one midwife, however, "pretended not to understand English in order to avoid answering questions" from Sheppard-Towner authorities.)[19]

While some distrusted outside interference, many midwives and expectant mothers welcomed the arrival of government health workers. Sheppard-Towner nurses and educators were not allowed to provide direct medical care; instead, they fanned out throughout rural areas to organize health conferences, "visited individual homes, advised mothers on basic health care and hygiene, instructed local midwives, and gave physical examinations to young children."[20] Midwife regulation was also part of their duties. In Arizona, Sheppard-Towner nurses were able to increase "the total of registered midwives in Arizona to 135, of which fifty-four were classified as white, seventy-three Mexican, six Negro, and one each Indian and Japanese." At the same time, "the field nurses were reporting that they had 'eliminated' some registered Mexican midwives because of old age or unfitness."[21]

Yet when Arizona's Sheppard-Tower program ended in 1929, it had not succeeded in bringing down the infant mortality rate in the state. Its Anglo director blamed this failure on "the unusually high death rate among Mexican American infants." She wrote, "As long as Arizona has its constantly changing and shifting Mexican population" and "large numbers of ignorant and constantly changing Mexican laborers," the state would not be able to improve infant survival rates. She did not mention that her program had hired only a single Spanish-speaking nurse to serve the entire state. Also, according to historian Mary Melcher, Arizona's Sheppard-Towner program had never even attempted to distribute health literature among the migrant laborer population and did not work with the mutual aid societies that could have helped reach more Spanish-speaking families.[22]

Even in states that did a better job of working with immigrant communities, Sheppard-Towner mostly imposed medical understandings from above without taking time to learn what patients needed and wanted. For example, many immigrant women held herbal medicine in high regard, but Sheppard-Towner registration rules banned midwives from carrying herbs and unapproved medicines in their bags. The regulations also forbid midwives from using skills that could save a mother's life, such as "version" (turning a baby in the uterus), and required them to call a doctor instead. Finally, Sheppard-Towner ended up eliminating many immigrant midwives from practice altogether. As historian Molly Ladd-Taylor writes, "Despite the good intentions of public health reformers and the benefits of their work," Sheppard-Towner midwife registration programs "deprived many women of experienced birth attendants without providing them with access to adequate medical and nursing services."[23]

Leaving women without other options for care was a political choice. Opposition from the American Medical Association (AMA) had ensured that Sheppard-Towner programs would be limited to health education and not actual medical care. And the entire program was ended by Congress in 1929 after intensive lobbying by the AMA and "patriotic" groups. Medical societies called Sheppard-Towner "socialistic" and "Bolshevistic," and a leader of Daughters of the American Revolution warned that the program was an effort to "place all children under Federal control." The arguments were very similar to the ones that had helped derail worker health insurance a decade earlier.[24]

The AMA also fought to replace midwives with physicians and to encourage women to give birth in hospitals instead of their homes, despite clear evidence that childbirth with a midwife was safer for both mother and baby and that many immigrant women continued to strongly prefer midwives.[25] By the end of the 1920s, far fewer midwives were available. In addition to the AMA's campaign, and Sheppard-Towner's attempts to eliminate unqualified practitioners, immigration restriction also reduced the number of midwives. A 1927 article on the drastic decline of midwifery in New York State noted that "the reason for the decrease lies in the fact that as midwives drop out of practice there are few to take their place, owing partly to restricted immigration." The New York City commissioner of health announced that "each year witnesses a decrease in the number of midwives. . . . To a large extent the decrease appears to be the result of restricted immigration . . . only patients of foreign extraction ask service of the midwife, and . . . she is employed to the greatest extent by native Italians."[26] Although midwives continued to serve Black and migrant communities in the South and Southwest, immigration restriction helped eliminate an important type of high-quality health care from a large part of the United States.[27]

Health under the Quota System

In New York City and other cities where southern and eastern Europeans had settled, immigration restriction did not eliminate the need for immigrant medical care. The Henry Street Visiting Nurse Association continued to work in the Jewish and Italian neighborhoods of the Lower East Side and expanded its work to the Bronx, where the nurses began using automobiles for home visits. As white immigrant groups "assimilated" after 1924, it became more difficult to attribute their health issues to racial differences. Henry Street nurses continued to see patients with problems clearly caused by poverty, crowded housing, and poor nutrition.[28]

In one eleven-block Lower East Side area served by Henry Street, the residents represented over forty nations. But between 1929 and 1933, only eight new immigrant families moved in. Henry Street workers reported, "The 'immigrant problem' as it faced the settlements and social agencies in the twenties and before the war seems over." Yet there was a new problem: many of the neighborhood residents did not take the steps needed to become US citizens. Older immigrants, especially, showed little interest in naturalization. Henry Street workers were concerned that the immigrants who did not naturalize "face discrimination, loss of jobs and security. Tomorrow, perhaps, persecution."[29]

Low levels of naturalization became a serious problem during the Depression because noncitizens were not eligible for New Deal jobs. In 1935 the Immigrants' Protective League in Chicago proposed opening a division entirely devoted to helping people naturalize. They were concerned that many poor immigrants did not apply for naturalization because of the hefty fees. They worked to provide funds for clients such as an Italian woman with six American-born children who needed to be naturalized to qualify for a state Mothers' Pension; she could not afford to "file a 659" (Declaration of Intent form to apply for citizenship).[30]

Not being naturalized also left immigrant residents vulnerable to public charge deportations. Social workers with the Immigrants' Protective League (IPL) took on the case of a German woman and her daughter, who had entered the US legally in 1929. The husband's visa was delayed, and when he finally arrived his visa was revoked "because there was a depression in the United States and because his wife could not furnish him with affidavits showing that he would not become a public charge." He was deported on August 9, 1932. "The wife was so upset at the deportation that she had a miscarriage, being pregnant when he left," according to the social workers. "Now she is destitute and sad."[31]

As this example indicates, one of the results of deportation was the separation of families. Health and health care continued to serve as a driver of immigration control that could lead to devastating consequences. In another case reported by the IPL, a Czech family immigrated to Chicago 1908 but left their child behind. When they finally were able to send for him, he was found to have "lung disease . . . was excluded at an American port and sent back to Czechoslovakia." The child partly recovered but was also diagnosed with tuberculosis of the skin. After the father naturalized in the US, he "again sent a steamship ticket, just before the boy became twenty-one years old. [But] by that time the United States immigration policy had changed and the boy was subject not only to medical tests, but to the rigid requirements of the quota act of 1924 . . . he was regarded by the Consul's doctor as afflicted with a chronic and perhaps contagious disease, and therefore refused a visa." Even minor health issues could lead arriving relatives to be labeled "likely to become a public charge" (LPC). Another problem noted by the Chicago social workers was that some immigrant families were required to pay for hospitalization or post bonds for their LPC relatives.[32] These costs could be so high that only well-off families could afford them, creating another barrier to family reunification for poor families.

Health Care Segregation and Exclusion

Some immigrant groups could accelerate their acceptance into American society by applying for naturalization and becoming US citizens, but all Asians (including, after a 1923 Supreme Court decision, South Asians) were denied that possibility. Banned from both further immigration and from naturalization, Chinese people remained shunned and stigmatized, but at the same time continued to strengthen their own communities and health institutions. For example, in 1925, Chinese mutual aid and political organizations in California successfully mobilized to defeat a bill that would have imposed federal drug restrictions on Chinese herbal medicines.[33]

San Francisco's Chinese Hospital, opened in 1925, provided both traditional and Western medicine, and remained under the control of Chinatown's civic organizations. According to historian Nayan Shah, "At first the hospital drew its staff of physicians from the city's white medical establishment, but within a couple of years several Chinese American physicians, trained at Stanford and the University of California, joined the staff." When San Francisco health authorities began directing some medical resources toward the Chinese community, including immunization campaigns and well-baby clinics, they utilized the Chinese Hospital as the best way of reaching the community.[34]

In Los Angeles, the Mexican population was growing dramatically due to increased immigration during and following the Mexican Revolution. By the 1920s, Los Angeles was home to thirty thousand people of Mexican origin. Natalia Molina writes, "it became clear that Mexican immigrants in the Los Angeles area were permanent settlers, not itinerant seasonal laborers." As Molina explains, the city began to establish separate health clinics for whites and Mexicans. The "Mexican" clinics offered only rudimentary services and received a tiny fraction of the funding allocated to white facilities. Los Angeles County health director John Pomeroy justified the discriminatory treatment by claiming it was "impossible to mix the Mexicans and the whites" in the same clinic because Mexicans' hygiene standards were so "appalling."[35] The county devoted fewer resources to the Mexican community even though rates of tuberculosis and some other diseases were dramatically higher for them.

Still, Los Angeles's clinic program was more generous than in other cities. In Chicago, which was opening several tuberculosis clinics for African Americans, sanatorium director Benjamin Goldberg argued that Mexicans should not receive similar resources. "The Negro" was an "essential element in our American population," Goldberg wrote, whose health would improve after adjusting to city life; "He is an American citizen, entitled to all the prerogatives and rights of such citizenry." Mexicans, on the other hand, are "a race that has no demand on us."[36] Rather than providing services to Chicago's Mexican population, he advocated restricting Mexican immigration, and for deporting those already in the country as public charges.

Goldberg's views were not widely adopted by the Chicago settlement movement. In the late 1920s, the University of Chicago Settlement started a "Mexican Club" that offered recreation, social activities, and English classes for Mexican migrants. As the name indicates, the club was segregated, but settlement leaders found this necessary because of rampant discrimination against Mexicans in the city. Mexican residents flocked to the club, and soon it became evident that many were suffering from serious problems related to unemployment and sickness.

Mexican Club leaders began referring sick people to Chicago clinics and hospitals and accompanying them to their appointments. They argued with local charities that were reluctant to give financial aid to Mexicans without legal residence. In contrast to Goldberg's rhetoric, the settlement house workers focused on the conditions that made people sick, including unemployment, evictions, and discrimination based on residency. They described

Mexican immigrants as eager to learn English, to participate in dances and social activities, and to utilize necessary medical services. In one memorable example of their eagerness for health, a group of "Mexican Mothers' Club" members gathered their children for treatment with diphtheria antitoxin, which could prevent this deadly childhood disease. "Not satisfied with this, one mother collected six children beside her own and also had them treated for the prevention of diphtheria," a social worker reported.[37]

Settlement workers noted that local charities and some medical facilities denied assistance to Mexicans because they were not legal residents. In addition, immigrants themselves could be reluctant to seek help because of the threat of deportation. Famed Hull House leader Jane Addams commented that Mexicans in Chicago "are afraid of being deported and are even afraid of receiving relief for fear of being sent back to Mexico as public charges."[38] A 1935 US Children's Bureau study of border health noted that "this fear of public services is especially dangerous when it affects accepted standards of health care." Most Mexican workers didn't make enough money to pay for private hospital care, "yet an alien fears the risk of being considered a public charge if he utilized the county or municipal free hospital." At least one county hospital on the border reported "all aliens to the immigration service for investigation," so Mexican residents in the area were "afraid to accept hospital care; mothers attending the prenatal clinics refuse[d] to go to the hospital" to give birth.[39]

Deportations of people for becoming a public charge were not yet common, but Mexicans were disproportionately affected by this practice. According to sociologist Cybelle Fox, "the sheer number of Mexicans deported for this cause . . . was higher than any other single nationality group." Between 1906 and 1932, "6,310 Mexicans were deported due to the public charge provisions . . . as compared to 4,106 people from England, 3,940 Italians, and 3,196 Germans."[40] Restrictionists pushed for the number of public charge deportations of Mexicans to be even higher. In Chicago, physician Benjamin Goldberg described Mexicans who got sick with tuberculosis as "subjects for charitable care and assistance" and lamented that "deportation legislation, unfortunately, is not utilized to the extent it should be."[41]

Mass Deportation, Health Care, and Health

That would change during the Great Depression, when the number of both deportations and extralegal repatriations exploded. The first wave of Depression deportations was not based on public charge accusations, but on the scapegoating of "aliens" as the cause of mass unemployment. In 1930, US secretary of labor William Doak announced a goal of expelling "four hundred thousand illegal aliens."[42] Agents of Doak's Immigration Service began conducting raids and rounding up suspects for deportations in workplaces, dance halls, and public gathering places. A notorious raid took place in February of 1931, when Mexican residents enjoying an afternoon at Los Angeles's La Placita park found themselves surrounded by armed agents who sealed off the park and demanded everyone's immigration papers. About thirty arrests were made, and following additional raids throughout Los Angeles, "the first official repatriation train left Los Angeles for Mexico with more than 400 on board."[43]

It would have been impossible to deport four hundred thousand people in a short period of time using required legal procedures. As the Depression deepened, local governments started their own "repatriation" campaigns. Federal deportation raids had sent a message to all Mexicans that they were not welcome and should not feel safe in the United States. Local governments exploited these fears to encourage or force Mexicans to leave the country. Using repatriation rather than deportation meant that officials could target US citizens and longtime legal residents, not just "illegal aliens." All Mexicans became subject to repatriation—especially if they used public services, including health care and unemployment relief, or if they were sick.

Gary, Indiana, was home to a community of Mexicans who had come for work in the steel mills. They were segregated in congested neighborhoods that did not receive municipal services. When the Depression hit, Mexican workers were the first to be laid off from the mills. The community suffered levels of pneumonia, tuberculosis, and rickets that reached "epidemic proportions." Gary newspapers and the steel companies launched a publicity campaign to encourage Mexican residents to return to their home country. But as the Depression continued, county welfare officials decided to make repatriation involuntary. They authorized "the removal of every Mexican family receiving public assistance." The county cut off unemployment relief to Mexican residents so they had no means of support and had no choice but to accept a ride to the border. According to observers, many of the deportees were suffering from tuberculosis "or otherwise diseased."[44]

The most extensive local deportation/repatriation campaign took place in Los Angeles, where charity agencies already had a tradition of cooperating with immigration agencies and reporting Mexicans as public charges. In 1931 the Los Angeles Department of Charities opened its own "Deportation Section."[45] Officials called for repatriation of Mexicans as a way saving money on "immense . . . costs" of "hospitalization, clinical and medical attention, and education facilities which this community is obligated to provide."[46] Between

1931 and 1933, Los Angeles deported over thirteen thousand people, putting them on trains to the Mexican border. Thousands of others left of their own volition. Most were longtime residents, and many were US citizens.[47]

The historian Emily Abel writes that Los Angeles officials seemed determined to "rid the county of clients with large medical expenses." In one example, county officials sought funds to take a mother with six children to Mexico via automobile, because the children had "numerous health problems which require costly medical care." The threat of deportation discouraged people suffering from tuberculosis and other maladies from seeking care in Los Angeles health facilities, but even that might not protect them from zealous officials. Abel writes of a family whose breadwinning father died at home of TB, and then his family members were repatriated for needing to go on relief.[48]

In order to round up Mexican people who tried to obtain health care, the Department of Charities located its Deportation Section *inside* the Los Angeles County Hospital. Going to the hospital was defined by the agency as "charity seeking." Instead of finding medical care, Mexican patients arriving at the hospital found themselves placed on deportation trains. In her research into a sample of 143 such cases, Natalia Molina discovered that Mexicans deported directly from the county hospital included patients suffering from tuberculosis, leprosy, syphilis, hypertension, arthritis, clogged arteries, mental illness, dementia, paralysis, blindness, and polio. One was a postpartum mother with a baby in an incubator. Molina notes that the deporting officials did not distinguish between citizens and noncitizens or legal and illegal immigrants.[49] Their criterion for deportation was being a Mexican who needed medical care.

The "cases where invalids are removed from the County Hospital and carted across the line" are among the most horrifying and tragic of the 1930s deportations. "Bedridden and terminally ill patients did not escape the repatriation dragnet," write historians Francisco Balderrama and Robert Rodríguez. They describe a group of deportees that included "tubercular Frank Sepulveda, paralyzed Fermin Quintero, and eighty-six-year-old Narcisa Renteria." Sick patients might be joined by their healthy family members who conceded to repatriation in order to travel with them. Los Angeles also sometimes provided medical workers to accompany the sick, but they had a carceral rather than a caregiving function: one patient's son "thought the hospital personnel were sent along as guards rather than as orderlies to assure they arrived at their destination."[50]

And repatriation itself was a threat to health and life. According to Balderrama and Rodríguez, "Deaths occurred daily along the way and in repatriation centers at the border. Too often, the forced repatriation of individuals not fit to travel became a virtual death sentence." A Mexican newspaper reported that "on board one repatriation train, twenty-five children and adults had died of illness and malnutrition during the trip to the border." In 1931 the *New York Times* published a story about twenty-six repatriated people who were left in Ciudad Juárez and then died of pneumonia and exposure.[51]

After the journey, inadequate health care and the weak condition of many repatriates led to additional tragedies. Mexico had only one tuberculosis hospital,[52] and the patients who made it there had little chance of survival. Interviews of deportees conducted by Balderrama and Rodríguez include many memories of poor health and even deaths following repatriation. Many repatriates were already sick, elderly, or babies. Never having been to Mexico, many were not immune to malaria or other local diseases and pathogens. Arturo Herrada contracted smallpox in Mexico as a four-year-old child and remembered there were "no doctors, no hospitals. . . . If you survived, you were lucky because ninety percent of the children died." José López, whose family was sent to Mexico by Detroit welfare officials when he was five years old, "felt that his health and physical development had been severely impaired as a result of the poor diet and lack of adequate medical care while in Mexico."[53]

The 1930s deportations and repatriations removed one million adults and children, the majority of whom were US citizens. Even those who left voluntarily found they had been misled by US and Mexican officials. They were promised farmland or health care in Mexico that turned out to be nonexistent. Repatriates were told that they could return to the US after the Depression was over, but if they had been removed by charity agencies, they were permanently labeled public charges and not allowed to return legally. US citizen children needed birth certificates to reenter, but many did not possess them.[54] For many, the exile was permanent. Those able to return faced family separation and illegal status.[55]

Compounding the trauma of expulsion, Mexican immigrants and Mexican Americans were mostly abandoned by potential allies. Charity and welfare agencies that had claimed to want to help their communities were the primary agents of deportation. Some churches cooperated, sometimes eagerly, in repatriation campaigns, and Los Angeles's Catholic archbishop was an enthusiastic proponent of expelling Mexicans.[56] Even mutual aid organizations participated in urging their compatriots to leave the country. The Los Angeles mutual aid society Comite de Beneficencia Mexicana defended Mexicans against public charge accusations and fought discrimination against Mexican workers, but also used its own funds to help pay for the repatriation expenses of at least 1,500 people.[57] The Cruz Azul also assisted with repatriations. These organizations and the Mexican consul worked to protect repatriates and make their journeys safer, but they were constrained by "the severity of the economic crisis," a lack of resources, and the sheer volume of need.[58]

There were some pockets of resistance. When it came to enthusiasm for Mexican repatriations, Chicago (apart from officials like Goldberg) was nearly the opposite of Los Angeles. As the sociologist Cybelle Fox has explained, Chicago and Cook County social agencies, including hospitals, had for decades shown a lack of interest in cooperating with immigration officials. When pressured to join deportation efforts during the Depression, Chicago welfare leaders objected that "the distrust raised by snooping immigration agents would be very detrimental to the welfare relief service" and "an examination of the people getting relief, to find out whether they are deportable aliens, would destroy faith in the community."[59]

One reason for Chicago's noncooperation, Fox argues, was its rule by the Democratic Party (the federal deportation campaign was run by Hoover Republicans) and its mayor Anton Cermak, who was himself an immigrant and continued to identify with the ethnic communities in the city. Chicago was also the cradle of the US settlement house movement. Jane Addams's Hull House, opened in 1889, had long been a defender of immigrants. The Chicago Federation of Settlements wrote a letter of protest against the deportation campaign to the US Department of Labor.[60]

During the Depression, the University of Chicago Settlement House workers who ran the Mexican Club argued against the stereotype of Mexicans as public charges. In 1930 they reported that "in spite of all economic disadvantages they are undergoing there is only a negligible number of Mexicans who apply to the welfare agencies for assistance," and in 1931, "the Mexican people ask for less and receive less than other families from charitable organizations."[61] In contrast, welfare officials in Los Angeles trumpeted the numbers of Mexicans using public services and even inflated those numbers.[62]

In 1932, as huge numbers of Mexicans in Chicago lost their jobs, Mexican Club members started an Unemployed Men's Club and participated in a May Day parade and several socialist-sponsored conferences. But when the communist-affiliated Unemployed Councils announced a march to protest relief cuts, the club voted not to officially participate; they were concerned that the police would target the march and put their members in danger of deportation. Despite their fears, forty-two members of the Unemployed Men's Club went ahead and joined the massive, peaceful protest, which presented demands to Mayor Cermak that included "deportations of foreign unemployed must be halted." The demands also called for "neighborhood medical, dental, and hospital care."[63]

A quieter resistance to deportations took place in Phoenix, Arizona. Initially, according to Fox, an attorney advised the county board against reporting relief recipients to the immigration authorities, "on the ground that many deserving aliens would be afraid to ask for help." Phoenix welfare authorities did eventually agree to appoint an official to "report deportable aliens to the Immigration Service." However, "Immigration officers later complained that the official, 'who was a citizen of the United States,' never reported a single relief recipient to the Immigration Service."[64] The appointed official was a leader of the Spanish-American Society, a longtime Arizona *mutualista* that enrolled both citizens and immigrants.[65] In failing or refusing to carry out his reporting duties, he clearly saw his role as quite different from the community leaders who cooperated with repatriations in Los Angeles.

Care for Migrant Workers

The Depression led to mass deportations and repatriations but also to new attention to the conditions of migrant workers. Migration for work became an important part of the US Depression economy, and the new, mostly white migrants became the subjects of government and societal interest. The health and living conditions of the nation's Asian, Mexican, and Black farmworkers had gone mostly unnoticed. It was only when the massive displacements of the Great Depression added thousands of native-born white workers to the migrant labor force that the government "focused unprecedented attention on migrant welfare issues," historian Michael Grey notes.[66]

At the height of the Depression, the new Social Security Administration conducted studies of farmworker health that revealed both devastating medical problems and severe obstacles to obtaining health care. Migrant farmworkers and their families suffered disproportionately high rates of malnutrition, tooth decay, tuberculosis, and especially infant mortality. In one California labor camp, "92 children under 15 had died in all of these families, or 13.1% of the total number born. . . . Proportionately, almost three times as many Mexican children had died as white children." The surviving children had many health problems, including dental caries, whooping cough, rickets, skin infections, inflamed tonsils and nasal passages, and tuberculosis.[67] The influx of new migrant workers and intense overcrowding was leading to outbreaks of infectious diseases, including smallpox.[68]

Health workers described the conditions that led to these problems among migrant workers. On California cotton farms, "The diet of these families consists principally of gravy, which is made with a little grease, flour, and either water or milk, biscuits, beans, and potatoes. This is the entire diet during the winter when rain and morning fogs prevent cotton picking for days at a stretch and between crops." Children especially suffered from the lack of milk and fresh fruit. "Fresh milk is relatively unobtainable, even in those counties where dairy herds adjoin the camp. . . . Very little fruit is eaten and is usually obtained while the family is working in the fruit. . . . The few oranges which were given them were cut into thin slices and devoured, skins and all." Toilet facilities and running water were inadequate or absent. Workers and their families crammed into tents set up alongside cabins "to accommodate overflows during picking." If there was no room left at the farms, they might move into nearby "auto camps" where they slept in their vehicles "or 'squat' along ditch banks by the roadside." According to one physician, such overcrowding was a primary reason for the large number of respiratory infections among migrants.[69]

Another set of health issues stemmed from the condition of transiency itself, of moving from place to place. Whether they started out in Mexico, Florida, Texas, or Oklahoma, migrant farmworkers and their families followed the harvest, in patterns sometimes called the "migrant stream." Workers in the stream were generally not eligible for local health services for the indigent poor because of county or town residency requirements. Some farmworkers were not eligible for assistance because their modest incomes put them above the level of extreme poverty, but they did not make enough to afford private doctors or hospitals. Even workers and families who were eligible for public medical care couldn't obtain it because of long waiting lists. If they were able to access treatment, the need to move on to the next job made any sort of continuity or follow-up care virtually impossible.[70]

As part of Franklin D. Roosevelt's New Deal, first the US Resettlement Administration and then the Farm Security Administration (FSA) funded programs to pay rural physicians to care for migrant workers and to set up clinics staffed by full-time public health nurses at farm labor camps. The FSA even ran two hospitals, one in Florida and one in Arizona. According to historian Verónica Martínez-Matsuda, the FSA decided to purchase its own hospitals to avoid the rampant discrimination against Black and Mexican migrant workers by local hospitals (although its Florida hospital was still segregated into Black and white wards).[71] At their height, FSA medical programs reached between seventy-five thousand and two hundred thousand migrants.[72]

The FSA's on-site public health nurses had a tremendous variety of duties at labor camps. These included, Martínez-Matsuda writes, "conducting thorough health examinations of each migrant seeking residence at the camp;

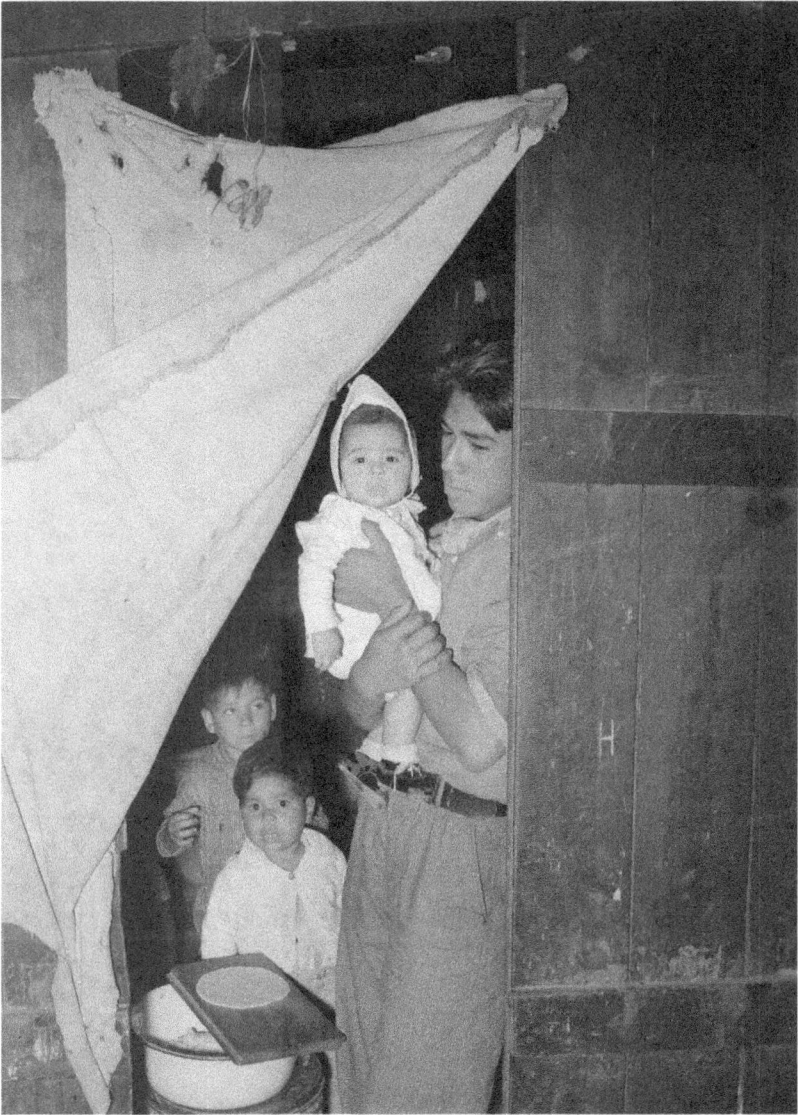

FIGURE 2.1. Migrant farmworker family in the 1930s. Original caption: "Mexican worker with children in doorway connecting two rooms of corral. Robstown, Texas." Photo by Russell Lee, 1939. Library of Congress Prints and Photographs Division.

deciding whether migrants required isolation, hospitalization, or a referral to an outside doctor; and providing minor medical or surgical treatments or, in emergency cases, triage care." Nurses provided medications, made follow-up and home visits, ran vaccination campaigns, and taught health education classes on nutrition and infant care.[73]

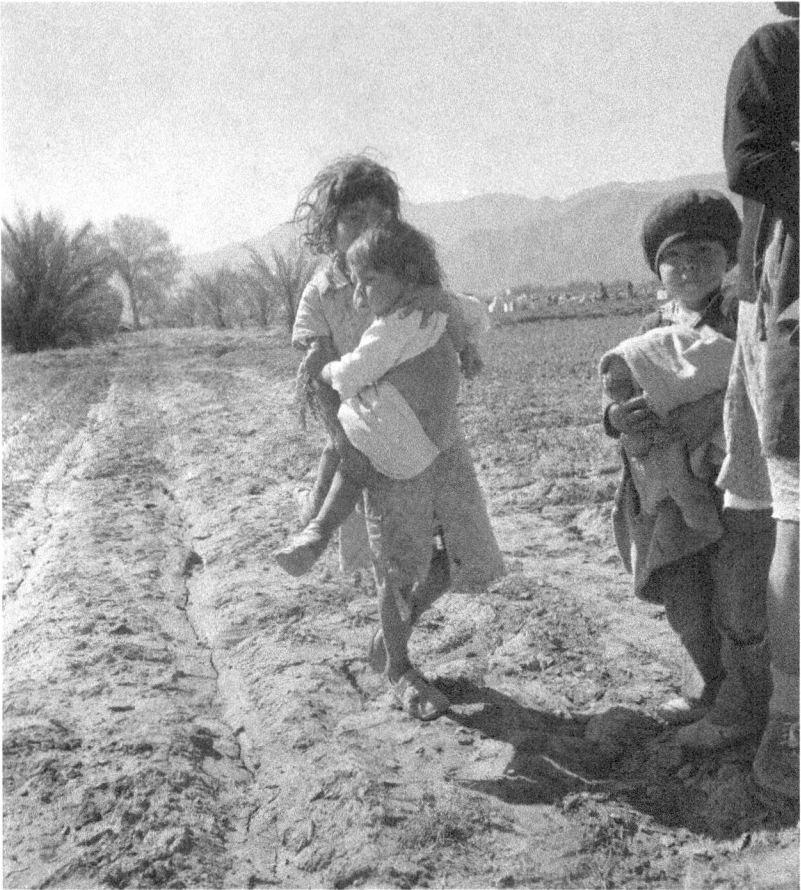

FIGURE 2.2. Original caption: "Children of migratory Mexican field workers. The older one helps tie carrots in the field. Coachella Valley, California." Photo by Dorothea Lange, 1937. Library of Congress Prints and Photographs Division.

Federal and state migrant health efforts during the New Deal were not primarily framed in terms of workers' rights to health protection or well-being. Rather, as Martínez-Matsuda argues, FSA programs emphasized the potential threat migrants posed as disease carriers and the benefit to the economy of a healthier labor force. While FSA publicity materials (including Dorothea Lange's famous photographs) portrayed migrants in a sympathetic light, some also perpetuated images of Black and Mexican farmworkers as ignorant about health and hygiene and thus partly to blame for their own medical problems.[74]

Yet evidence from migrant health programs shows that immigrant and migrant farmworkers were vitally interested in protecting and improving their health and that of their families. When two nurses and a doctor trav-

eled around California migrant camps in 1936–37 offering well-baby talks and
exams, workers eagerly offered their homes for the gatherings. Sometimes,
the doctor reported, "an intelligent Mexican mother would act as interpreter."
At one of the camps, "mothers began to congregate at seven in the morning
waiting for the conference to start." Families stood "in the sweltering heat"
until "the very end" of the conferences, which included lectures and demonstrations on "importance of diet, regularity in feedings and elimination, need
for adequate rest, fresh air and sunshine, posture exercises," and "child behavior." According to the physician, "Sometimes the conference was not finished
until night and kerosene lights or even headlights from automobiles were
used for illumination." In addition, "the Mexican families respond readily to
an immunization or vaccination program." (White migrants in the camps—
the "Okies" described by John Steinbeck—were terrified of the shots and "said
they'd rather have smallpox than be vaccinated," but they did become more
accepting when educated about the benefits of vaccines.)[75]

New Deal efforts on behalf of farmworkers clearly provided medical attention to families who both needed and desired it. However, all of the medical
care programs for migrants, along with the rest of the Farm Security Administration, were ended by a conservative Congress in 1947 as part of its backlash
against the New Deal. A newspaper reporter dramatically described what the
end of the FSA camps meant for migrant potato workers in Morehead City,
North Carolina. In 1947, workers lived "in orderly columns of homes" built by
the FSA. "One year later, the Republican 80th Congress toppled this simple
but efficient structure, and with it vanished the health clinics, the washhouses,
bathhouses, sanitary privies, and recreation facilities. . . . Now . . . the migrant
worker lives in subhuman squalor appropriate to the station of the despised,
disinherited American."[76]

To complete the abandonment of migrant workers, the Social Security
Act and the Fair Labor Standards Act both excluded farm laborers from their
protections. Domestic workers (who worked in people's homes) were also
excluded. These exclusions were in part at the behest of southern Democratic
legislators who wanted to avoid covering Black workers but were also supported by some western Republican congressmen who represented agricultural regions heavily dependent on Mexican farm labor. As a result of their
exclusion, farm- and domestic workers were not covered by the new federal
minimum wage requirements or unemployment insurance, and they still
lacked the right to organize unions.[77]

Even so, New Deal medical programs had planted new ideas about migrants' and immigrants' rights to health and health care. Martínez-Matsuda
argues that the FSA programs attempted to create "migrant citizens" who

could exercise democratic rights regardless of their immigration status, and, at least briefly, "forced U.S. society to see migrant workers beyond their economic value."[78] This was seen in the pleas of a California public health department director, who wrote to the farm employers in his district, "The laboring man does not ask for a luxurious home in which to live. He does ask for decent housing and sanitary conditions for himself and his family. Give these things to him, they are his just due."[79]

Another opportunity for the expansion of immigrant and migrant rights came with the explosion of labor union organizing during the Great Depression. Thousands of workers in the vegetable, fruit, and cotton fields of California boldly conducted strikes in the early 1930s, but they had few victories, mostly because of increased organizing by employers that included violent vigilantism and anticommunist repression.[80]

Labor activism was also extensive in the food processing industry, in which Mexican American and Mexican immigrant workers predominated. In San Antonio, Texas, the young Mexican American organizer Emma Tenayuca led militant strikes in the pecan-shelling factories. Women workers in California fruit packing successfully organized locals of the United Cannery, Agricultural, Packing, and Allied Workers of America. By the early 1940s, organized cannery workers in Southern California had won a hospitalization plan for their members.[81]

The cannery workers' victory was a rare example of advancement for immigrant workers' health rights. The organizing of immigrant and migrant workers was hampered by employer and police violence and the deportation and repatriation campaigns. Mexican workers joining the 1937 Republic Steel strike in Chicago were beaten and shot alongside many others, and police also threatened them with deportation. The San Antonio pecan strike ended when employers decided to mechanize the industry rather than pay higher wages. The traditional labor movement was mostly uninterested in interracial organizing, and they launched anticommunist attacks on the new CIO industrial unions that did try to organize Black and immigrant workers.[82] Even unions that included Mexican workers, such as the International Ladies' Garment Workers' Union (ILGWU), did not prioritize them. Russian Jewish ILGWU organizer Rose Pesotta was enthusiastic about Mexican workers' active participation in garment workers strikes in Los Angeles but was disappointed when the union decided not to create a Mexican local.[83]

The failure to unionize some of the nations' most exploited workers was also a loss for immigrants' and migrants' health care. In previous decades, garment unions enrolling mostly Jewish and Italian immigrants had brought about extensive improvements in workplace conditions, "practically eliminated sweat shops" in the Northeast, and, in the case of the ILGWU, created medical services for their members.[84] Without unions, and without the protections offered by New Deal labor legislation, newer immigrants and all migrant workers were left with fewer tools to protect and improve their health. In the Southwest and California, as well as the entire US South, poll taxes and school segregation further eroded Black and Mexican residents' ability to fight for better conditions.[85] And starting in the 1940s, contract labor programs created a new class of deportable workers with no enforceable rights at all.

3

Insuring, Exploiting, and Caring for Migrants

Health Insurance for Braceros

During World War II, the US and Mexican governments created the Emergency Farm Labor Program to bring Mexican laborers to work for US farms and industries experiencing labor shortages. It was supposed to be a temporary wartime measure, but the "bracero program" (as it came to be known) proved so beneficial to US businesses that in 1951 Congress created a law to codify it (Public Law 78) and continued to reauthorize it for over twenty years. Eventually, over four million Mexican men worked as braceros (the term derived from the Spanish word for "arm"; the closest equivalent in English was "farmhand"), primarily in agriculture. Braceros were given temporary work permits and expected to return to Mexico at the end of their contracts.

To entice the continued participation of Mexico and to calm opposition from American labor unions, the US government promised to enforce some basic standards for bracero labor. Employers of braceros were supposed to pay no less than the prevailing wage of local workers; provide decent housing, food, and medical care; and provide return transport to Mexico at no charge. However, these requirements were frequently not enforced. The bracero program actually led to more undocumented immigration, as workers "skipped" their contracts or remained after they ended, and employers continued to seek cheap labor in addition to or instead of braceros. When the bracero era came to an end in 1964, overall farmworkers' pay in the US had declined compared to wages in manufacturing. Most devastating to individual workers, many braceros were not paid in full and waited years for back wages that never came.[1]

After expelling Mexicans in the 1930s, the US wanted them back in the 1940s, but only under controlled conditions and always with the assurance that they would return home. Control of braceros included, once again, la-

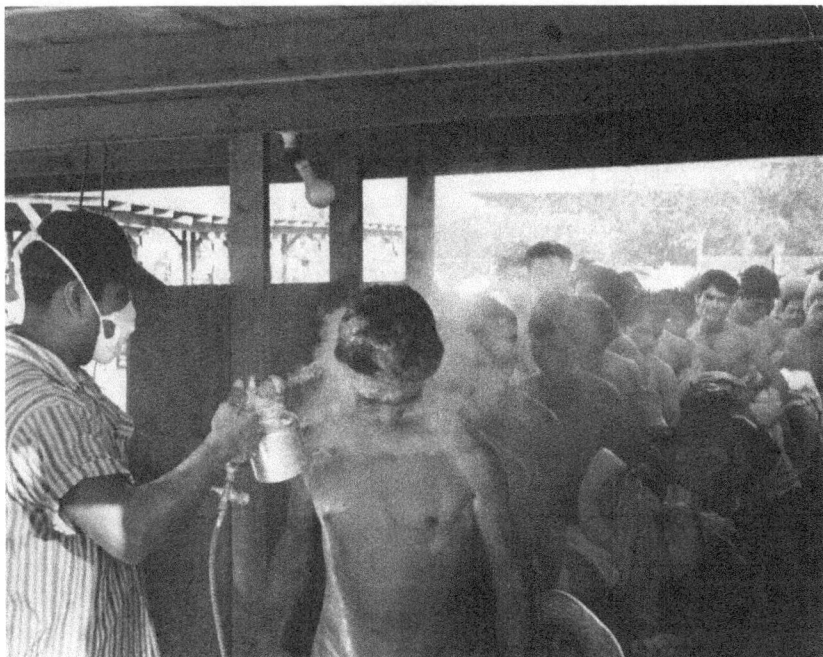

FIGURE 3.1. Bracero workers being sprayed with pesticides at Hidalgo Processing Center, Texas, 1956. The person doing the spraying is masked, but the braceros are not. Leonard Nadel Photographs and Scrapbooks, Archives Center, National Museum of American History, Smithsonian Institution.

beling Mexicans as potential carriers of disease. To be accepted as a bracero laborer, men (women were not allowed into the program) had to undergo medical inspections at recruitment centers in Mexico. Applicants were crammed together in waiting rooms and required to publicly undress and undergo tests for tuberculosis, sexually transmitted diseases, and psychological defects. If they passed these inspections, a second medical examination awaited them on arrival in the US, where a delousing process included spraying the workers with DDT and other dangerous chemicals. One bracero recounted that "men would come in with masks, and they'd fumigate us from top to bottom. Supposedly we were flea-bitten and germ-ridden." The braceros were not offered their own masks to protect themselves against inhaling the chemicals. While the exams could be humiliating, alarming, and dangerous, some of the men who made it through also expressed pride that their health and fitness had passed the scrutiny of modern medicine.[2]

Braceros were required to arrive healthy, but many of them ended up getting sick or injured in the US. As historian Mary E. Mendoza describes it, "Braceros' health began to decline almost as soon as they crossed into the

United States." Their housing conditions were extremely crowded and created breeding grounds for tuberculosis and other respiratory diseases. Bracero contracts required employers to provide them with food, but often the quality was horrible and led to malnutrition, intestinal parasites, and outbreaks of food poisoning. In the fields, workers became sick from heat, dehydration, exposure, pesticides, and overexertion. Braceros were injured or killed in work accidents and, frequently, automobile and truck crashes.[3]

Officially, braceros were supposed to have some insurance protection for illness and accidents. Starting in 1949, braceros were included in workers' compensation for on-the-job injuries, and in 1953 the program added a requirement for life and health insurance.[4] But in practice, braceros' access to medical services varied widely and was sometimes nonexistent. Employers and the government found ways to limit or deny their access to care, including pocketing workers' insurance payments, denying that they were covered, and deporting them if they needed medical care.

Whether or not they had insurance, workers might need to depend on the generosity of their employers. Some braceros recalled that when they got sick or injured, the *patrón* (boss) or *mayordomo* (field manager) would drive them to the doctor or hospital and take care of the bill. But one told an interviewer that when he injured his leg and asked the foreman to get a doctor, the foreman refused, saying, "it would be a bad example because all the men would be asking to see the doctor."[5]

Employers and recruiters did little or nothing to inform braceros about their health and accident coverage, whose premiums the workers were required to pay themselves via payroll deductions. When scholar and labor organizer Ernesto Galarza interviewed 345 braceros in the mid-1950s, not a single one was able to describe "even one provision" of their insurance policies. Galarza deduced that they had never been shown their own insurance contracts. They definitely knew, though, that thirteen cents a day was deducted from their wages for the insurance premium.[6]

Most of the braceros interviewed by Galarza never sought medical care. Of those who did, "some reported that they had been well cared for; others complained of delays in being taken from the camp to a physician." The bracero insurance didn't allow for doctors and nurses to make "camp calls," and "since camp managers do not feel responsible for maintaining what they commonly call a 'taxi service' for their men, it is up to the sick bracero" to find transportation. "Often the sick man walks. During the course of this study," Galarza reported, "eighteen (Mexican) Nationals, singly or in pairs, were picked up along main highways and country roads going to a nearby town to visit a doctor or to buy medicine."[7]

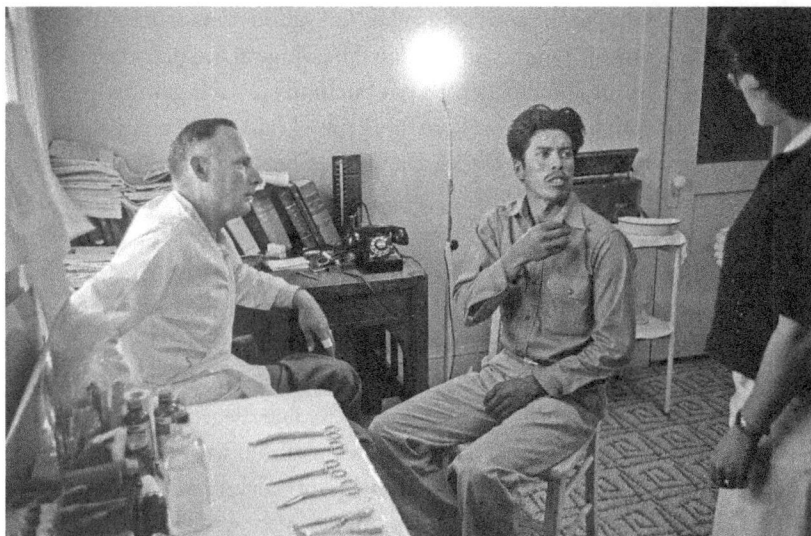

FIGURE 3.2. A bracero speaks to a nurse during an appointment with Dr. Stanley Savoy, Salinas Valley, California, 1956. This image illustrates both the agency of braceros in seeking medical care and the importance of bilingual nurses in doctor-patient communication. Neither the bracero nor the nurse are named. Leonard Nadel Photographs and Scrapbooks, Archives Center, National Museum of American History, Smithsonian Institution.

Galarza found numerous violations of workers' rights to utilize their insurance. He reported that sick workers "who are paid up on their insurance premiums" were still billed for their medical care. Braceros who were denied reimbursement had little recourse; neither the US government nor the Mexican consuls devoted resources to investigating compliance with bracero labor contracts. "With no official check," Galarza concluded, "it is small wonder that braceros are often denied the medical care to which they are entitled and for which they have paid."[8]

Ben Yellen, a doctor in Brawley, California, was so disturbed by what he saw of bracero health coverage that he brought a lawsuit against the insurance company that he believed was stealing workers' money. Braceros, Yellen asserted, "are paying for first class adequate medical care" but not getting it. Men kept coming to his office because the insurance company's doctor only had office hours when workers were in the fields. Like Galarza, Yellen reported that workers were not informed about their benefits: "Many do not know that they are entitled to weekly disability payments," and the insurance company didn't give copies of their policies to the workers "(so) they know nothing. . . . The laborer often does not know that he should have been sent to the hospital."[9]

Gabriel Mondrajon Gomez, who came to California as a bracero in 1957, told his health care story to a congressional hearing on the bracero program. He reported, "Around November 1, I got pneumonia from getting wet while working. I was sick for 22 days. The whole time I had to keep paying for my board out of my own pocket. The insurance paid nothing. Finally, on November 20, my contract expired. I was sent back [to Mexico], although I was still sick."[10] "This trick of sending the sick workers back to Mexico," Yellen wrote in one of his many complaints, "and thereby avoiding the payment of medical expenses and avoiding the payment of disability payments . . . is really slick." Braceros who got hernias and other injuries on the job "were kicked back to Mexico without operation," Yellen claimed, and "back in the isolated valleys they came from where there were no doctors," some died.[11]

Far from passive victims, braceros spoke out about their conditions. This had been true since the earliest days of the guest worker programs in World War II. As the historian Chantel Rodriguez has shown, wartime braceros working on US railroads collaborated with local advocacy and church groups to publicize exploitation and abuse and even held protests demanding reimbursement for medical care.[12] In the subsequent farm labor programs, braceros continued to speak out. In 1950, for example, 7 percent of the forty-six thousand braceros in Texas filed some sort of complaint or claim against their employer.[13]

Bracero complaints were supposed to be investigated by the US Department of Labor, but, one observer noted, "Within the compliance system were provided built-in mechanisms for systematic evasion of the law." Grace L. Wiest, a researcher who studied the bracero program, wrote that "Mexican workers would remain in the United States too short a time to pursue legal channels in the event of disputes, and the budget was not provided to operate an adequate surveillance program." In addition, she made the crucial point that "the initiative for making complaints rested, primarily, on the individual who was least able to protect himself from retaliation by the growers, since the person complaining was a Mexican national, on a temporary visa in a non-unionized occupation."[14]

Retaliation often took the form of sending workers back home. The greatest obstacle to braceros' claiming their rights was their deportability. Studies of the program and congressional testimony are full of examples of braceros being returned to Mexico if they got sick. Yellen charged that employers colluded with insurance companies and immigration agents to remove sick and injured workers so that they would not have to pay insurance claims. In one example described to researcher Harry Anderson, a bracero broke his collarbone on the job and was supposed to be awarded $500. According to Anderson's informant, who was a federal agent, the worker "was asked to sign a statement saying that he had received two hundred dollars, and was told that the other three hundred would be sent to him after he returned to Mexico. He complained that he wanted to wait for the whole five hundred dollars. He was advised to sign. He refused." The informant then "witnessed two other agents violently force [the] bracero into a car and drive off toward the border. After the truck got back from the border, some of the employees at the center saw blood on the upholstery. [The agent] said the bracero had cut his finger."[15]

Deportation was also used as retaliation against workers who complained about their treatment. Yellen tells of one bracero who went to small claims court "to sue his exploiters, but the big farm corporations got the U.S. Border Patrol to catch the bracero and run him out of the U.S." Another worker was hospitalized but then "forced out" of the Brawley hospital when the insurance company refused to pay for his care. This man was supposed to serve as a witness for lawsuits against the growers, but, Yellen alleged, "the defendants acted to eject [the bracero] from the United States to Mexico where it would be impossible to find and return [him] to be a witness in time for these two lawsuits."[16]

By 1963, thanks to bracero complaints and the efforts of civil rights groups, labor unions, and researchers like Anderson and Galarza, opinion in Congress began to turn against the program. US unions argued that contracted Mexican labor constituted unfair competition, depressed the wages of local workers, and weakened organizing efforts. Small farmers complained that the program was a direct government subsidy to large growers, who utilized the vast majority of bracero workers. Opponents accused employers of flouting the contracts by using braceros to performed skilled labor and of "systematic evasion" of the benefits they were supposed to provide.[17]

Health insurance and other benefits played a role in Congress's decision to end the bracero program. In 1960, the Joint United States–Mexico Trade Union Committee had recommended "that domestic [US] workers be covered by the same . . . Worker's Compensation as the braceros in California, which had compulsory Workmen's Compensation Laws." Pressure from the AFL-CIO then forced Congress to double the injury compensation amounts in the 1961 bracero program reauthorization. Employers, especially smaller farmers, became alarmed that "should the bracero program continue, a 'fair labor standards act' would be effected for domestics, using the bracero program as a base." Their fears seemed to be validated when Senator Eugene McCarthy proposed a bill requiring employers to provide "the same benefits for domestic farm workers as those provided for braceros," including medical insurance. Researcher Grace Wiest argues that the prospect of being forced to provide coverage to US farmworkers "finally created farm opposition to the bracero program" and led to its demise in 1964.[18]

Even though braceros were often denied what they had been promised, bracero labor contracts provided far more protections than US farmworkers ever had. The bracero program offered an opportunity to make the case for similar benefits for domestic laborers. Instead, those very guarantees led to the program's end, before US workers were able to claim similar rights. By requiring insurance coverage, the bracero program actually gave temporary Mexican workers more health protection, at least on paper, than US citizen workers, most of whom were entitled to none. As the program ended, the California state senate held a hearing to discuss how the state would now "be dependent on out-of-state workers for its farm harvesting" rather than Mexican workers. One concern expressed at the hearing was "medical care for farm workers whose income from seasonal employment is not enough for such care. It was pointed out that under the Mexican labor (bracero) program medical care is provided for. There is no such provision for domestic workers."[19] There was even less protection for the undocumented Mexican workers who continued to arrive.

With organizing curtailed, wages depressed, and undocumented migration unabated, the bracero era left the US farm labor movement weakened. But the persistent efforts of unions, civil rights leaders, and braceros themselves to expose the program's abuses did lead to increased attention to the health problems of agricultural workers, which would culminate in a Migrant Health Act in 1962.

Japanese American Internment and Health Care Activism

In the earliest days of the bracero program, not all of the unfree workers on US farms were from Mexico. In Oregon, Idaho, Utah, and Arizona, Japanese Americans could be found laboring in fields of sugar beets and other crops. They were prisoners of the US government, labeled "enemy aliens" due to their national origin. When their work was finished, they had to return not home, but to internment camps—also accurately called concentration camps.

In February 1942, after Japan attacked Pearl Harbor, President Franklin D. Roosevelt ordered the evacuation of over 110,000 West Coast residents of Japanese origin, the majority of whom were US citizens. The evacuees were detained in ten hastily built camps in remote interior areas of the western US, Arizona, and Arkansas. Responding to demands from agricultural employers, in May of that year the federal government established the Seasonal Leave

Program, allowing Japanese and Japanese Americans to be released from detention to assist in "essential war work." Between 1942 and 1944, about thirty-three thousand detainees were taken from the camps to work on farms. They lived in labor camps supervised by the Farm Security Administration, the New Deal agency, which at least ensured that their conditions were less abusive than for braceros. Although they were clearly exploited for their labor, some Japanese farmworkers felt that their position was an improvement over internment and even petitioned to continue working in the fields rather than return to the camps.[20]

Their reluctance to return was understandable, for health conditions in the internment camps were atrocious. Gwenn M. Jensen's extensive study concludes that "a number of factors compromised health care in the concentration camps: poor planning and design, adverse environmental conditions, the contamination of food and water, overcrowding, inadequate staffing, and racism." Most of the camps were located in dry areas, where their construction stripped all vegetation, leading to continual dust storms that tormented the detainees and seared their eyes and lungs. The sand blew through the flimsy buildings into the tiny rooms where they slept crowded together. The two camps in Arkansas were built on swamps, leading to constant flooding.[21]

Over two hundred babies died in the concentration camps, and many of these deaths were due to dehydration and heat. The medical officer at Rohwer camp in Arkansas reported that "the temperature in the nursery for hours at a time was above 104 degrees." Detainees also suffered in the cold, which at one camp in Wyoming dropped to thirty below zero. Contaminated food and water led to many illnesses. Inmates suffered from food poisoning and dysentery, and thirty-nine diabetics died due to inadequate diets. Tuberculosis, polio, and typhoid also spread through the overcrowded camps.[22]

The prisoners were supposed to be provided with medical care, but it took months or even years for adequate facilities to be set up. There was a shortage of medicines and basic equipment such as X-ray machines. In one camp, detainees even took up a collection to buy medical equipment with their own money. So few trained personnel were available due to wartime shortages that the camps employed their own prisoners as medical staff. Jensen writes that "nurse's aides, all of Japanese descent, provided the bulk of patient care." Interned nurses and physicians were still treated as prisoners and experienced racial slurs and abuse from the white medical staff, as did patients.[23]

Raising money for medical supplies and working as medical practitioners were types of detainee collective action on behalf of their community's health. Some of the imprisoned Japanese and Japanese Americans went even further

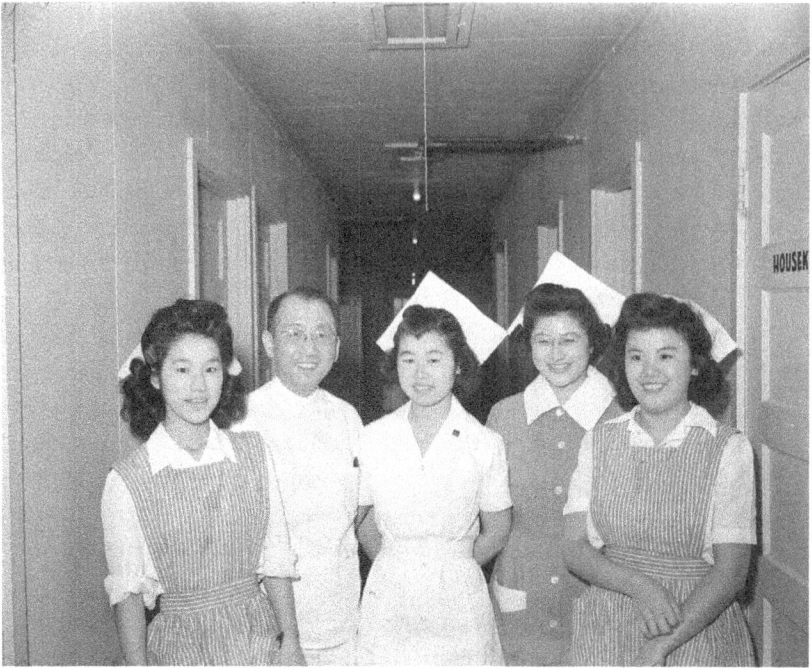

FIGURE 3.3. Unidentified Japanese and/or Japanese American doctor, nurses, and candy stripers, Tule Lake Relocation Center, Newell, California. Their smiles belie their imprisonment and the involuntary conditions under which they worked. Photo by Pete O' Crotty, 1943. Library of Congress Prints and Photographs Division.

by actively protesting against medical abuse and neglect. At Tule Lake detention center in California, internees pushed for the resignation of the "autocratic" white medical officer, Dr. Pedicord, who called all his medical staff "Japs." Pedicord persisted in his ways, until a group of young men "pulled him out of his office" and beat him up. In another, less violent type of resistance, the detainee medical staff at Heart Mountain camp in Wyoming staged a walkout to protest inadequate hospital facilities.[24]

These activities were part of the collective actions of detainees to establish schools, farms, and other enterprises that helped them survive the camps. They also engaged in lawsuits, draft resistance, and strikes. When faced with deadly conditions, people of Japanese origin imprisoned in the camps used many methods to fight for better medical care, including actually providing that care. As historian Susan Smith writes, the internment "produced a health care crisis of enormous proportions that was averted only because of the efforts of Japanese Americans themselves."[25]

Exploiting and Deporting "Wetbacks"

Most interned Japanese American farmworkers left the fields after their release in 1945, but braceros remained, alongside another type of Mexican worker whose numbers were rapidly growing: the "wetback." This derogatory term, used as early as 1920, was coined by Texas employers to describe workers who crossed the border without permission. Since they had to ford the Rio Grande, they arrived "wet" (*mojado*).[26] The height of the bracero era coincided with a significant growth in the numbers of undocumented migrants. Far from reducing incentives to enter without papers, the bracero program instead encouraged more workers to risk an unauthorized border crossing, since there were far more jobs available than official openings. Also, many braceros stayed after their contracts expired, thus becoming "illegal" themselves. Some even "skipped out" of abusive contracts, preferring to take their chances as undocumented workers.[27]

Some Americans feared that the influx of undocumented workers constituted a threat to public health. A presidential committee noted that, unlike braceros, "the wetback undergoes no health or physical examination as he illicitly enters the United States.... Moreover, while he is here ... the wetback will not ordinarily risk the chance of apprehension by seeking medical or health assistance." Undocumented workers could also be turned away from public medical care due to their nonresidency.[28]

Yet, in the eyes of some farm employers, these workers' lack of a right to medical care helped make them desirable employees. "Some farmland owners appear to prefer the wetback to the bracero," reported the *Arizona Republic* in 1953. To hire a bracero, "the employer must agree in advance on hourly rates of pay, on housing, on medical attention.... But to employ a wetback, a farmer offers little or no housing—some sleep in the fields—a wage below that given braceros, no medical care, and no transportation." (Some employers who hired both bracero and undocumented workers did provide them with the same or comparable wages and benefits.)[29]

"Legal" and "illegal" workers shared the condition of deportability. Both ex-braceros and illicit border crossers were swept up in "Operation Wetback," the Eisenhower administration's 1954 mass deportation campaign. Attorney General Herbert Brownell initiated the operation following a wave of media reports and complaints from officials in California and the Southwest about the influx of undocumented migrants. They alleged that "wetbacks" led to a rise in crime and venereal disease, and—echoing the repatriation campaigns of the 1930s—that they drained local resources, including medical and hospital care.[30]

In "Operation Wetback," the Immigration and Naturalization Service (INS) conducted raids, demanded papers, and (they claimed) deported over a million people. A militarized immigration service used cars, helicopters, and airplanes in their roundups. In Los Angeles, detainees were held in pens awaiting deportation. In Chicago, captured Mexicans were loaded onto airplanes and flown to the Mexican border, then put on ships to be taken further south. As in the 1930s deportation drives, legal residents, family members, and US citizens were also caught up in the raids.[31]

Also like the earlier repatriations, Operation Wetback proved devastating to health. Mexican border towns again "swelled by the arrival of thousands of Mexicans who had either been apprehended and sent there or who had fled across the border to avoid capture. A great many of these people were without food and shelter." In the "hot-foot lift," agents dropped deportees in the middle of the desert, "deliberately hauling them to one place where there is no food, water, or shelter." A newspaper reporting on this practice called it "a revolting operation that attempts to strip the last shred of human dignity from oppressed peoples and treats them as worse than animals."[32]

Operation Wetback also led to fatalities. In Texas, a man was decapitated by the propellers of a Border Patrol plane searching for Mexican workers to deport. To prevent deportees from quickly recrossing the border, US officials conducted a "boat lift" to take them halfway down the Gulf Coast of Mexico. In 1956, deportees on the ship *Mercurio* mutinied to protest horrific overcrowding. Dozens jumped overboard as part of the protest, and four men drowned.[33]

There were other examples of resistance to Operation Wetback. Jesus Morales was in his Los Angeles barbershop when he and his customers saw several agents pulling up "with carloads of Mexicans they had already caught." As agents approached the shop, customers began "cussing them out loud" and one of his customers "yelled, 'You are like a pack of mad dogs the way you go around stopping people!'" The agents left without entering the shop. A group of women workers in a factory being raided "escaped the dragnet" when their boss hastily led them out a back exit.[34] Also in Los Angeles, Japanese Americans joined in protests against the "undemocratic herding and fencing of human beings." An Arizona resident wrote to the governor to protest the misery caused by the deportations and argued that the Southwest's prosperity was a product of the "patient, willing labor" of Mexican workers.[35]

The INS claimed that the Operation Wetback resulted in 1,300,000 deportations. This was undoubtedly a gross exaggeration. But the campaign did have serious repercussions for both deportees and local communities.

"'Operation Wetback' had a significant impact on the people of Mexican descent in the United States," writes historian Juan Ramon García. It "once again attested to the fact that Mexicans were welcomed here only as long as there was a need for their labor." In addition, it was clear that Operation Wetback "was aimed at only one racial group."[36]

Mexican American Rights, Health Rights—but Not Yet Immigrant Rights

In the 1920s, as immigration from Mexico had started to increase, Mexican Americans in Texas began to form a new kind of organization. The new clubs all had the word "America" in their names: Sons of America, Knights of America, the League of United Latin American Citizens (LULAC). Unlike the *mutualistas*, which welcomed both long-term residents and immigrants, these clubs were open only to US citizens.[37] Texas was experiencing an upsurge in discrimination against people of Mexican descent, and Mexican Americans wanted to protect their communities by distinguishing themselves from the masses of unwanted, "foreign" Mexicans.

Increasingly, Mexican Americans were subject to "Juan Crow" discrimination in schools, restaurants, and the courts. Rather than making common cause with the African Americans who were fighting for their civil rights, most Mexican American organizations from the 1920s through the 1950s chose a "whiteness" strategy. They argued that US citizens of Mexican descent should not be identified as a race of their own but instead should be included in the "white" racial category. This strategy met with mixed success, since even if they were officially designated white, the dominant society still viewed all Mexicans as racially distinct.[38]

The new Mexican American organizations joined US labor unions in opposing the bracero program. In Texas, they managed to prevent the establishment of the guest worker program for several years by publicizing the harsh racial discrimination there and convincing Mexico that Texas would never protect braceros' rights. When they lost the battle against the bracero program, Texas activists turned their attention to opposing undocumented "wetbacks."

Mexican American organizations saw their fight against immigrants as inseparable from the struggle to improve the conditions of life for US citizens of Mexican descent. Alongside their anti-bracero and anti-immigrant campaigns, these groups worked to end hospital discrimination against Spanish-speaking people and to attack the terrible health conditions that led to high mortality among the Mexican population in Texas. The most prominent

Mexican American organization to engage in health-related activism was the American GI Forum, founded in 1948 by thirty-four-year-old physician Hector P. García.

As its name indicates, the GI Forum was created primarily for veterans of World War II. García was born in Tamaulipas, Mexico. His family emigrated to Corpus Christi, Texas, during the Mexican Revolution, and he earned his medical degree at the University of Texas–Galveston. After serving in the Army Medical Corps in Europe during the war, García returned to Corpus Christi to set up a medical practice. He began hearing many complaints about the unfair treatment of Mexican American veterans who were being denied their full pension and education benefits. García founded the GI Forum to address this injustice. At the group's first meeting in 1948, seven hundred veterans showed up, and by the end of the year, there were forty GI Forum chapters in Texas.[39]

As a physician with a local practice, García daily witnessed the intolerable health conditions suffered by Mexican American communities. In Corpus Christi and around the state of Texas, Mexican Americans had disproportionately high rates of infant mortality, dysentery (due to unclean drinking water), and tuberculosis. García was infuriated that Nueces County, where Corpus Christi was located, had only a single twenty-bed tuberculosis hospital "but 7,000 TB cases." García's GI Forum also demanded that the US government establish a veterans' hospital in South Texas. García repeatedly complained that Mexican American veterans had to travel hundreds of miles to San Antonio to receive care.[40]

In denouncing the deadly health conditions plaguing Mexican Americans, García put the blame squarely on poverty and discrimination. "Poor housing, slum areas, a low standard of living leads to poor bodily resistance which in turn opens the door to all kinds of diseases," and "too many people do not have a decent wage," he declared in a 1948 speech. Yet the state government neglected the health problems of the poor. "It has always been rather peculiar that when a disease like 'Polio' strikes the upper class, everybody concentrates their efforts in stopping the disease," García noted, "and yet 'Polio' accounted for only 29 deaths in Texas last year," while in that same year 2,740 people died of tuberculosis in the state and diarrhea killed 1,100 babies. García concluded that "officials are not as interested in protecting the health of the poor people as they are in the higher income group."[41]

García clearly defined health disparities as a product of racial and class discrimination. The GI Forum fought against the same kinds of public accommodations segregation that Black civil rights groups were protesting. In 1948, Corpus Christi organizations called a meeting to protest "the segregation of our people at Memorial Hospital." This public hospital designated certain wards for Mexicans only. The following year García went to see a patient at Memorial and found him on a gurney in the hallway because the "Mexican Ward for Males" was full. García called the superintendent and—invoking the "whiteness" strategy—insisted that the patient be placed on the Anglo (white) ward. Perhaps due to García's clout, the superintendent complied.[42]

The GI Forum investigated discrimination at other Texas hospitals, including a complaint about the treatment of newborn Mexican babies at the county hospital in Bay City, near Houston. According to Bay City resident Carmel Zarate, after his wife gave birth there in November 1953, he asked to have the baby placed in the hospital nursery, since he had to get back to work and the new mother was exhausted. After making several excuses, a nurse finally told Zarate that "Latin-American babies are not placed in the nursery." He complained that the baby "remained" with his wife "in her room" for her entire three-day stay.[43] Zarate's response was a protest against blatant racial discrimination, and also an example of Mexican American patients' desire for "modern" skilled hospital care rather than traditional postnatal practices. In the eyes of medical modernizers like García, the denial of such care was an especially egregious form of racism.

Also in 1953, the GI Forum chapter in Colorado City, Texas, complained that several medical clinics in the city were discriminating against Mexican patients. The clinics "follow the practice of segregating of Mexican descent or nationality in separate waiting rooms with Negro people." The GI Forum was not objecting to the principle of segregated waiting rooms, but to Mexicans being classified as nonwhite. As the historian Brian Behnken has shown, due to their anti-Black racism the GI Forum and other Mexican American organizations resisted joining the struggle against Jim Crow, leaving Black Texans to "fight their own battles." García even insisted that he disliked the term "civil rights" because of its association with Black organizations.[44]

Rather than fighting discrimination on the basis of civil rights, García insisted on health rights earned through veteran status or US citizenship. It would be years before mainstream Mexican American organizations like the GI Forum moved away from acting on their racism and embraced civil rights coalition politics.[45] They would also have to undergo a similar journey away from their anti-immigrant stances. Around the same time Operation Wetback was launched, the GI Forum copublished a pamphlet with the Texas State Federation of Labor entitled "What Price Wetbacks?," arguing that both braceros and their undocumented counterparts displaced US workers, drove down wages, and "damaged the health of the American people."[46]

But there were a few Mexican American organizations and leaders that defended the rights of immigrants as well as citizens. Labor organizations in the Southwest like El Congreso and the Asociación Nacional México-Americana, which arose out of the militant strikes of the 1930s, welcomed noncitizens into their ranks, although by the start of the 1950s they were decimated by anticommunist attacks.[47] Labor leader Ernesto Galarza, while strongly opposing the bracero program and the exploitation of undocumented workers, also "advanced arguments that increasingly diverted blame from individual braceros and wetbacks while pointing a finger at government and business," historian David Gutiérrez writes. Gutiérrez also notes that, dismayed by the abuses of Operation Wetback, some members of the mainstream LULAC began "explicitly linking the issue of immigrants' rights to their own campaign to achieve civil rights for American citizens of Mexican descent."[48]

When Mexican American political activists founded the Community Service Organization (CSO) in Los Angeles in 1947, they "actively encouraged" noncitizens to join. The CSO engaged in voter registration and helped elect Edward Roybal as the first Spanish-surnamed member of the city council since 1888. They pushed for immigrants to become citizens, while also arguing that noncitizens deserved a place in the community.[49] The CSO was also the training ground for a young Cesar Chavez, future founder of the United Farm Workers of America, who started working for them as an organizer in 1952.

The Road to the Migrant Health Act

In 1947, two nurses wrote, "John Steinbeck's *Grapes of Wrath* vividly depicted the lives of migrant farm workers during the Depression years. It seems inconceivable that ten years later, despite our high level of prosperity, the social and economic status of most migrant workers has not changed essentially."[50] When it canceled FSA medical care for agricultural workers, Congress had "ended the program but not the problem."[51]

That same year, a group of advocates formed the National Citizens Council for Migrant Labor (NCCML). The council, led by a Congregational Church minister named Thomas Keehn, fought to add farmworkers to the minimum wage and child labor requirements of the Fair Labor Standards Act. In 1949, Keehn testified to Congress, "Agricultural labor generally and migrant workers in particular represent the most forgotten group in our society. . . . Surely it is time to begin to count these workers in the fields."[52]

The NCCML also discussed proposing a bill that would focus specifically on migrants' health care. Since a conservative Congress always shot down legislation it deemed "socialistic," the advocates decided that a plan solely for medical care would be more palatable. "There is widespread Congressional interest in the health field," a NCCML memo noted, and "Of all types of social legislation, health bills—other than those with compulsory insurance features—are the least controversial." Even the American Medical Association might not be threatened by a migrant medical care program, since they were "on record as favoring tax-supported programs of medical care for the indigent in which category farm migrants certainly fall."[53]

But far more modest proposals than this were failing to sway Congress in favor of migrant worker protections. In 1950—the same year that he gave up his proposal for national health insurance—President Harry S. Truman established the President's Commission on Migratory Labor in American Agriculture, "to investigate the social, economic, health, and educational conditions among migratory workers, both alien and domestic, in the United States." The commission held hearings around the country, where speakers made arguments both for and against the bracero program and improved housing and working conditions for domestic farm laborers. In its final report, the Truman commission recommended easing the importation of contract laborers, greater use of domestic (citizen) labor, the adoption of housing and minimum wage standards for domestic migrants, and penalties for employers who hired undocumented workers. But Congress adopted exactly none of the commission's recommendations and instead renewed the bracero program again. The failure of the commission attested to both Truman's weakening influence and to the increasing political power of consolidated agribusiness, which had strong representation on Capitol Hill.[54]

Even so, the Truman commission hearings and reports did begin an accounting of the health problems of agricultural laborers that would, right before the end of the bracero era, lead to a new federal program to provide medical care to domestic migrant workers. The 1950 report noted, "State after state, from North to South and from East to West, reports similar stories of the close relationship between migratory farm labor, sickness, disease, and death. Tuberculosis, infant mortality, maternal mortality, dysentery, enteritis, smallpox, typhoid: all are more prevalent among migratory workers than among the general population."[55]

According to most accounts, migrant workers deserved improved conditions not because of their human right to health, but in order to protect the general public. Migrant workers brought "a cargo of sickness" wherever they went, according to a Texas newspaper, stating that "Texas exports to at least 31 other states a deadly cargo of virulence" via migrants, including tuberculosis, venereal disease, typhoid, dysentery, and even leprosy. "All these people are sick. You name it, they got it," reported a Texas health official.[56] A North Carolina newspaper warned, "the venereal (sexually transmitted disease) rate among these workers, who handle our food, is 11 percent." The rural schools director of the National Education Association commented, "It is unfortunate, but understandable, that local parents sometimes resent the migrant child's attendance in the local school because of the danger of communicable diseases."[57]

But arguments for protecting the public health were no match for conservative opposition to government involvement in labor conditions. In 1956 the Colorado state senate killed a bill that would have required better sanitation in migrant worker camps. Legislators argued that it was the workers themselves, not their conditions, that led to their bad health and that "if they ha[d] modern facilities, they [wouldn't] know how to use them." Lamented the bill's sponsor, "The whole thing boils down to the fact that migrants don't vote and employers do. . . . These are the most tragically neglected people in the entire population. They frequently live under conditions which imperil the health of the entire community. But they're impotent, politically, and no one does anything about it."[58] Employers, on the other hand, were far from politically impotent. A similar bill in Texas was voted down in 1959; legislators complied with the "farm groups" who "worried that such requirements under the control of 'centralized government' would increase the costs of migrant labor."[59]

Legislation proposed in North Carolina to improve migrant camps where workers lived "in subhuman squalor" repeatedly failed. In that state, only a few church volunteers made an effort to assist the migrants who traveled annually from Florida to work the potato fields, and who were primarily African American US citizens. There was little interest in passing legislation for a group that was only in the state for part of the year, and especially not for Black migrants. Grotesque, open racism underpinned this neglect. The sanitation officer of Carteret County, North Carolina, told a reporter that the workers "don't appreciate what the growers do for them. We are dealing with the scum of the earth. Animals . . . What can you do about it?" He placed the blame for their sickness on the migrants themselves: "If they had the intelligence to be sanitary they wouldn't be migrant workers."[60]

But gradually, at the federal level, there were signs of a shift. Along with the NCCML, groups like the Young Men's Christian Association, the Parent Teacher Association, and the National Consumers' League put pressure on Congress to pass legislation for migrant health and education. President Dwight D. Eisenhower showed some openness to reform by establishing a Committee on Migratory Labor in 1954. In amendments to the Social Security Act in 1954 and 1956, Congress made certain categories of farmworkers eligible for federal old-age pensions. And during the perennial debates over

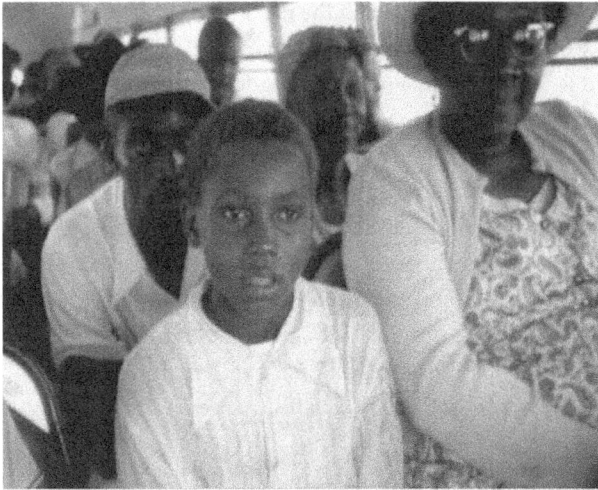

FIGURE 3.4. "The long journey begins." Migrant farmworkers on a bus traveling from Belle Glade, Florida, to "the fields and orchards of America." From the 1960 TV special *Harvest of Shame*. CBS News/Getty Images.

renewing the bracero program, congressional liberals regularly added amendments to require employers to provide better conditions for all farmworkers.[61]

Such amendments were always "torn out" by the time the bills reached the pro-agribusiness Senate.[62] But by 1960, a movement toward migrant health legislation finally gained traction. A Pennsylvania congressman proposed an omnibus migrant health bill, and the Senate Committee on Appropriations asked for a report on "services for migrant mothers and children."[63] In November, John F. Kennedy was elected president, and just a few days later, millions of Americans turned on their television sets and learned about migrant workers for the first time.

On the day after Thanksgiving, 1960, CBS broadcast the documentary *Harvest of Shame*, produced and narrated by the esteemed journalist Edward R. Murrow. The program focused on the horrific conditions experienced by Black and white US citizen migrants from Florida who followed the harvests along the eastern seaboard. Viewers witnessed migrants packed into open trucks, labor camps with no toilet facilities, families sleeping on straw, and children left on their own all day while their parents worked in the fields. They heard from a white migrant mother who only could give her children milk once a week, and from Jerome, a nine-year-old child of Black migrant workers, who showed the camera a nail stuck in his foot that his mother had tried to treat with alcohol since no doctor was available. The show also condemned the bracero program, with the narrator noting that "the constant flow of foreign workers . . . depress[es] the wage scale of the domestic migrant."[64]

Edward R. Murrow was a popular broadcaster, and *Harvest of Shame* generated significant publicity. Many viewers were moved by the depiction of the migrants' plight, but the program angered farm employers and their congressional supporters. The Florida Citrus Commission threatened to sue CBS and the show's sponsors, and Florida senator Spessard L. Holland accused the program of multiple inaccuracies and exaggerations. But in his counter-attack, Holland ended up painting an even more damning picture of migrant conditions. He pointed out that one of the mothers interviewed on *Harvest of Shame* said she had fourteen children, but in reality "seven of her children were dead."[65] This was not exactly an effective defense of agricultural employment conditions.

By early 1962, there were seven migrant health bills being discussed in Congress. Multiple proposals to improve migrant conditions were nothing new, but this time the Senate would actually pass one of the bills. On February 15, the House Committee on Interstate and Foreign Commerce held hearings on "An Act to Amend Title III of the Public Health Service Act to Authorize Grants for Family Clinics for Domestic Agricultural Migratory Workers." It would become known as the Migrant Health Act (MHA).

The hearings on the proposal repeated perennial findings about migrants' terrible health conditions. One sponsor of the House bill announced that farmworkers' lives were "a paradox of poverty amidst plenty, preventable disease in the midst of one of the most highly developed health care systems in the world." Migrants harbored diseases "that medical science has conquered and controlled," including diphtheria and typhoid. The health director of Palm Beach County, Florida, described "tragic stories of sickness, suffering and death. . . . The pregnant woman who has had no prenatal care and for whom there is no place to deliver her baby; the child whose teeth are already rotting away; the baby dying from filth borne dysentery." Again, Congress needed to act not to alleviate migrants' suffering, but to protect the general public. Speakers at the hearing agreed that migrant families "constitute a menace to the permanent residents."[66]

The migrant health bill proposed to allocate $3 million in federal grants to public and private agencies to set up migrant clinics that would provide "health care, preventive medicine, immunization, and some health education." At the hearing on the bill, Dr. Donald Harting of the National Institutes of Health, who had worked with a migrant clinic in Fresno, California, emphasized that the clinics would provide comprehensive services; they would "make it possible with one trip in an evening to get care for the family's problems." Part of the funds would go to setting up a system to coordinate migrant health efforts across state lines, which, according to Harrison Williams, the bill's Senate sponsor, will "enable continuity of health care" for migrants "no matter where they travel."[67]

As an indication of the relative lack of controversy the proposal generated, the hearings on the migrant health bill only took two and a half hours and included no negative testimony. (By contrast, congressional hearings on renewing the bracero program lasted multiple days and were highly contentious.) The bill was supported by Kennedy's Department of Labor and Department of Health, Education, and Welfare. Its sponsors preempted Republican criticism by emphasizing that the cost would be modest and justified federal involvement because "the scope of the migratory health problems are interstate and can only be handled properly and effectively by Federal and State cooperation." The bill's House sponsor, Herbert Zelenko, a New York Democrat, also couched the proposal as a Cold War measure. "There has been a growing public awareness in recent years that the plight of the migrant worker is foreign to our American institutions," Zelenko declared. "This long-festering sore in our society and in our economy provides a propaganda weapon for those who oppose our traditions and ideals. . . . Failure to take prompt remedial action may be viewed as a repudiation of our moral responsibility to our own people, thereby abetting our adversaries in the struggle for the minds of men."[68] Also, the proposal did not include health insurance coverage, so no alarms would be raised about "socialized medicine."

The Migrant Health Act was constructed to avoid opposition from agribusiness. It did not require employers of migrants to pay into their health care or to make any sanitary or housing improvements at all. Sponsors of the bill thought medical care would be the least controversial of all possible reforms, especially if employers were not required to provide it themselves. In fact, the legislation would benefit "farm groups" by subsidizing their employees' fitness to work. Neither would it threaten the medical profession or hospital industry, since it would prevent "unpaid doctor or hospital bills left at the end of a crop season by a migrant whose illness might have been prevented by routine health care and early detection."[69]

Another major reason for congressional support for the Migrant Health Act, and for a lack of employer opposition, was that it preempted arguments that US citizen workers should have the same benefits guaranteed in the bracero program. All of the reform groups testifying at the hearing brought up the bracero medical benefits as an example of the neglect of American workers. The American Public Health Association stated, "Informed people in all groups feel that the difference between the health services provided foreign farmworkers under Public Law 78 [the bracero program], and the services available to domestic workers and their families who are citizens, are indefensibly great." The National Sharecroppers Fund announced, "We find it hard to believe that foreign farmworkers, imported under Public Law 78 and the Puerto Rican worker program, are entitled by the conditions of their contracts to free or inexpensive medical care, while American citizens are forced to suffer disease or even death because of the lack of proper treatment." (The speaker failed to acknowledge that Puerto Ricans were US citizens.)[70]

Only one of the organizations testifying at the hearing made an argument for full equality of benefits. The Friends (Quakers) declared that "domestic migrant workers should receive at least the same assurance of safe transportation, adequate housing and pure water and sanitary facilities, and working conditions guaranteed imported laborers."[71] But the Migrant Health Act was careful *not* to provide these benefits. The bill reflected a strategy of providing modest federally funded services to workers instead of insurance coverage and instead of requiring agribusiness employers to improve conditions.[72] When Congress ended the bracero program two years later, it left zero migrant workers in the US with guaranteed health coverage—and no example of covered workers that could be used as an argument to extend benefits to everyone.

The Migrant Health Act passed with bipartisan support, and the president signed it into law in 1962. In his February 1963 address to Congress on the "health needs of the nation," John F. Kennedy mentioned the passage of the act as an example of his administration's progress in community health. He called the health of migrant workers "deplorable" and announced that he would be requesting supplemental appropriations from Congress to get the program "under way at the earliest possible date."[73]

By May of 1964, the new Migrant Health Unit of the Public Health Service had disbursed federal grants to fifty-five projects "providing health services to migrants in 163 counties scattered over 27 states. Most of the funds were allocated to areas with 3,000 or more migrants at the peak of the crop season." The most common type of local project were evening clinics, which were set up in "township halls, school buildings, church basements, or other improvised space located near large farm labor camps." The clinics primarily offered screenings and minor services and were supplemented by referrals to local doctors.[74]

In Florida—perhaps still smarting from its role in *Harvest of Shame*—public health officials moved quickly to establish a statewide program. They used the federal funds to hire a migrant health coordinator, two health officers, twelve public health nurses, nine sanitarians, two health educators, a nutritionist, a dental assistant, and six clerical and technical personnel. But the staff was stretched thin over Florida's sixty-seven counties. Some counties weren't able to get anything up and running because they couldn't find enough nurses.[75]

But other Florida counties were able to set up successful clinics. Usually they were run out of a county health department building. Where the program was most active, local physicians cooperated with state officials and provided services at the clinics. In some areas of the state, however, doctors refused to work with the MHA. Although the act did not initially provide funding for hospitalization, a few counties negotiated a reduced fee schedule with local hospitals for emergency room visits, which, state officials reported, resulted in fewer inpatient hospitalizations.[76]

Transportation was still a major problem. Florida MHA personnel had trouble finding volunteers willing to drive migrants, due to worries about accident liability. Some growers brought workers to the county health department for clinics, "but this was an infrequent event. . . . A sprinkling of the more enlightened migrants, including some pregnant women, walked or 'thumbed' their way for several miles to clinic locations."[77]

Florida's clinic program fared better than its sanitation and housing efforts. They hired sanitarians who did not speak Spanish, who reported that "several factors hampered their effectiveness. The language barrier and lack of literacy prevented them from conveying instructions to some migrants. Apathy on the part of migrants was considered a hindrance to improving conditions in housing areas." In addition, "Absentee landlords delayed the progress of needed repairs and renovations in housing, due to their unavailability for contact. Many units that were condemned as unfit for human habitation were reoccupied by the evicted migrants soon after the sanitarian left the premises." Growers argued that they needed federal funds to construct sanitary housing for migrants. But the MHA only designated funds for housing inspection, not for actual housing.[78]

By the end of the 1960s, the program was providing grants to fund clinics, public health nursing services, and (starting in 1965) hospitalization coverage in 317 counties in thirty-six states.[79] But the Migrant Health Act continued to fall far short of need. "Hundreds of the Nation's communities with an annual influx of migrants still lack an organized program to provide health services to workers and families," announced Texas senator Ralph Yarborough in 1969. "Every year the migrant health grant funds available are inadequate to respond to the need and requests from communities for grant assistance. As a result, the present program has temporary contact with only about one-third of the Nation's migrants each year," and "funds for hospital care are often exhausted before the season is over." Congress considered and rejected making migrants eligible for the new Medicaid coverage, so workers had to rely on scattered MHA clinics rather than carrying their own insurance with them.[80]

While its reach remained limited, the Migrant Health Act was more transformative even than its supporters gave it credit for. Several years before Lyndon Johnson launched the War on Poverty, the Migrant Health Act created a federally funded program that included both preventive and curative services. It was thus "a precursor to . . . the consolidated community health center program" and "the oldest of all laws that have come to comprise the modern health centers program."[81] Local program reports noted that Migrant Health Act funds acted as a "catalyst" that sparked local communities' and health workers' interest in serving migrants. In Florida, for example, some public health nurses working with the program started taking Spanish classes.[82] Program officials also kept asking Congress to expand the definition of who could be served by the MHA. In 1970, "seasonal farmworkers," workers who did not migrate but who "lived and worked in the same areas as migrants," were added to the MHA's purview, expanding its potential client base from one million to 3.5 million people.[83]

And, quietly, the word "domestic" was dropped from the law. According to MHA administrator Helen L. Johnson, the original act had specified "domestic migrants" in order to ensure that braceros would not be eligible, since they had their own medical program. Apparently, the qualifier "domestic" was not intended to exclude all foreign workers, only those in contract labor programs. With braceros no longer potential competition for other workers, the Department of Health, Education, and Welfare "ruled that Migrant Health Program services should be open to all receiving care regardless of their point of origin."[84] This was especially remarkable since other federal welfare programs began specifically excluding noncitizens in the 1970s.[85] Yet the migrant health programs managed to remain insulated from the politics of immigration. This may have been because migrant health advocates, including some in Congress, were committed to providing access to all farmworkers regardless of their status. Even more likely, it was a matter of realism: by the 1970s, undocumented immigrants were approaching a majority of the migratory farm labor workforce—although this fact was never mentioned in congressional discussions of migrant health.

Citizen Foreigners: Puerto Ricans and Urban Health Care

Although they were by far the most numerous, Mexican braceros were not the only Spanish-speaking contracted workers in the nation's fields. Puerto Ricans had been recruited for US farm labor by private companies ever since the Caribbean island was taken over by the US in 1898. The first government-sponsored labor migration program for Puerto Rico started in World War II, when US officials pushed to utilize more Puerto Rican workers because they were citizens, unlike the contract workers from Mexico, Barbados, Jamaica, and the Bahamas who were also laboring on US railroads and farms. In 1947, Puerto Rico created its own Farm Labor Program, which gave Puerto Rican contract workers similar protections (on paper) to braceros. In addition to protecting workers, the Puerto Rican government's motivation for continuing and expanding the program was to alleviate seasonal agricultural unemployment on the island.[86]

In 1952 Puerto Rican workers were officially defined as "domestic" migrants, which should have given them preference over foreign guest workers. However, as scholar Ismael García-Colón shows, Puerto Rican workers were less desirable to farm employers because they were not deportable. The US government, too, worried that migrants would stay in the US rather than return home. Although they were citizens, Puerto Ricans spoke Spanish and were of mixed racial backgrounds, marking them as foreign and racially inferior. As a colonized population, they occupied a "particular place . . . between minorities and immigrants," writes García-Colón.[87]

Starting in the 1950s, far more Puerto Rican migrants were heading to the cities than the countryside. The island's labor migration program had begun recruiting workers for low-wage industrial jobs in New York and Chicago. In addition to these contracted migrants, hundreds of thousands of Puerto Ricans moved to the US mainland in the two decades after World War II. They were encouraged by their own government to leave, as a way to address continuing high unemployment on the island, the displacement of agricultural workers by its economic modernization campaign (Operation Bootstrap), and so-called overpopulation. Their migration was facilitated by newly affordable flights between San Juan and the mainland.[88]

Most Puerto Rican migrants headed to New York City, and many of them to the Lower East Side. The Henry Street Settlement still sat amid the largest immigrant enclave in the world, but the composition of the neighborhood was changing. The health needs of long-term Jewish and Italian residents had shifted from childbirth and infectious diseases to aging and chronic illness. Fewer neighbors required the services of visiting nurses, since more of them were covered by Blue Cross or HIP, New York City's own prepaid health insurance plan. There were more medical institutions in the neighborhood, including outpatient clinics at Gouverneur Hospital and Beth Israel Hospital, where many Henry Street clients went for care.[89]

Puerto Rican migration created the next wave of newcomers on the Lower East Side. In a twelve-block area surveyed by Henry Street in 1954, nearly 20 percent of the households were from the island. Commenting on the new arrivals, the writer of the survey report mused, "It has been so many years since New York has been forced to bestir itself to consider the problems brought on by a great wave of immigration that it has nearly forgotten how."[90] (This writer fails to mention that Puerto Ricans were citizens, not immigrants.) The settlement house again adjusted to address the needs of younger people, families, and non-English speakers.

Some of the problems experienced by the Puerto Rican newcomers were strikingly similar to those Henry Street witnessed earlier in the century. The tenements had improved, but they were still tenements. A quarter of the housing inhabited by Puerto Rican families in the survey only had toilets in the hall, not in the individual apartments. Fifty-nine percent did not have heat included in the rent. There was still an acute housing shortage on the Lower East Side, and overcrowding in both homes and schools led to "resentment against newcomers." Even though their experiences had so many similarities, older neighborhood residents felt they had little in common with Puerto Ricans, who differed in language, religion, and "national background." Also, although the report did not mention it, Jews and Italians were now able to uphold their white identities as equal to or more important than their ethnicity or immigrant backgrounds, which may have contributed to what Henry Street saw as their lack of welcome for Black and Brown Puerto Ricans.[91]

Although it was no longer providing much direct care, Henry Street carefully studied the health situation of Puerto Ricans on the Lower East Side, especially their access to medical services. In the 1956 survey, they found that 74 percent of Puerto Rican residents utilized a free clinic at Gouverneur Hospital, in contrast with only 54 percent of the older immigrant groups. Many older immigrants detested the clinic and complained about poor treatment there, but Puerto Ricans, according to the report, "Evidently . . . expect very little and are always pleased with the clinic's treatment."[92]

A more complex picture of Puerto Ricans' experiences with neighborhood health care emerged in detailed case studies compiled by Henry Street in the early 1960s. Some Puerto Rican residents did express dissatisfaction with Gouverneur Clinic, which was affiliated with the public Gouverneur Hospital, just a couple of blocks from Henry Street. One family avoided the clinic because their son was treated "in a not nice way" by a doctor there. They "think that most doctors (except Dr. Paymen, the pediatrician at Gouverneur Clinic) are 'bulldogs.' They do not go to the clinic more often because they are frightened of doctors." An older Puerto Rican woman "chose a private physician who speaks Spanish" instead of the clinic "because the doctor does not speak Spanish at the clinic." She expressed that she "wants a doctor 'who tells her the truth in Spanish.'"[93]

Puerto Rican residents with steady jobs—especially union jobs—had more health care options. One man worked as a mechanic for the city transit authority, so his entire family was covered by Blue Cross, "which comes out of union dues paid by Mr. C. . . . The insurance paid for Mrs. C's delivery and [their toddler's] two hospitalizations." The L family had to take their sick children to Beth Israel, the neighborhood's private nonprofit hospital, and ended up with a bill of $200. Fortunately, the father, a shipping clerk, "belongs to a union health plan which paid the entire amount."[94]

But for most Puerto Rican residents, their health care choices were constrained by poverty, sporadic employment, lack of childcare and transportation, and language barriers. One woman was afraid to enter the hospital for a needed hysterectomy because "the Welfare told her they would put her children in a shelter because she had no one to care for them," stated a Henry Street report. "Also she did not get kids vaccinated because welfare did not provide a baby carriage or carfare." Mrs. P's family was able to go to a union health doctor "during periods of employment," but for her last pregnancy, she "went completely without pre-natal care." The S family used Gouverneur Clinic in emergencies, but they "have never had a complete checkup. . . . No member of the family has ever received a chest x-ray, and the last laboratory tests (blood counts and urinalysis) were taken 5 years ago in Puerto Rico." Only the youngest children had up-to-date immunizations, and that was because their mother made the "self sacrifice" of a full day's pay to bring them to the vaccination clinic.[95]

The Right to a Hospital: The Battle for Gouverneur Begins

Gouverneur Hospital's outpatient clinic was the only free clinic within walking distance for most Lower East Siders, and despite its flaws, it did provide some adequate and even excellent care. Puerto Rican residents went there for TB screenings, children's vaccinations, and regular diabetes treatments.[96] Yet, like all of New York City's public hospitals, Gouverneur suffered from deteriorating facilities, increasing expenses, and staff shortages. In 1956, a private advisory board, the Hospital Council of New York, proposed closing

Gouverneur and shifting its patients to Bellevue Hospital, over two miles to the north.[97]

Two years earlier, neighborhood leaders, including Helen Hall of Henry Street, had formed the Lower East Side Neighborhood Association (LENA), an advocacy coalition for the community. LENA refused to acquiesce to the hospital's closing and instead demanded that the city build a new Gouverneur Hospital. They wrote to New York mayor Robert Wagner that "the vast majority of our neighbors cannot pay anything like the full cost of adequate health care. . . . All of these, except the few who are covered at their place of employment by broad-scope health insurance, need the services of a City hospital and its clinics." LENA said the new hospital should be located more conveniently than the current, "obsolete" one; it should provide four hundred beds and a clinic equipped to handle two hundred thousand visits a year, and, to ensure quality of care, it should be affiliated with a medical school.[98]

But in 1961, the city announced that Gouverneur, along with several other public hospitals, would be closed—with no plans for a replacement. LENA launched a campaign of petitions, letters, and picketing to protest the closure. The protests, and the case for better health care on the Lower East Side, were impressive enough to wrest the promise of a new hospital from city officials. Yet, six years later, LENA was again rallying its members, for the old hospital had been closed, and the new hospital was not yet opened.[99] This second campaign for Gouverneur Hospital would look different from 1961, since the old-time Henry Street advocates would be joined by a new, vigorous, multiethnic health rights movement (a story to be continued in chapter 4).

Toward Migrant Empowerment?

In a speech to the American Public Health Association in 1961, Los Angeles City Council member Edward Roybal argued that that a necessary precondition for health was a political voice. Mexican migrants and Mexican Americans lacked such a voice. "Some cities in the Southwestern United States have as high as 90% of their residents Spanish-speaking," Roybal said, "and still do not have [a] Spanish-speaking elected representative." He found it unsurprising that populations who were forced into segregation and "excluded from democratic participation" suffered disproportionately from infectious diseases, infant mortality, crowded and unsanitary housing, and lack of services. "Personally," he told the public health professionals, "I look on the problems inherent in segregation as the most challenging in the field of public health."[100]

Leaders like Roybal, and groups like the GI Forum and the Community Service Organization, engaged in the fight against anti-Mexican segregation and for a political voice for Mexican Americans. Church groups and labor unions succeeded in ending the bracero program and passing the Migrant Health Act. But these reforms did not alleviate the exploitation of farm laborers or the medical neglect of Spanish-speaking communities, nor did they bring political power to migrant workers or the increasing numbers of undocumented immigrants entering the US. To advance those goals, the struggles of workers and immigrants had to be joined with the fight for civil rights.

From Access to Rights

In February of 1962, thirty-five-year-old organizer Cesar Chavez resigned from the Community Service Organization of Los Angeles. He was frustrated that the CSO had decided not to get involved in organizing farmworkers. Chavez had himself grown up working the fields, after his parents lost their Arizona farm during the Depression and had to go on the road as migrants. After leaving the CSO, he moved with his family to Delano, his wife Helen's hometown in California's Central Valley, and started the National Farm Workers' Association (NFWA). He had no money or official support, but thanks to his CSO work he had many allies across the state. Chavez devoted himself to organizing farmworkers from early in the morning to late every night, driving from one community to another, often going without food if he needed the money for gas instead.[1]

Slowly, the NFWA built a base of dues-paying members. Most were local seasonal farmworkers, not migrants. They were Mexican Americans whose families had lived in the Central Valley since the Mexican Revolution or newer immigrants who got green cards or temporary work permits after the end of the bracero program.[2] When Filipino workers went on strike in the grape fields around Delano in 1965, AFL-CIO organizer Larry Itliong asked Chavez if his members were ready to join them. After a rousing vote on September 16—Mexican Independence Day—the NFWA (later renamed the United Farm Workers of America) joined the grape strike.

The struggle for union recognition that followed would last five years and would become the most successful agricultural organizing campaign in US history. The United Farm Workers (UFW) became famous for their nationwide grape boycott and Chavez's magnetic, heartfelt leadership. It's less remembered that the UFW also built its own health care system.

Medical Care Controlled by Farmworkers: From Trailers to Clinics

As word of the strike spread throughout California, church and student volunteers headed to Delano to help. They found a community long accustomed to not only exploitative working conditions in the fields, but also a lack of medical services. The private Delano Hospital demanded cash deposits before admission. The county hospital was thirty-five miles away in Bakersfield and had restrictive eligibility requirements and long waiting lists. Farmworkers shared horror stories of negligent treatment by the hospital, including accident victims who died without adequate care, a woman who gave birth unattended in the delivery room, and a diabetic man who was told his case was hopelessly fatal (he survived after receiving a leg amputation at another hospital).[3] Some private doctors in the area reportedly sent injured workers back to the fields without treatment. There was no migrant clinic in Delano, and since most of the local farmworkers were settled residents, they were not eligible for federal migrant care anyway.

After witnessing these barriers to health care, UFW organizers added a new goal to their demands: "to prevent the suffering which all farm workers had to endure when they were sick."[4] Just one month after the grape strike began, a nurse and several volunteer doctors who had been providing first aid on the picket lines set up shop in the kitchen of a home in Delano. This first UFW clinic, just "a sheet over a kitchen door and three cardboard boxes of drugs," was supported entirely by donations. As it grew, the clinic moved into another house and then into a trailer that was a gift of the International Ladies' Garment Workers' Union, which also donated medical equipment. Soon the trailer clinic was treating hundreds of workers and their families.[5]

Cesar Chavez was acutely aware of local medical neglect of farmworkers and saw it as reflecting "the arrogance of the Delano power structure." Even as they devoted their limited resources to the uphill battle of the grape strike, UFW leaders decided that workers needed a permanent medical clinic at Delano. As the union organized a nationwide boycott of grapes and grape products in 1965 and a march to the California state capital the following year, they also began a campaign for medical donations, supplies, and volunteers. Soon the UFW obtained a second trailer for the clinic and added another full-time nurse and additional doctors. The volunteer medical staff provided farmworkers and their families with home visits, medications, lab tests, and monthly pediatric and obstetrics and gynecology clinics.[6]

As the strike dragged on, the trailer clinic became a focal point for the union.[7] It addressed a seemingly inexhaustible demand. "There is a constant stream of people moving through the clinic," reported El Malcriado, the UFW's newspaper, "bringing the health problems which were never solved in the past by the medical men of Delano. . . . No union member is ever turned away, appointment or not." By 1970, the paper noted, "More than 10,000 farm workers and their families have been provided with health care and limited medical service" in the trailers.[8]

The strike, boycott, and national attention finally led to some victories for the farmworker's struggle, as a majority of California grape growers began signing union contracts. In their contracts, alongside wage increases the UFW won employer contributions for worker medical care.[9] In Delano, the members voted to use the new funds to finally open and operate a permanent outpatient clinic. They argued that a union-run clinic would allow both "maximum utilization of the money" and "community control."[10] On October 21, 1971, six years after nurses and doctors began providing first aid on the Delano picket lines, the medical trailers were replaced by the UFW's Terronez Clinic. The new facility was named after Rodriguez "Roger" Terronez, a farmworker and strike organizer who had died due to medical negligence after a car accident.[11]

The clinic opened in two "barracks style" buildings, which were converted into a "modern attractive facility" by volunteers, "with adobe brick walls and a mission-style tile roof." The opening of the clinic was cause for celebration and a turning point for the union. "This clinic is unlike any other," UFW literature asserted. "It was founded in protest of the inadequate medical care available to farm workers and the indifferent treatment and discriminatory practices of [health care] institutions. . . . The sacrifices made to build this health center reflect the sentiments of farm workers that their ethnic and economic backgrounds are no excuse for delay, indifference or mistreatment in health care."[12]

Terronez Clinic was unique in other ways as well. It was staffed by four physicians, three RNs, and one nurse practitioner, all of whom had been recruited in a national campaign "that emphasized the clinic's philosophy" of empowering farmworkers. According to clinic doctor Peter Rudd, the medical and nursing staff at Terronez "all shared the belief that the clinic was an organizing tool for the union. . . . Most of them, in fact, received only room and board and a stipend."[13] The absence of professional salaries was one reason the clinic could run on a shoestring budget. Its dedicated physicians, fresh out of medical school, "all had to learn Spanish, and we all had to learn a lot of medicine as we went along," recalled volunteer MD Dan Murphy, who was a conscientious objector to the Vietnam War.[14]

Terronez Clinic did have a paid administrative staff, which it recruited from the local farmworker community. The employees were all bilingual in

English and Spanish or Tagalog. The paid staff members, the union believed, were crucial to the overall goal of empowering farmworkers and needed to be offered "the education and training which is the real reason for having the clinic at all." They were trained in medical casework and health promotion and encouraged to take college classes; Rudd reported that at least one Terronez staff member showed "strong potential and desire for medical school."[15]

Also reflecting the union's philosophy of health, Terronez Clinic emphasized preventive and outpatient care. Thanks to nonstop fundraising, the clinic was able to purchase an X-ray machine, defibrillator, and laboratory equipment, and to open a pharmacy. It provided twenty-four-hour emergency care for workers who could not come during the regular opening hours of 11 a.m. to 7 p.m. and a full labor and delivery service with two beds.[16]

Abby Flores Rivera, the daughter of a Delano striker, spoke about what the Terronez Clinic meant to her. "My family never had a family doctor when I was growing up. Aside from births, only twice did we see a doctor and that was at the hospital for emergencies," Rivera remembered. At school, she and her siblings were embarrassed when they filled out emergency forms and had to leave the space for "family doctor" blank. After the clinic opened, "I felt such pride the day that I was able to write Dr. Murphy, Delano Clinic on my school emergency card." Her family used the clinic often, and "We felt proud having farm workers on clinic staff, too."[17]

The UFW saw its health care efforts as essential to workers' pride and empowerment, but also as a strategy for strengthening the union and recruiting new members. Dr. Sheldon Rosen, one of the Delano volunteer physicians, wrote to Chavez that the Terronez Clinic could serve as a crucial organizing tool: "If farmworkers see *results*"—meaning the provision of high quality medical care to workers—"they will become interested [in the union]."[18]

But medical care was also part of what made the UFW *more* than a union: its broader vision for social change. Health care was not just a union benefit, but a right of workers and the poor. "Farm Workers supply us with most of the food we daily consume," a UFW fundraising letter noted, "and have a right, not only to organize into Unions and bargain collectively for fair wages and other benefits but, also to receive not adequate but good medical and dental care for themselves and their families."[19] Farmworker Richard Chavez told *El Malcriado*, "I feel our clinic will provide the care and medical assistance deserving of all human beings, whether rich or poor."[20]

Cesar Chavez himself was vitally involved in creating Terronez Clinic and expanding the UFW's health programs. UFW volunteers remember that Chavez "was upset at how ill served campesinos (farm workers) were when they had medical problems" and how Delano Hospital "turn[ed] away farm-

VOTE ☒ 🦅 UNITED FARM WORKERS
AFL-CIO

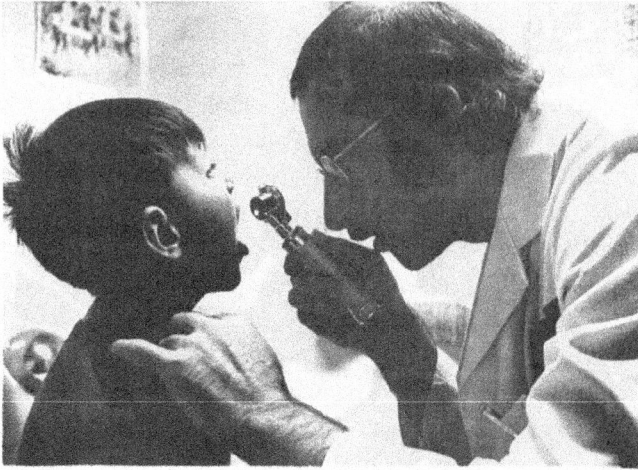

FIGURE 4.1. "Dr. Dan Murphy at work in the UFW clinic in Delano." This undated election pamphlet shows how the UFW portrayed its medical programs as a major benefit of union membership. Farmworker Movement Documentation Project, University of California, San Diego. The image is property of the United Farm Workers of America and is used with permission. For more information about the United Farm Workers, please visit www.ufw.org.

workers in need of emergency care."[21] As doctors and nurses developed ideas for the permanent clinic, "Cesar wanted to know every detail of every plan," and Chavez took "many walks around the clinic site" as it was being constructed.[22]

Chavez saw the clinic, union organizing, and the right to health care as inextricably connected. "The same struggle and sacrifice that goes into building a union goes into organizing a clinic," he told volunteers. "That struggle . . . will go on until every farm worker is protected by a contract and until every farm worker family is assured of decent medical care." He ended this speech with "VIVA LA CAUSA—VIVA LA HUELGA—VIVA LA CLÍNICA"—long live the cause, long live the strike, long live the clinic.[23]

Terronez Clinic placed heavy emphasis on preventive care, follow-up, and health education. Nurses made home visits for prenatal and postnatal care, and for all types of patients who didn't return to the clinic for their recommended follow-up. A doctor-nurse team conducted childbirth classes for both expectant mothers and their partners. Clinic nurses and health volunteers also held meetings in workers' homes "on basic health care concepts" and well-baby care. But farmworkers would not be denied specialist care if they needed it. Local doctors shunned UFW patients, but the Terronez Clinic developed a network of specialists who would visit Delano or accept patients at major medical centers, including UCLA and Stanford.[24]

The UFW's expansive vision for its clinics was starting to be realized. Clinic staff "have learned the necessary ingredients for administering a quality health care system for the multi-national, multi-lingual population," according to El Malcriado in 1972. "The clinic's success is based on direct participation of the people. They trust the clinic because they know it is run by themselves, for themselves."[25] In addition to providing a model for a new type of health care system, the clinic embodied the ways in which the UFW was a new type of union, one that sought long-term improvements in the lives of working people. It was a "dream come true for farm workers," said El Malcriado,[26] and a model that the union wanted to replicate elsewhere. Chavez envisioned "a network of clinics throughout California and in other areas of large union membership."[27] By 1973, the UFW had opened three more clinics in California, in Calexico, Sanger, and Salinas.[28] In addition, the UFW operated a health insurance program called the Robert F. Kennedy (RFK) Memorial Plan, which farmworkers could take with them wherever they traveled. (The plan's name honored Kennedy "because he gave our Cause his unfailing support and gave his life in the defense of the poor."[29])

Initially, the RFK Plan was wildly popular among UFW members, who were thrilled to have medical coverage for the first time. However, a portable health insurance plan proved to be extremely complex to administer. Workers had to file paperwork to be reimbursed for care. Paperwork delays—due in part to reliance on overworked volunteers—increasingly kept the funds from reaching workers in a timely manner. Some members were pursued by collection agencies due to unpaid hospital bills, and physicians in some areas began to refuse to accept RFK insurance. By the late 1970s, member complaints about reimbursement far outweighed their praise.[30]

Instead of considering proposals to redesign their health programs to better meet workers' needs, the UFW leadership dug in, taking any criticisms as an attack on Chavez himself.[31] Inflexibility and a rejection of criticism also characterized another damaging internal controversy related to health care. In the mid-1970s, the union tried using health and medical issues to justify its campaign targeting undocumented farmworkers for deportation.

While he repeatedly proclaimed his sympathy for the undocumented (whom he often called "illegals"), Cesar Chavez insisted that they were used by employers to compete with union members and to undermine union organizing. The UFW did at times quietly organize undocumented workers, who were already becoming a majority of the California farm labor force, but the union also sought to purge workers "without papers" from the fields and especially to prevent undocumented migrants from acting as strikebreakers.[32] In the spring of 1974, Chavez contended that undocumented workers were to blame for a series of failed strikes in central California grape and lettuce fields. He said that that the union "had identified twenty-two hundred" undocumented farmworkers "in Fresno alone."[33] In what became known as the "Campaign against Illegals," he called on UFW members to identify undocumented workers and report them to immigration authorities. "If we can get the illegals out of California," Chavez promised, "we will win the strike overnight."[34]

UFW staff used arguments about undocumented workers' danger to health in support of this campaign, and they relied on familiar stereotypes linking immigrants with disease. A UFW letter to boycott leaders around the country alleged that, in addition to breaking strikes, "illegals . . . bring in diseases from other places which are not prevented, detected or cured because the illegals do not seek treatment for fear of being caught and deported."[35] In press releases about the campaign, Chavez described undocumented migrants as health threats who were "bringing in disease which is neither detected nor cured."[36]

The increase of undocumented workers in the Central Valley would undermine not just wages and organizing, the UFW leader argued, but also public health. Undocumented migrants threatened to bring sickness, and, because of their poverty and poor health, they would overrun local medical facilities and burden county health resources—a reiteration of the "public charge" accusations wielded against immigrants for over a century.

In June 1974, two UFW staff members conducted a survey of Fresno-area health providers in an effort to confirm the union's claims. But their search for diseased and medical care–seeking "illegals" did not yield what Chavez expected. When the staff interviewed a Fresno County public health official, she told them that county communicable disease statistics showed "no significant deviation from median rates" elsewhere in the state. The county health clinic, which did not ask patients for immigration status, likewise showed no spike in disease rates, even while the administrator did note an increase in undocumented people using the clinic.

As for "illegals" flooding the health system, a public health nurse told the UFW staffers that "in general illegals avoid going not only into Valley Medical Center [the main hospital in Fresno, which was known to report all patients who lacked immigration papers], but to all public health agencies because of greater chance for exposure of their status. They generally prefer to be seen by private physicians which will usually protect their residential status in the

name of doctor-patient confidence." After examining additional statistical reports, the UFW staffers concluded that "they do not lend support to an argument that illegal aliens cause an increase in disease, at least as far as is seen by
the Public Health Sector."[37]

Committed to eliminating unfair labor competition, Chavez continued with his campaign anyway, even though it not only failed to link the
undocumented to an increase in health problems, but also alienated many
UFW supporters around the country. These included Mexican American civil
rights groups and church allies dismayed that the union was targeting the
most vulnerable workers. UFW headquarters received dozens of letters and
petitions from boycott committees and other union supporters, protesting
that the union's drive to report the undocumented "is against workers and
therefore against ourselves," that it "takes the focus off the real enemy of the
farm workers—the growers," and that "this campaign appeals to the national
chauvinism and racism of the public." Many of the letter writers urged that
the union should instead organize all workers, regardless of nationality or immigration status.[38] Chavez was infuriated by the protest, widening a damaging
fissure in his organization.

By the late 1970s, the UFW was under tremendous external pressures and
suffering from internal strife. In 1978, Cesar Chavez and the UFW Executive Board issued an agonizing order to close all of the clinics.[39] The strain
on union resources due to its fight against the competing Teamsters Union
and the expiration or loss of many of its labor contracts meant that the UFW
could not consider providing salaries to physicians and nurses, which made
it increasingly difficult to retain and recruit medical staff.[40]

But Chavez's withdrawal of support from the clinics was even more closely
related to the internal strife that led to purges and the mass exodus of volunteers from the UFW in the late 1970s. Scholars and former volunteers agree
that Chavez and the union executive board responded to tension between
members and the leadership, including over the Campaign against Illegals,
with increasing authoritarianism. Delano physician Dan Murphy remembered that "more and more people were told not to question anything and to
do just what they were told. In the end this attitude made it almost impossible to function in the clinic." Murphy, the last doctor remaining at Terronez
Clinic, resigned in 1977.[41]

That year, Chavez issued a directive to stop giving clinic access to workers
who were no longer working under union contracts. This seemingly arbitrary and self-destructive move would affect many union members whose
contracts had expired. Salinas Clinic physician Marc Sapir recalled, "We . . .
told Cesar we would not agree to cast out from the clinic rolls hundreds or

thousands of patients, loyal to the UFW and Cesar." Sapir was told to leave, Salinas Clinic closed, and the UFW Executive Board decided to end the entire clinic program at its meeting in March–April 1978.[42]

UFW organizer Dan Spelce was working in the lettuce fields near Salinas when word reached him about the executive board's action. He and his fellow farmworkers were devastated by the news. "That day, when my . . . crew learned that the Union health clinics were to be closed," Spelce remembered, "the air began seep out of the balloon of my hopes for the UFW as a leading transformative social force."[43]

Spelce's fears were partly correct. The UFW's extraordinary efforts did not end up leading to long-term unionization of farmworkers or significant improvements in their health or health coverage. Its most significant legislative victory, the 1975 California Agricultural Labor Relations Act, gave some protection for farmworker organizing in the state, but was not duplicated elsewhere in the country; farmworker unionization, even in California, has dropped significantly since 1980.[44]

But in other ways, the organization's impact was profound. Despite their sadness about the UFW's decline, former volunteers continue to express admiration for Chavez and the union's accomplishments. Dan Spelce, for example, followed his story of the clinic program's ending with the comment, "Still, I feel a simple reverence for Cesar and the UFW." Scholar Randy Shaw argues that the UFW's David versus Goliath example led to activism "beyond the fields" that affected millions of people, including the struggles for Chicano/Latino rights, immigrant rights, and a labor movement more inclusive of, and often led by, the lowest-paid workers and workers of color.[45]

Shaw's analysis does not mention health care, but the UFW medical programs must be recognized for the ways they contributed to some lasting changes. Starting at around the same time as the nationwide community health center movement, the Delano clinic "provided inspiration" for "a surge in community health centers" in California during the 1970s, a former UFW nurse argues, especially in their "focus on Spanish-speaking and rural populations." The UFW's contribution to subsequent health centers was also a material one, since many "employ (and employed) a number of veterans of the union."[46] And the Campaign against Illegals, paradoxically, led to an explicit and public defense of immigrant workers by UFW volunteers and supporters by bringing the topic out of the shadows. "Even if the UFW clinics were not sustainable in the long run," said former UFW nurse Khati Hendry, "the union deserves credit for organizing around health issues, and the clinics for providing a vision of what health care should be."[47]

From Migrant Clinics to Community Health Centers

Clinics funded by the 1962 Migrant Health Act were *for* workers; the clinics operated by the UFW were *by* workers. Although they were short-lived, the democratic aspect of UFW medical programs would be reflected in calls for "maximum feasible participation" during President Lyndon B. Johnson's War on Poverty. Starting in the mid-1960s, the idea that poor people should not just receive services but should have a voice in their operation began to influence the federal migrant health programs, and also the new community health centers movement.

The federal government's interest in "maximum feasible participation for the poor" began, one story goes, early in the presidency of John F. Kennedy, when a Native American activist allegedly told Attorney General Robert F. Kennedy, "Plan it with us and not for us." "Economic opportunity" was another watchword of the Kennedy administration, and in 1964 the new Congress overwhelmingly passed the Economic Opportunity Act to honor the assassinated president's legacy. The act created the Office of Economic Opportunity (OEO) to oversee antipoverty programs and fund "community action" projects. The OEO was required to ensure that "all community action grantees would hire and train citizens from the local area served" and would include poor people in project governance.[48] This notion was nothing new to grassroots organizing groups such as the Community Service Organization, but its arrival in Washington signaled a major rethinking of the top-down approach of government efforts to address poverty.

The civil rights movement had also advanced the idea that the poor deserved not just programs, but democracy and justice. Some historians locate the beginnings of the community health center movement in 1964, when physician Jack Geiger went to Mississippi with the Medical Committee for Human Rights to provide first aid to nonviolent protesters who were being attacked and beaten during the Freedom Summer voter registration drives. He and other volunteers started a small clinic in the Mississippi Delta, where the connection between poverty, powerlessness, and poor health was glaring. A year later, Geiger went to Washington and proposed to OEO staff the idea of community health centers: medical facilities that would serve the poor but also empower them. To Geiger's surprise, they awarded him $1.3 million to expand the clinic in Mississippi and start one at a housing project in Boston. OEO staff were enthusiastic about the health center concept, and by 1968, they were funding thirty-three such centers. The federal Department of Health, Education, and Welfare (HEW—a different bureaucracy than OEO) also began funding community health centers—a total of twenty-four of them by 1969.[49]

HEW already oversaw the clinics funded by the Migrant Health Act. It quickly became evident that the migrant health programs fell far short of the new goals of the War on Poverty. In addition to being underfunded and only reaching a tiny percentage of migrants, the programs did little to empower the poor they served. Federal migrant health grants were controlled by public health departments or medical societies that tended to defer to local power structures. Migrant clinics focused on health education and screenings, but "provided little in the way of primary care." In 1969, new agency guidelines encouraged migrant health projects to begin operating on the same principles as community health centers: "comprehensive primary care and consumer involvement in program governance."[50] HEW followed its own guidance by adding five former migrant workers to its National Migrant Health Advisory Committee in 1971—"the first time that migrant farmworkers will be directly represented."[51]

The new guidelines were transformative for some local migrant health programs. In Washington State's Yakima Valley, Migrant Health Act projects had been controlled by the county health department and medical society, and local farmworker activists were frustrated that the funds were perennially underused. They would get "like $30,000 a year," recalled organizer Tomás Villanueva, and "spend $15–20,000, like maybe $15,000 on hiring a nurse and maybe $5,000 buying aspirin or prescriptions, and usually send the rest of the money back." When they heard that federal funding was available for consumer-controlled projects, Yakima Valley farmworkers held meetings and concluded that "what the community demanded was primary care." Organizers went to Washington, DC, to meet with HEW officials, and in April of 1970, they were awarded the jaw-dropping amount of $365,000.[52]

The Yakima organizers called their project the Farm Workers Health Center, and it embodied the principles of community participation. Twelve out of the twenty-seven slots on the center's governing board were reserved for workers, and the board was "elected in community elections in which only the farm workers could vote." The program began training both Mexican American and Anglo farmworkers to be community health workers. This was "to give disenfranchised persons an opportunity to gain some marketable skills" and "to expose the minorities to the health disciplines." They operated a full-time outpatient primary care center, not just evening clinics, and charged patients on a sliding scale, with the goal of eventually becoming self-supporting. Apart from its federal funding and ability to pay professional staff, the Yakima migrant health center operated on many of the same principles that drove the UFW's clinics: delivery of primary care, worker governance, financial contributions from patients based on ability to pay, and vocational training for community members.[53]

The federal health center programs gave hope to communities that were desperate for medical services. Most US counties still did not even have a migrant health program. In their application for community health center funding in 1974, residents of Roosevelt County, New Mexico, east of Albuquerque, described the severe shortage of care in their area, which was home to many Spanish-speaking, first-generation farmworkers. The county had only two doctors who took pediatric and obstetric cases, and they were "so swamped . . . that they are turning away patients who cannot pay in advance. They are now asking expectant mothers to pay $300 in advance or they will not be accepted as patients for pre-natal care." The local health department also refused to hold prenatal clinics. Local activists reported that at least one baby, "the child of a Chicano farmworker family," had died because of being denied medical care. At a community meeting "to discuss the health problems of the poor, the people themselves outlined what they wanted in health care. They felt that above all they needed a good doctor who cared about them. They need a caring nurse who speaks Spanish. They need a home health aid[e] who can make home visits to teach them about good health. They need a clinic where they can make arrangements to pay according to their ability to pay."[54]

Federal health centers funding allowed places like Roosevelt County to increase access to medical care for the poor. Also, unlike the migrant health programs, grants were not restricted to rural areas. In Los Angeles, community activists formed the East Los Angeles Health Task Force to apply for funding to open a health facility "controlled by community residents." In the late 1960s, the Health Task Force used federal grants to organize neighborhood health councils, start a youth health education program, and open a treatment center for alcoholism.[55]

In Tucson, Arizona, physician Herbert K. Abrams, fresh from organizing with Martin Luther King Jr. in Chicago, arrived in 1968 to open an OEO neighborhood health center in the El Río barrio. "Most of the doctors in the community had moved to the East Side where the more affluent and middle class people were," Abrams recalled, "and there were very few doctors left in the old neighborhood." With federal funds, activists converted an old juvenile jail with "eighteen cells" that "became doctors' offices." The program's "number one objective was comprehensive care to a poverty population. And secondly, the hiring and training of people from the neighborhood in health skills." The El Río clinic's first board of directors "was composed of 21 people, of whom sixteen were elected in the barrios, and five were professional people from the community," according to Abrams.[56]

Federally funded health centers faced opposition from the same local power structures that had worked to limit the reach of migrant health programs. In Tucson, "We encountered some significant hostility" against the El Río Health Center, said Abrams. "The concern there was mainly from a few doctors in the community in private practice who thought it was a 'comminist' [sic] enterprise, and they were afraid of competition from the health center." Even the nuns at Tucson's Catholic hospital "were concerned because they were serving an indigent population and they wondered why we were moving in to serve what they thought would be the same population." Abrams "simply had to reassure them that we'd work in collaboration with them. I thought that the need was so great that there was room for both our organization and theirs."[57]

In the Yakima Valley of Washington State, activists had bitter fights with growers who opposed the new Farm Worker Health Center because they feared it would be used for union organizing. One of the valley's largest employers, an asparagus grower, yelled at a meeting, "Farm workers don't need a medical clinic! They have pretty strong backs. All they need is a box of aspirins," organizer Tomás Villanueva remembered. The local congressional representative, with a nod to the employers, tried to block the health center's funding. Opponents finally agreed to accept the clinic if it would be controlled by the county health board, with farmworkers serving on an advisory committee. Villanueva replied, with the strength of farmworker organizing behind him, "No. How about you guys be the advisory committee and we be the policy-makers?"[58]

As farmworker clinics moved from the top-down migrant health model to more democratic community health centers, the transformation could be too much for the local medical establishment to bear. In a bizarre example, physician Ben Yellen, who had earlier been a champion of bracero rights, led a campaign against the new community health clinic in the California Imperial Valley town of Brawley. In 1970, Casa Amistad, a farmworker community center in Brawley, won a $375,000 grant from HEW to start a health clinic. According to its organizers, "the basic concept for a clinic was formulated by the farmworkers themselves" and it would be governed by a board directly elected by workers. But Yellen and a handful of other Imperial Valley MDs filed a lawsuit (Yellen's specialty) against Casa Amistad. The suit argued that the federal funds would be used fraudulently because they were intended for "domestic, migratory, agricultural workers and their families" but "agricultural work in Imperial County is performed by residents of a foreign country who are neither migratory nor domestic." Yellen, who had long opposed the "importation" of Mexican laborers, was now making an early objection to using federal funds for the health care of undocumented workers.[59]

HEW officials defended their funding of the Casa Amistad clinic. They dodged the issue of "foreign" labor, arguing instead that "the need for better health services for migrant workers has been clearly demonstrated in all of the grant areas."[60] Indeed, like the migrant health programs, the community health center guidelines never mentioned a citizenship requirement for the people to be served. If Yellen was concerned that the new federal funding would be an opening wedge for provision of health care to the undocumented, he was correct (even if HEW never explicitly stated this). The Brawley doctors' other concern, that failing to restrict the clinic to "domestic migrants" meant that "the general public will use the clinic," was also prescient. Rather than applying limited, "categorical" eligibility standards, federally funded health centers were beginning to serve the whole community.[61] But when federal officials organized a conference to assess the achievements of the migrant and community health center programs, they were surprised to learn that still more was demanded of them.

The Chicano Rights Challenge

The Southwest States Chicano Consumer Conference on Health, held in 1972 in San Antonio, Texas, brought together a constituency unheard of when the OEO began less than a decade earlier: the Chicano movement (*El Movimiento*). The organizers who had fought for and won federal funding for clinics were no longer just church volunteers, social workers, or local public health officials. They were also representatives of a new civil rights movement on behalf of Mexican Americans. The terms Chicano and Chicana designated a Mexican American identity focused on ethnic pride and a critique of US colonialism. Rooted in the years of struggle by groups like the CSO and UFW, and inspired by the Black civil rights and antiwar student movements, Chicano activists fought for equal rights, cultural autonomy, and community empowerment.

Chicano organizers whose projects had received migrant health grants were well placed to criticize the program. At the San Antonio conference, a group gathered to discuss the topic declared that "Migrant Health is tokenism, a payoff to Chicanos to keep them quiet."[62] They argued for federal funds to be increased to meet actual demand. The Migrant Health Act's "fourteen million in fiscal year 1971 for an estimated one million migrants means less than fourteen dollars per person per year; this sum is not only inadequate but obviously unrealistic," participants pointed out. They resolved that "federal regulations should include [a] minimum service package," so that programs would provide actual medical care—not just education and prevention— and that health projects should serve populations regardless of municipal or county boundaries. "The Migrant Health Program, even with new regulations and the trend toward larger centers, has too limited resources to meet the health needs of all rural people," they declared. "Other programs must direct their efforts to meeting this need."[63]

Conference attendees argued that, as well as falling short on providing medical care, migrant health guidelines to increase consumer participation were insufficient, since they only required projects "to appoint migrant representatives, rather than democratic election." They passed resolutions demanding "at least 51% representation of workers and community" on the boards of migrant health projects and "that the next director of the [federal] Migrant Health Branch . . . be a Chicano." In addition, "Programs must recruit Chicanos at all levels to make them responsive and sensitive to the Chicano community."[64]

Chicano activists' criticisms of the migrant health programs were echoed in their frustration with other federal antipoverty initiatives that failed to provide actual medical services. A resolution passed at the San Antonio conference declared, "we the Chicanos of the Southwest are tired of Federal lip service and want health care NOW!"[65] Speaker after speaker inveighed against federal funding that went to studying communities' problems rather than actually solving them. Another resolution insisted that "the monies being used to fund feasibility studies be stopped and put into actual delivery of care."[66] Erasmo Andrade of the Crystal City, Texas, health department claimed that "La Raza [the Chicano population] had been studied so much that we were beginning to suffer from statistical indigestion; why not provide the money to representatives from an actual community and allow them to develop their own solutions."[67]

The discussions at the Southwest Chicano Consumer Health Conference produced an outpouring of creative ideas. The conference resolutions reflected some common themes: demands for Chicano representation in decision-making bodies; support for the farmworkers movement, including a demand that the federal government provide medical aid for workers on strike; and even a demand for a national "Chicano Commissioner of Health."[68] But hopes were quickly deflated when the same agencies that called the conference announced that the Nixon administration was scaling back its direct support for community health projects. HEW representatives told the Chicano activists that they needed to work on getting their clinics and projects to become self-supporting, and to convert their reliance on federal support to various types of private funding, especially third-party reimbursement using a new model called the health maintenance organization.[69] (In 1973, Nixon's head of OEO would try unsuccessfully to eliminate the Migrant Health Program and replace it with grants to the states. His reason: too many MHP grantees were supporting causes "inimical to the administration"—specifically, the United Farm Workers movement.[70])

So, as many activists (including the UFW) had been arguing all along, the road to community health empowerment would not be through the federal government. "The only way the Chicano could effect change," one conference resolution concluded, "was to acquire more political power."[71] As a step in achieving this goal, the Chicano health movement turned its attention to the center of power in the health care system: the medical profession.

Becoming Chicano Doctors and Nurses: Representation and Language

The Chicano rights movement gained national attention in 1968 through the actions of young students in Los Angeles, who walked out of their high schools to protest a segregated and underfunded educational system. The student movement spread to universities and then to health professional schools. In 1970, medical students in California founded the National Chicano Health Organization (NCHO). The NCHO soon had branches at medical and nursing schools throughout the Southwest.[72]

Announcing the opening of an NCHO office at the University of New Mexico in 1972, medical student Stan Padilla condemned US health care as "motivated by profit and not by people's health . . . perpetuated by racism, and . . . carried out by the fragmentation of the delivery of health care. What totally inadequate health care is available in the United States has been systematically excluded from Chicanos." The NCHO would work to increase the number of *Raza* (Chicanos) entering the medical profession. Members pointed out that "there are about 430 physicians in Albuquerque and less than 10 of these are Spanish surnamed. Out of 13,000 people taking admission tests required for entrance into medical colleges two years ago, only 48 were Chicanos." Traditional medical school requirements were inherently discriminatory and favored applicants from high-income backgrounds; the NCHO proposed "that the criteria for admittance should also reflect the community's need for physicians and the desire of the student to serve people." To achieve their goals, the Albuquerque office was developing a summer program for high schoolers to prepare for entering the health professions and projects to retain Chicano students admitted to the UNM medical school.[73]

Chicano medical students converged on the 1972 Student Health Manpower Conference in Chicago, which had been organized by the federal Bureau of Health Manpower to discuss the national shortage of health professionals. They joined with Black, Puerto Rican, Asian, and Native American students in a "Third World Caucus" that denounced the meeting's paternalism and federal health planning's neglect of poor communities. "White people who think they are liberal CANNOT solve the health problems of minority people," they said in their hastily mimeographed manifesto. "They cannot solve the problems of minority health science students. Minority people alone, when they gain control of their own communities and resources, can solve their problems." The time had come "for a unified attack against our common oppressor" and "to direct and rebuild *our* health system for *our* people."[74]

For the NCHO, attacking the "common oppressor" meant going after the medical school establishment. The Albuquerque students charged that "the University of New Mexico School of Medicine and the College of Nursing have done little to insure equal representation of Chicanos and other minorities in the health education field." They pointed out that health education programs relied on poor patients as teaching material: "Our communities have served as a training ground for future Anglo private physicians and WASP oriented nurses" who would not end up serving poor communities but rather the "White portion of society, who can afford their services." The University of New Mexico students' list of demands included a civil rights investigation of medical and nursing school admissions policies, admitting Chicano students in proportion to their 40 percent share of population in the state, and recruiting Chicano faculty. Their demands also extended to patient care, including transforming curricula to emphasize "Chicano health and illness" in "a course planned and instructed by Chicano community people"; transportation to health facilities for all people in the county, including "the surrounding Indian pueblos"; and provision of "Chicano and Indigenous translators" at the county medical center to ensure "maintenance of the patient's rights and dignity."[75]

The national NCHO decided to primarily focus on the goal of increasing the number of Chicano health professionals by recruiting young people to enter medical and nursing education. A pamphlet produced by the organization's Los Angeles headquarters implored, "Prepare for Medical School: LA RAZA Needs You."[76]

Another NCHO pamphlet displayed the invitation "Wanted: Chicano and Chicana Nurses . . . Reach Your Potential Caring for the Community." It

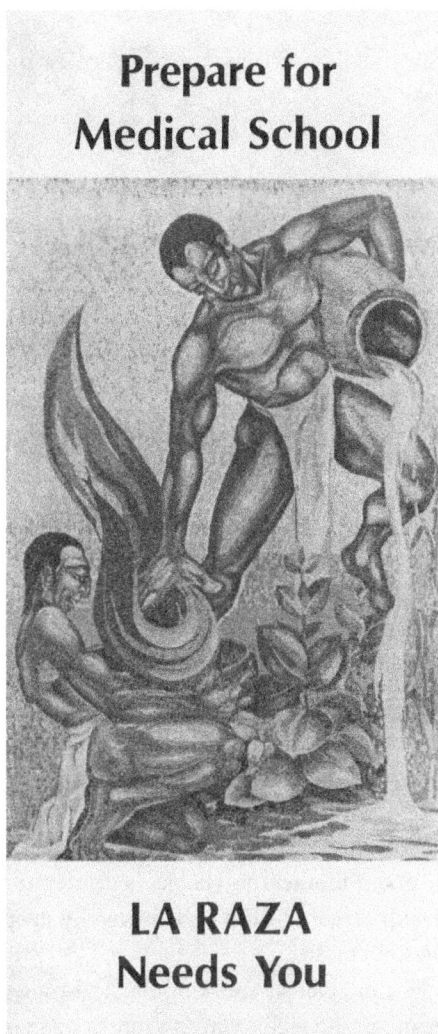

FIGURE 4.2. "Prepare for Medical School: LA RAZA Needs You," cover of National Chicano Health Organization pamphlet. Box 21, Folder 7, Frank I. Sanchez Papers, MSS 612 BC, Center for Southwest Research, University Libraries, University of New Mexico.

encouraged students, starting in middle school, to resist being tracked into vocational programs and to take math, lab sciences, and other preprofessional subjects. It placed the struggle for medical care in the context of broader rights mobilization: Chicano youth "have had their heads busted and have been put in jail because they tried to publicize the appalling conditions in our barrios. . . . What they did was open the door for all of us . . . let's open that

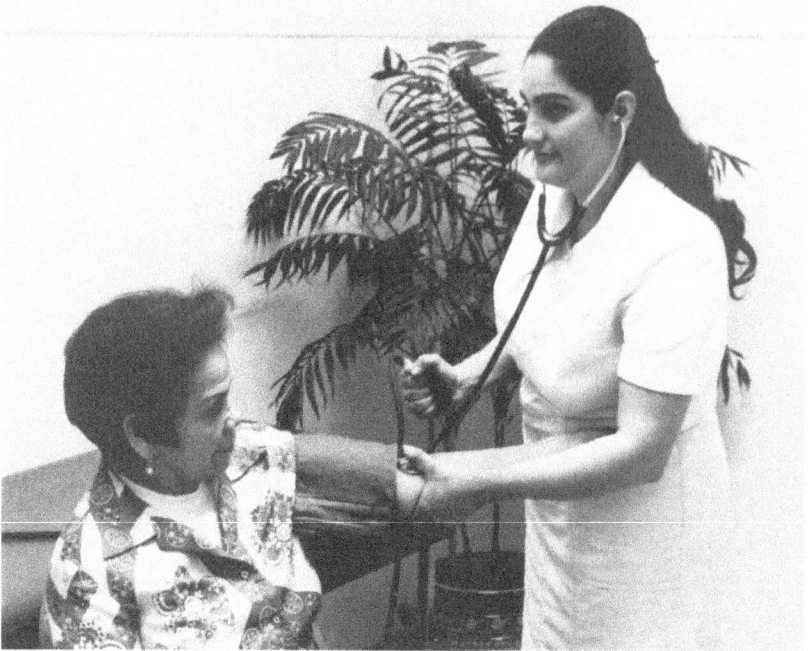

FIGURE 4.3. Image of nurse and patient from "Wanted: Chicano and Chicana Nurses," National Chicano Health Organization booklet, ca. 1972, Box 1, Folder 1, Gloria Arellanes Papers, California State University, Los Angeles, Special Collections.

door even wider." By becoming a nurse, "you and your friends . . . can change the high death rate of our mothers and babies, a death rate that is preventable if mothers seek health care early, if it is delivered by people who speak her language and know her culture."[77]

The egregious lack of Spanish-speaking medical professionals was a rallying point of Chicano health rights activists, one they shared with the growing movement for bilingual education. The inability to be understood was a daunting barrier to access for immigrant and Spanish-speaking patients. A welfare worker, describing a hospital waiting room in East Los Angeles, noticed "the terrible, rude service and attention they give to the Spanish-speaking people. I have seen 'Chicanos' crying in desperate anxiety after waiting four or five hours to relate their problem as best they could to a rude receptionist, nurse, or doctor in their broken English." The GI Forum protested the low number of Spanish-speaking nurses at a Texas hospital, asking, "Is it ethical and fair to deprive unilingual Spanish speaking Mexican American patients of comprehensive and quality nursing care because of inadequate assessments and histories obtained from poor linguistic communication?" It was also unfair, they noted, that the few nurses who did speak Spanish had to serve as unpaid translators.[78]

Multilingual Health Rights: Chinese and
Puerto Rican Activism in New York City

As the Chicano movement in the West and Southwest brought to light the relationship between provider diversity, language, and health care access, activists in New York City's immigrant and migrant neighborhoods were making similar arguments. The battle to save Gouverneur Hospital on the Lower East Side, which had begun in the late 1950s, grew into a broader movement that demanded not only a local hospital, but also health professionals and staff who spoke Chinese and Spanish and who would be representative of the entire neighborhood. It also became a fight for a community-controlled clinic.

New York City had closed the public Gouverneur Hospital in the early 1960s, but thanks to a compromise with the Henry Street–affiliated Lower East Side Neighborhood Association (LENA), it continued to operate Gouverneur's outpatient clinic under a new partnership with the private Beth Israel Hospital. The arrangement was not to the neighborhood's satisfaction. Beth Israel, a 1969 LENA broadside charged, was run by "a rich group of people . . . who don't live on the Lower East Side or know its problems and needs." Neighborhood residents without health insurance were regularly turned away from the hospital, even when private beds were available, and "patients have died because of these discriminating practices."[79]

Although Beth Israel received taxpayer dollars for the Gouverneur affiliation, it failed to recruit medical staff from the local population, LENA claimed. The clinic had a few "token" Black staff, but "*No* Puerto Rican doctors, social workers or administrative personnel, and very few Chinese personnel. Therefore the lower level bi-lingual personnel, in addition to their regular tasks and responsibilities, have the additional burden of translating for professional personnel. Yet . . . they do not receive any compensation for these tasks."[80]

The promised new Gouverneur Hospital kept being delayed. Neighborhood activists, now organized in the Lower East Side Health Council, increased the pressure on the city. In the summer of 1971, Chinese members of the health council and other groups organized the Chinatown Health Fair. The fair provided health screenings and education materials and raised "community awareness of minority employment issues at the new Gouverneur Hospital being built east of Chinatown."[81] The health fair lasted ten days and was attended by 2,500 people. Near the end, the fair was visited

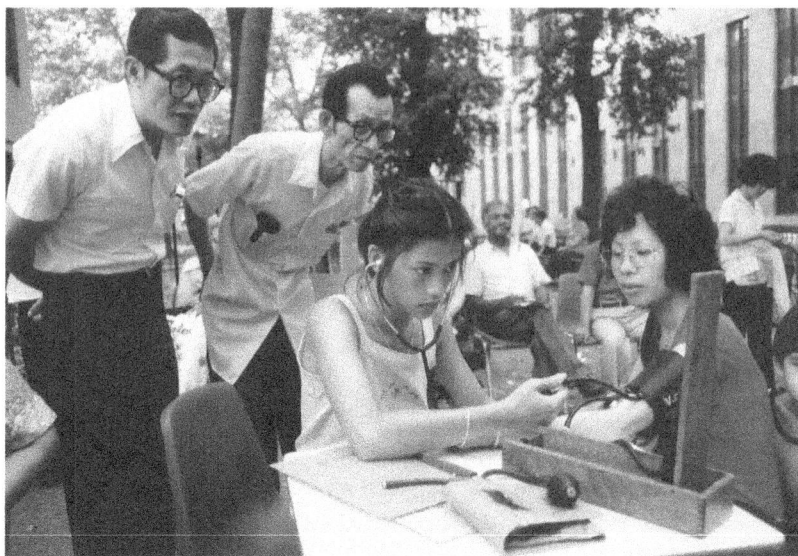

FIGURE 4.4. Taking blood pressure at the Chinatown Health Fair, New York City, 1971. Photo by Corky Lee, used with permission of the Corky Lee Estate.

by Joseph English, who headed the New York Health and Hospitals Corporation (HHC), the umbrella organization governing the city's hospitals. He was greeted by residents waving posters and shouting slogans in Chinese. As they chanted their demand to hire more Chinese staff at the hospital, English "sheepishly" had to ask what they were saying. His bewilderment "was exactly the point of the mini-demonstration," health fair organizer Thomas Tam later said. "Nobody in the hospitals understands what Chinese patients are saying. This is why Chinatown has such a health crisis."[82]

Emboldened by the success of the health fair, organizers held a protest on November 16, 1971. About 150 neighborhood residents marched, many of them Chinese senior citizens. There were also Puerto Rican and Black demonstrators demanding the opening of the hospital and that the new facility be representative of the community. They carried signs reading "Gouverneur Serve the Chinese Community Now" and "Give Chinatown Equal Health Services." After marchers arrived at his office, HHC head English announced that the new hospital would open the following July. He also agreed that the hospital would hire nineteen bilingual staff, including patient advocates for the Chinese and Puerto Rican communities.[83]

But Chinatown organizers wanted more than just a hospital provided by the city; they wanted to establish a community-run health clinic. Thomas Tam, the young Chinese immigrant who was also a leader of the health coun-

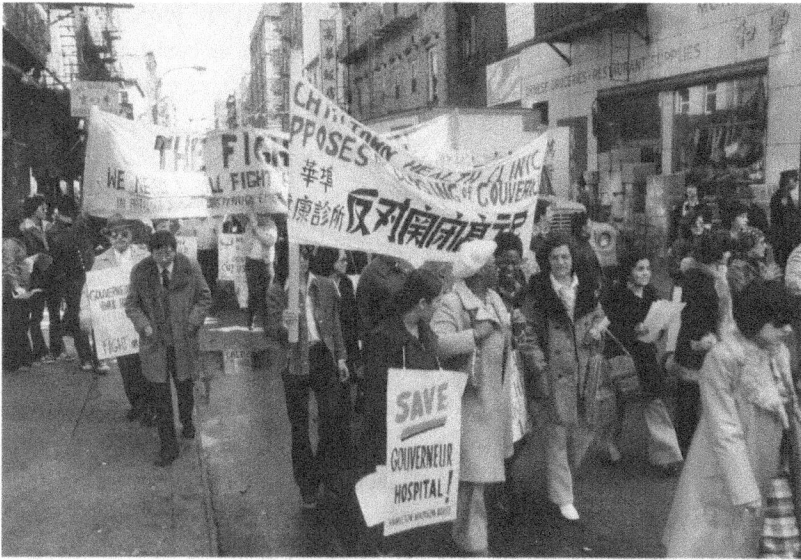

FIGURE 4.5. Multilingual protest against the closing of Gouverneur Hospital, New York City, 1971. Photo by Corky Lee, used with permission of the Corky Lee Estate.

cil, pushed the group to open a clinic in Chinatown. The health fair screenings had brought to light widespread medical problems in the community, especially high levels of tuberculosis and venereal disease. In December 1971, the Chinatown Health Clinic opened, with two volunteer doctors, donated supplies and equipment, and space provided by a local Episcopal church. Other volunteers worked as interpreters to aid communication between a Mandarin-speaking doctor and Cantonese- or Toisanese-speaking patients. They also accompanied patients who were referred to Bellevue or other hospitals. Word of mouth about the clinic soon attracted other physicians and lab workers, including from prestigious Manhattan hospitals. The Chinatown clinic became known as a place to receive excellent medical care, at no charge.[84]

Chinatown's extraordinary health activist movement thrived and made connections with other movements, including the women's health movement, unions, and Puerto Rican activists. At the 1973 Chinatown Health Fair, volunteers translated the radical feminist medical guide *Our Bodies, Ourselves* into Chinese. Chinatown clinic volunteers "went to Chinatown's many garment factories and discussed health issues with the workers during their lunch breaks. They gave out information on women's health issues, including family planning and birth control." The International Ladies' Garment Workers' health center (founded in 1913) formed a partnership with the Chinatown Health Clinic and "agreed to do all the Clinic's lab work for free."[85]

The Chinatown clinic also collaborated with Puerto Rican activists in the neighborhood. In September of 1970, Black Puerto Rican community activist Paul Ramos had opened a mobile clinic in a trailer donated by a local church. The Betances Health Unit, named for Ramón Betances, a nineteenth-century Puerto Rican physician and advocate for Puerto Rican independence, raised funds to purchase a larger trailer and began offering free immunizations, Pap smears, and extensive disease screenings for residents of the Lower East Side. Chinatown clinic workers "recalled borrowing the Betances mobile van from Paul Ramos and parking it in various locations around Chinatown." They sang Chinese songs through a loudspeaker to encourage residents to take blood pressure tests in the van.[86]

Puerto Rican and Chinese activists had also worked together in the Lower East Side Health Council and in the fight for a multicultural Gouverneur Hospital. In 1969 the health council used federal OEO funds to hire a full-time health advocate at Beth Israel Hospital to represent the community. The advocate was a woman named Gloria Cruz, whose appointment was controversial because she was connected to the Health Rights Revolutionary Movement, a group of activist workers employed at New York public hospitals. Cruz was also a leader of the Young Lords Party, a militant Puerto Rican organization.[87]

The Young Lords Party had been started by Puerto Rican student activists in New York's East Harlem in 1969. They modeled themselves on Chicago's Young Lords Organization, which was a youth gang until its leader, Cha Cha Jiménez, transformed it into a Puerto Rican rights and service organization. In both Chicago and New York, Young Lords members occupied churches in Puerto Rican neighborhoods to demand, among other things, free health clinics. In East Harlem, New York, the Young Lords became involved with health rights activism when they protested budget cuts and fought for community control at the public Metropolitan Hospital. They ran projects to bring better trash collection to the neighborhood and to screen residents for lead poisoning.[88]

In 1970 the New York Young Lords conducted a dramatic twelve-hour occupation of Lincoln Hospital in the South Bronx. Joined by radicalized physicians, the young Puerto Rican activists announced free health screenings and childcare at the occupied hospital. Their demands to hospital leaders included no budget cuts, an increase in staffing, better wages and conditions for workers, and "self-determination" through a "community-worker board." The occupation ended peacefully, with only two arrests.[89]

Health care for the people was a central demand of the era's militant movements. The Black Panthers required every one of its chapters to open a free clinic.[90] Like the Panthers, the Young Lords adopted a radical analysis of health under capitalism and colonialism. East Harlem was home to several prestigious and wealthy hospitals, but neighborhood residents had high levels of disease and little access to preventive care. Tuberculosis was a major problem in East Harlem, as it was in Puerto Rico, where mortality from TB was "the highest in the world." According to historian Joanna Fernández, in 1970 the Young Lords began administering TB tests to residents of East Harlem and the Bronx.[91] When the New York City health department refused to expand their TB screenings to include times that working people could attend, a group of Young Lords hijacked the city's mobile chest X-ray van and began screening hundreds of people in East Harlem. The city agreed to pay for the Young Lords to operate the clinic "twelve hours a day, seven days a week."[92] It was the Young Lords' takeover of the mobile clinic that inspired a young radical activist and photographer, Corky Lee, to come up with the idea for the Chinatown Health Fair.[93]

Health Care as Liberation: Militant Clinics

In northern New Mexico, activists in the mid-1960s began a campaign that focused not on civil rights, but on land rights. The people of this mountainous region were known as Hispanos, and included Spanish-speaking families who had arrived in the late 1600s and retained much of their culture even after the border crossed them in 1848. Due to the protection of Spanish and Mexican land grants guaranteed by the Treaty of Guadalupe Hidalgo, the Hispanos were supposed to retain rights to ownership of their land, but it was taken from them through a combination of fraud, economic pressure, and violence. The region had long been a center of resistance to Anglo control, where secret organizations in the nineteenth century launched campaigns of sabotage against white-owned ranches on the territory of the original land grants. In 1967, a group known as the Alianza Federal de Mercedes (Federated Alliance of Community Grants) announced an occupation of the Tierra Amarilla land grant. The "land-grant wars" came to national attention when the Alianza's leader, Reies Tijerina, and several others were arrested after attempting an armed raid on the local courthouse.[94]

In Tierra Amarilla, in Río Arriba County near the Colorado border, the people who used to own the land lived in extreme poverty. Per capita income in the county was around $2,000 per year. There was only one doctor, and in 1967 he left to serve in Vietnam. "It was strange to see front page pictures of this doctor treating Vietnamese children, while Chicano children back in Tierra Amarilla had no doctor at all," recalled community leader Maria Varela. The nearest hospital was seventy-five miles away, which led to tragedies: "Among other things, two people bled to death on the highway waiting for an ambulance. . . . Modern medicine is killing our people. It does not worry about problems in the rural areas because there is no money in the rural areas. As a result, there are no physicians in rural America," Varela said. Varela was a member of the Cooperativa Agrícola del Pueblo de Tierra Amarilla, a farm co-op that was part of the land-grant movement. When the doctor returned from Vietnam but put up his practice for sale, "La Cooperativa decided to buy the clinic from the doctor," Varela recounted.[95]

With fundraising help from the activist physicians' group the Medical Committee for Human Rights, the new Tierra Amarilla clinic opened in 1970 and was named La Clínica del Pueblo de Río Arriba. Initially it provided just first aid and dental care, but soon expanded to offer maternity care, emergency services, and health education.

La Clínica did not apply for federal funding. Instead, organizers raised money from churches, foundations, and "wealthy individuals." Like the UFW, Tierra Amarilla activists believed that accepting government funds meant losing grassroots power. They were skeptical of the OEO bureaucracies: "We who believe in community control are the ones who have to stop this practice of professionals making money from poor people's programs," stated the clinic's newsletter. They were able to hire outside physicians but avoid the need for government funds "by working ourselves on a subsistence salary," and also by charging some patient fees. Another source of clinic revenue was to get as many local people signed up for Medicaid as possible—a way of channeling federal dollars to their care without requiring federal control.[96]

Within a few years, the clinic became a point of pride for the community. "Traditionally our people planted, harvested, built houses, cut firewood and grazed animals together. Now," said the cooperative's newsletter, "people born and raised in this high mountain valley are training themselves to fight the infant mortality rate, save the lives and limbs of accident victims . . . (and) build the health of our children." By 1972, the clinic was credited with a sharp drop in the county's infant mortality rate: "It is now nearly half of what it was in 1960," said organizer Varela. "We feel that this is because of the quality of care given at La Clínica as well as the fact that women no longer have to travel 70 miles to have their babies." Although the clinic was not free, its sliding-scale fees made medical care affordable for local families for the first time.[97]

The ultimate goal of clinic activism, according to La Cooperativa, was for "La Raza [to] really build its own system of health, education, welfare, and economic development. Only then will we have a system that our young Chicano doctors, dentists, nurses, and other professionals can work in without becoming anglicized or without being forced to become profit hunters. . . . A health clinic is an important step for our community people to learn about how to own something of our own . . . about how to build the clinics, stores, and food production that we need to run our own lives."[98]

Self-determination was a central value of the militant Chicano movement, which included the land-grant efforts and, in the cities, the Brown Berets. The Brown Berets were started in Los Angeles in 1968 by young activists who had joined the high school walkouts and protested police brutality. Like the Young Lords, they were inspired by the Black Panthers and adopted a stance of self-defense, which included quasi-military drilling and outfits. While the Panthers wore black berets and the Young Lords purple ones, the Chicano group chose a moniker and headgear to reflect "brown power." Also like the Panthers and the Young Lords, the Brown Berets saw community services, including health clinics, as a central part of their mission to empower the people.

Chicanos needed their own "free clinic concept," according to Brown Beret member Gloria Arellanes, different from California's free "hippie" clinics (most famously in San Francisco's Haight-Ashbury neighborhood) that focused on "V.D., freaked out acid trips etc. . . . We knew we would be dealing with our people, a people who had been traditionally alienated by Anglo ran health institutions, health facilities with their over crowded conditions, dehumanizing environments and the lack of real humanitarian values. A people who could not afford private medical care and a people who were not aware of their basic human health rights." In 1969, the Brown Berets opened a clinic in East Los Angeles with private funding from the United Way and the Ford Foundation (militant clinic organizers seemed less concerned with private foundation influence than government regulation). The new clinic was on Whittier Boulevard, in the heart of the *barrio*, "between two bars, so it reached people's attention." Arellanes remembers that neighbors were suspicious at first, asking, "why were we doing this, doctors didn't work for free, no one provides free medical services, what was expected in return?" But soon "there were long lines" at the clinic, of people "waiting patiently for the most modest forms of health care," said clinic worker Castulo de la Rocha.[99]

Variants of the Brown Berets sprang up around the nation, with some calling themselves Black Berets ("Gorras Negras") in honor of Cuban revolutionary Che Guevara. In Albuquerque, the Black Berets opened a medical clinic in 1971. After the landlord evicted them after only four months, the clinic reopened in a space donated by the local Catholic parish. The Albuquerque Berets decided to name their clinic after Bobby Garcia, a Chicano student activist who had been mysteriously murdered. It was open three nights a week and served between twenty and thirty patients each night (occasionally closer to fifty). Although the clinic clientele was primarily Chicano,

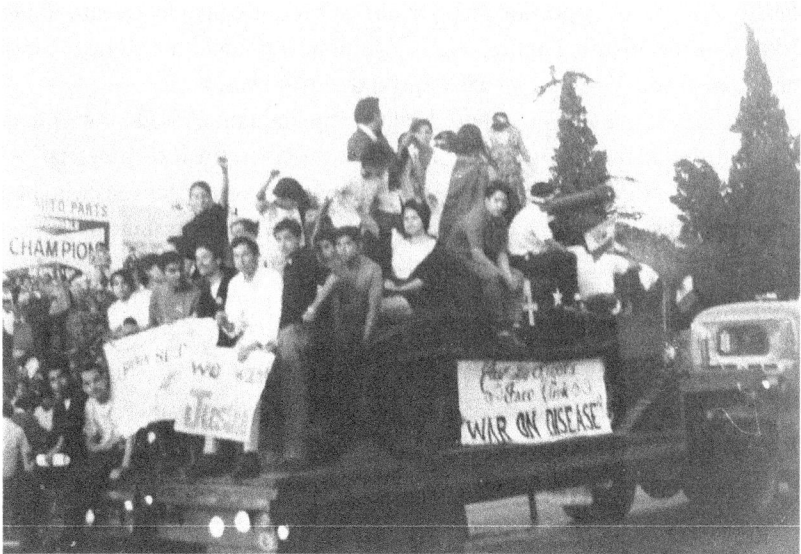

FIGURE 4.6. Brown Berets riding in a Mexican Independence Day parade with banner reading "East Los Angeles Free Clinic 'War on Disease,'" Los Angeles, ca. 1969, Box 5, Gloria Arellanes Papers, California State University, Los Angeles, Special Collections.

it also served Black and Anglo patients. One of its first successes was controlling an epidemic of strep throat in the neighborhood. In addition to providing medical care, the Bobby Garcia Clinic trained local high school students in first aid and bought a van for mobile medical care, including bringing assistance to striking city workers in the eastern New Mexico town of Artesia.[100]

The doctors, nurses, and lab workers at the Bobby Garcia Clinic were all volunteers, and the staff were paid workers from the local community. The Albuquerque clinic provided inspiration for some activists and community people to pursue health careers. Black Beret member Marvin Garcia enrolled in a laboratory sciences course at the University of New Mexico so that he could start serving the clinic as a lab technician. Staff member Cecilia Garcia started training to become a paramedic. According to the Black Berets newspaper, clinic staff "were becoming professionals—not like those who acquire education and then forget their communities, but in the spirit of building community self-reliance."[101]

The independence and self-reliance of the militant clinics made them threatening to both the traditional medical establishment and local power structures. Shortly after the northern New Mexico activists opened their clinic in 1969, it was burned down by arsonists. The community suspected that "certain ranchers" were to blame, but there were no prosecutions. They were able to reopen thanks to a donation from the Presbyterian Church (another source of private funding apparently less threatening than the government). Clinic leader Maria Varela explained, "You can see why we in Tierra Amarilla try to steer away from any kind of money or resources that politicos, ranchers or bankers could put their fingers into."[102]

Police and political repression of militant activist movements also targeted clinics. The New Mexico land-grant movement was extensively surveilled by the FBI and the state police. The Tierra Amarilla sheriff, who headed an entrenched political machine in the county, was particularly hostile to the Clínica del Pueblo. In 1975 his deputies broke into the clinic and the house of its board chairman, allegedly searching for marijuana and guns. "Overzealous officers picked through the contents of cabinets in the laboratory," the clinic's newsletter reported sarcastically, "as culture plates, incubators and various small chemical bottles are, of course, natural hiding places for rifles." The raids did not uncover any drugs or weapons. La Cooperativa joined with the civil rights group La Raza to sue the sheriff and held press conferences and protests against police brutality and local corruption.[103]

In Albuquerque, the Black Berets were subject to surveillance and death threats from local right-wing groups who were allied with law enforcement. In 1972, an informant lured two Black Berets leaders to a location where they were killed in a shootout with police. Clinic namesake Bobby Garcia had been found dead with a bullet in the back of his head. Although the Bobby Garcia Clinic was not physically attacked, the Albuquerque archdiocese evicted the clinic from its building in 1974 and refused to provide a promised renovated space.[104] Another example of violent backlash occurred in Mathis, Texas, where an outspoken physician who ran a federally supported clinic for the poor was shot to death by an Anglo police officer in 1970. This killing occurred against the backdrop of extreme racial tensions following the rise of Mexican American political organizing in the town and resentment by local Anglos against federal poverty programs.[105]

In Chicago, the medical clinics run by the Young Lords and the Black Panthers were both harassed and finally shut down by city officials. Shortly after the Young Lords opened their Betances Health Center in a church they had occupied, police regularly drove by, parked in front of the clinic, and even took photos of the patients coming and going. The Chicago Board of Health participated in the campaign against the militant clinics by trying to use an old licensing regulation against them and by conducting repeated, intrusive inspections. In 1971 Chicago mayor Richard J. Daley introduced, and the city council passed, a new law to require a license for any health center that was not owned or operated solely by physicians. By 1972, both the

Betances Health Center and the Black Panthers' Spurgeon Jake Winters clinic had closed down.[106]

Women's Health Activism and the Campaign against Forced Sterilization

In East Los Angeles, the Brown Beret's El Barrio Free Clinic also imploded—but would soon be reborn. In 1970, the female Brown Berets who ran the clinic resigned from the organization, accusing the male members of sexism and of refusing to allow women into leadership roles. They formed a new group, Las Adelitas de Aztlán (inspired by the name given to female soldiers in the Mexican Revolution), and focused both on organizing against the Vietnam War and on creating a new clinic. In 1971 they opened another East Los Angeles clinic under a similar but new name, La Clínica Familiar del Barrio. As the name indicated, the clinic focused on family medicine and women's health care. Volunteer pediatricians and ob-gyns offered their services. La Clínica Familiar emphasized family planning education and offered birth control counseling, although at one time staff were cautioned not to explicitly discuss abortion. (It's unclear how serious this restriction was; Gloria Arellanes remembers that abortion advice was provided at La Clínica Familiar.)[107]

La Clínica Familiar represented a new Chicana health movement that fought against the entrenched male supremacy of Chicano organizations and worked to empower women through a feminist approach to health care. Unlike their counterparts in the Anglo women's health movement, however, some Chicana health activists were wary of abortion advocacy. This was partly due to the Catholicism of communities they served (and occasionally funding from the Catholic Church), but also because of concerns that family planning programs were targeted at women of color, particularly Mexican women, who were accused of having too many babies. In addition to fighting the stereotype of the overly fertile Mexican woman, Chicana activists argued that women's right to have children was just as important as the right not to.[108]

The Puerto Rican Young Lords also advocated for a woman's right to bear children, but they included abortion in their definition of full reproductive rights. The Young Lords joined the Black Panthers in attacking sterilization campaigns that targeted women of color, especially since coerced and involuntary sterilization of women on the island of Puerto Rico was rampant. But while many Panthers condemned abortion as a form of genocide, feminist leaders of the New York Young Lords insisted that the right to terminate a pregnancy was inseparable from the right to be free from involuntary sterilization. All types of family planning, the Young Lords argued, had to be wrested from governments and the medical profession and placed under "community control."[109]

Involuntary and coerced sterilization had long been used in the US as a tool of eugenics, to prevent "undesirables" from having children. In Los Angeles in the 1960s and early 1970s, it was used in the service of "population control" and even of immigration policy. Mexican American and Mexican immigrant women were its targets. Alongside the stereotype of having too many children and thus contributing to overpopulation, Mexican women were accused of crossing the border to give birth so their children would be US citizens. And if they had a baby in a public hospital, they were also tarred with "public charge" accusations. If Mexican women using public hospitals were US citizens, they were a burden on the welfare system; if they were immigrants or migrants, they were deportable. Regardless of immigration status, they were seen as targets for sterilization.[110]

In the fall of 1974, physician Bernard Rosenfeld walked into the Los Angeles County Center for Law and Justice, a legal aid office, with a box full of records documenting involuntary sterilizations at Los Angeles County–USC Medical Center. The records showed that large numbers of Spanish-speaking women who came to the public hospital were coerced into having their "tubes tied" after giving birth. Doctors convinced the women to sign a form consenting to the surgery by giving them false information, including telling them that the operation was required by law, that it was necessary for their health, or that it could be easily reversed. Sometimes doctors refused to assist with childbirth or pain control until the laboring woman signed a sterilization consent form. Women who could not understand English signed forms without knowing what they were agreeing to, and in some cases, no consent was secured at all. Between 1968 and 1974, at least 240 women underwent coerced or involuntary sterilization while under the care of Los Angeles County.[111]

As scholar Elena Gutiérrez explains, the doctors justified their actions by stating that they were fighting overpopulation or protecting taxpayers from the burden of paying for welfare for large families. They argued that since the women were receiving public medical care, physicians had the right to impose controls on their fertility. Some used racial slurs and described Mexicans as ignorant and impoverished. Doctors also used sterilization as a form of immigration enforcement. In one San Diego hospital, if a Mexican woman declined sterilization the resident would tell her, "We know you're here illegally and if you don't consent to have a tubal, we'll call the feds and get you deported."[112]

Legal aid attorney Antonia Hernández interviewed hundreds of women who had been sterilized at Los Angeles County Hospital. For some, it was the first time they learned what had happened to them. Ten of the women agreed to join a class-action lawsuit, *Madrigal v. Quilligan*, against the hospital, twelve doctors, the State of California, and the federal government. They lost. The judge ruled that the hospital and doctors had not violated the women's civil rights and had not conducted a systematic campaign against Mexican women's fertility. Instead, the sterilizations were a result of a "communication breakdown." It was not the hospital's fault that the women could not understand the consent forms or communicate with their doctors in English, according to the judge.[113]

Even though the legal case was not successful, *Madrigal v. Quilligan* was a milestone for health rights activism. The publicity surrounding *Madrigal* occurred around the same time that the federal government was adopting ethics standards for medical research following revelations about the abuses of Black communities in the Tuskegee Syphilis Study. The Mexican women's class action induced the State of California to hold public hearings and to create stricter regulations for consent. These new requirements included a waiting period for hospital sterilizations and bilingual consent forms written at a level that patients could understand. The case galvanized the Chicana feminist movement, which defended women's right to "have as many children as we want when we want to have them," in the words of activist Esther Talavera, "for that is an integral part of our decision to determine our destinies." The head attorney in Madrigal, Antonia Hernández, went on to lead MALDEF (the Mexican American Legal Defense and Education Fund). When she looked back on the sterilization battle, Hernández remembered how "the case became an organizing vehicle for the Chicano community . . . a rallying force . . . improving the quality of healthcare for Latina women and for all women."[114] The women who spoke out about their coerced sterilizations ensured that considerations of communication and bilingualism would continue to be central demands of health rights movements.

Legal Action, Legal Change: A Migrant Worker and His Doctor Create an Interstate Right to Health Care

Henry Evaro, a US citizen of Mexican heritage and a resident of New Mexico, was a welder by trade. In the summer of 1971, he traveled to Phoenix, Arizona, to take a job there. Evaro was asthmatic, and on July 8, about six weeks after arriving in Phoenix, he had a bad attack that left him "gasping for breath." He went to a neighborhood clinic, and the doctor who examined him was so concerned that he sent him to the nearest hospital, Phoenix Memorial.

Evaro was so sick that Memorial, a private, nonprofit community hospital, admitted him immediately. But at the same time, staff got on the phone to Maricopa County Hospital, which was the only public hospital in Phoenix. The county hospital was required by law to treat indigent people who had no health insurance, so Memorial told them that they were going to send Henry Evaro over.

But Maricopa County Hospital said that they wouldn't accept him. The reason was that Evaro had only been in Phoenix for six weeks. Under Arizona law, patients had to have lived in the state for one year before becoming eligible for treatment at the public hospital. Like many states, Arizona had "durational" residency requirements, which were supposed to deter poor people from traveling to a state to obtain welfare or medical services. Many such laws originated during the Depression when millions were migrating for work. They also had deeper historical roots in the colonial-era poor laws that mandated "warning out" of impoverished nonresidents.[115]

Evaro ended up staying at Memorial as a patient for eleven days. During his entire stay, the hospital staff kept trying to get him transferred to the county hospital, and the county kept refusing. When he was discharged, a now-unemployed migrant worker with no health insurance, he could not pay his bill. But instead of suing Henry Evaro for payment, Memorial Hospital sued Maricopa County Hospital for the cost of his care.

This unprecedented move happened because the doctor who had first seen Evaro at the neighborhood clinic was a man named Augusto Ortiz. Ortiz was a Puerto Rican migrant who had attended medical school in Illinois. After he completed military service in Arizona in the 1950s, he set up a private practice in central Phoenix that expanded into a clinic, primarily serving the poor Mexican migrant workers who populated that neighborhood. Evaro was not the first of Oritiz's patients who had been refused at the county hospital because of residency requirements, but his case was the last straw. Ortiz told his colleagues at Memorial Hospital, "This time we take them to court."[116]

Their lawsuit, *Memorial Hospital v. Maricopa County*, went all the way to the US Supreme Court. In 1974, the court ruled in Memorial's favor, agreeing that durational residency requirements for medical care were a violation of the equal protection clause of the Fourteenth Amendment that protected the right to interstate travel. In his opinion, Justice Thurgood Marshall wrote that "the State of Arizona's durational residence requirement for free medical care penalizes indigents for exercising their right to migrate to and settle in that State." The Supreme Court had also relied on the Fourteenth Amendment when it ruled five years earlier in *Shapiro v. Thompson* that states could not impose durational residency requirements for welfare benefits. *Memorial v.*

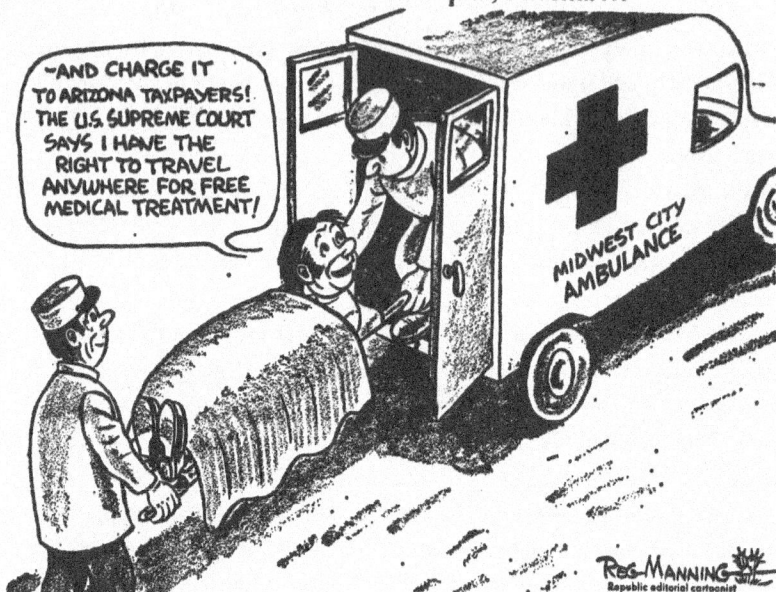

FIGURE 4.7. "Take me to Memorial Hospital, Phoenix." *Arizona Republic* cartoon reacting to the Supreme Court decision in *Memorial v. Maricopa*, March 2, 1974. © Reg Manning/Arizona Republic-USA TODAY NETWORK.

Maricopa extended the *Shapiro* ruling to include medical care. Indigent US citizens who traveled between states or were recent arrivals could no longer be denied access to public medical and hospital care based on how long they had been in the state.[117]

The historical record does not reveal what became of Henry Evaro. But Augusto Ortiz went on to found health clinics throughout rural Arizona and become a professor at the University of Arizona Medical School. In 1972, Ortiz served as Cesar Chavez's physician during the UFW leader's hunger strike in Phoenix. One day when Ortiz was speaking to Chavez about the difficulties of getting health care for farmworkers due to residency requirements, Chavez replied, "We have the same problem in some counties in California. But you know, we take them to court, because there is a precedent on the books, a man from Arizona . . ." The Supreme Court decision in *Maricopa* was still two years away, but news of the "welder who had asthma" who took a hospital to court had already reached the United Farm Workers in California.[118]

Although it defined the use of public medical care by interstate migrants as protected by the Fourteenth Amendment, *Memorial v. Maricopa*'s reach was limited. It did not prevent states or counties from denying care to non-citizens. And at the same time, the federal government would begin creating regulations to ensure that undocumented migrants would not have rights to public services (see chapter 5).

By the end of the 1970s, the radical democratic medical care programs of the United Farm Workers, the Young Lords, the Brown Berets, and other groups had come to an end due to internal strife and external repression. But some of the clinics founded by activist organizations continued under somewhat different forms. Ironically, considering the movement's distrust of government control, most of the clinics that survived and thrived did so because they ended up accepting support from Washington, DC. New Mexico's Clínica del Pueblo, New York City's Betances and Chinatown Health Centers, and Los Angeles's Clínica Familiar del Barrio all continued to grow as federally funded clinics. This blunted their radical edge, but federal health centers became crucial providers for underserved communities, and they are one of the few types of care accessible to undocumented immigrants.[119]

Los Angeles clinic founder Gloria Arellanes remembers how La Clínica Familiar del Barrio, which replaced the Brown Berets' clinic and accepted federal funding, expanded its clientele to include undocumented people. A Clínica Familiar poster from around 1980 announced that "¡Ningún Papel, Identificacíon, o Visa!" (No paper, identification, or visa!) was required to receive care there.[120] The 1972 Chicano Conference on Health had included virtually no discussion of care for undocumented immigrants. But when the 1980 health conference of the Chicano Federation of San Diego passed resolutions on bilingual and bicultural medical staffing and affirmative action for medical and nursing schools, they also included a demand that "local, state and Federal programs providing health services stop requiring proof of citizenship before rendering services."[121]

The growing embrace of the rights of undocumented immigrants reflects the change in both militant Chicano organizations and mainstream civil rights groups described by historian David G. Gutiérrez. He explains how the Chicano movement increasingly defined Mexican immigrants and Mexican Americans as "one people" and also developed critiques of US exploitation of immigrant labor. As immigration debates heated up in the 1970s, more mainstream groups like the GI Forum began to see crackdowns on immigrants as threats to Mexican American US citizens, who were subject to racial profiling. By the late 1970s, even the United Farm Workers was moving away from its anti-undocumented stance.[122]

Health activists in the 1960s and 1970s fought for farmworkers' empowerment, created a clinic movement, and pushed for multilingualism, representation, and equity in medical care. The movement around *Madrigal v. Quilligan* broadened the definition of informed consent, and *Memorial v. Maricopa* ended durational residency requirements for public medical services. The next step for the civil rights, workers' rights, and health rights movements was to include undocumented people in their demands.

Health Politics as Immigration Politics

The Creation of the Undocumented "Crisis"

In 1965, the US Congress ended the discriminatory national origins quotas for immigration. This change was the result of decades of pressure by Jewish and Italian American organizations, buoyed by the civil rights commitments of the Kennedy and Johnson administrations. The new Immigration and Nationality Act of 1965, also known as Hart-Celler, equalized national quotas across the globe. It also replaced country preferences with preferences for family reunification and skilled occupations. Although President Lyndon Johnson remarked that Hart-Celler was "not a revolutionary bill," it had unintended consequences that were transformative. Especially, it changed the demographics of legal immigration, so that within a couple of decades the vast majority of immigrants admitted to the US came from non-European countries, primarily because of family preferences.[1]

The Hart-Celler Act also unintentionally created new generations of undocumented migrants. The law was pro–civil rights, but it was not pro-immigration. It continued the policy of restriction by putting a low ceiling on the overall number of immigrants admitted. In addition, numerical caps and country quotas were imposed on the Western Hemisphere for the first time. Included as a compromise with opponents, the new restrictions on legal immigration from the Western Hemisphere—the first in the nation's history—would have devastating consequences. Equalizing national quotas meant that a country like Iceland got the same number of legal immigration slots as a country like Mexico. Since US demand for Mexican workers and poverty in Mexico both continued unabated, the new Western Hemisphere quotas ended up forcing large and increasing numbers of Mexican migrants to become undocumented immigrants.[2]

"The imposition of a 20,000 quota on Mexico," Mae Ngai writes, "recast Mexican migrations as 'illegal.'" Between 1964 and 1972, the number of INS arrests of unauthorized immigrants increased from eighty-two thousand to more than 465,000, and 97 *percent* of those apprehended were from Mexico. By 1973, Congress estimated that there were between one and two million undocumented people living in the United States (and sensationalized media reports claimed that there might be up to ten million).[3] In 1974 Nixon's INS commissioner Leonard Chapman testified in Congress about a "silent invasion" of "illegals," and Attorney General William Saxbe called for mass deportations.[4]

Congress would not pass new immigration legislation until 1986. But at the local level, governments began to look to welfare and health care policies as a way of doing something about the undocumented "invasion." States had no control over immigration policy, but they did control their Medicaid programs, and cities and counties ran public hospitals and indigent health clinics. Local governments couldn't prevent immigrants and migrants from coming, but they could impose restrictions on their programs that sent the message that undocumented people were not welcome.

Undocumented Health and Welfare Exclusions

In 1961, former Hollywood movie star Ronald Reagan recorded a speech for the American Medical Association in which he attacked John F. Kennedy's plan for Medicare as "socialized medicine" and "the end of freedom in America." Six years later, he was elected governor of California. Reagan promised to crack down on student antiwar protests and to cut welfare costs. One of his first acts as governor was to implement reductions to California's Medicaid program, known as Medi-Cal, which provided medical coverage for the poorest people in the state. Reagan insisted that Medi-Cal, a federal-state program that was only two years old, was on the verge of bankruptcy and was an unsustainable burden on taxpaying citizens.[5]

One woman who relied on Medi-Cal was a young mother in East Los Angeles named Alicia Escalante. Right after Reagan took office, Escalante's doctor told her that he would no longer be able to care for her and her five children if Medi-Cal were cut. He suggested that she join him in a protest downtown. Escalante remembers this as the moment she became a welfare rights activist. She went on to start the East Los Angeles Welfare Rights Organization, which also became known as the Chicana Welfare Rights Organization.[6]

As Reagan sought deeper welfare cuts, local governments began lobbying for immigrant exclusion as a way to save money. California welfare officials insisted that the ending of residency requirements for welfare by the US Supreme Court had left them without ways to keep immigrants off the aid rolls. Reagan listened, and the California Welfare Reform Act of 1971, in addition to instituting widespread cutbacks in services, banned public assistance to "illegal aliens and temporary foreign visitors." It also encouraged county welfare offices to report noncitizen applicants to the federal INS.[7] The California State Welfare Board continued to publicize the notion that immigrants abused medical services, producing an anecdotal report claiming that people crossed the border "with deliberate intent" to obtain free medical care and to give birth in public hospitals.[8]

Alicia Escalante was a social worker as well as a welfare rights organizer. She and her fellow case managers were told to start implementing the new exclusions, which required welfare applicants to complete an "Alien Status Verification Form" to be shared with the INS. Escalante was furious, calling the new requirement "one of the most discriminatory directives ever to come out of the State." She argued that most of the people affected would not be the undocumented, who rarely applied for assistance, but rather would be long-time residents and even citizens. Los Angeles County was "cutting off people who have been here 15 to 20 years, paid their taxes, send their sons to . . . school and war, but may have no papers, due to many reasons." Escalante also charged that "this directive is geared toward the deportation of Chicanos" and warned that anyone's "*abuelita* or *abuelito*, *tío* or *tía*" (grandma or grandpa, aunt or uncle) who may have been "here for a long period of time, that may not have citizenship paper or proof of local residence," could become vulnerable to deportation.[9]

As a leading figure in *El Movimiento*, Escalante saw the 1971 welfare restrictions as part of the overall oppression and dispossession of Chicanos in the US. "The public may scream, why should we aid the illegal alien," she said, "but the question to me is who is the illegal alien . . . when you are in fact in occupied Mexico[?]" She noted the racial and political bias of the exclusion: "Why does the State not question the Cuban refugee program, the Hungarian program?" Those categories of Cold War refugees were guaranteed both asylum and federal financial assistance, while Mexicans were targeted for exclusion and deportation. Escalante denounced Los Angeles County acting in "the role of Immigration" and warned officials that "we intend to appeal" the welfare exclusion "and fight it throughout the Southwest."[10]

In March of 1971, the California State Department of Social Welfare held a hearing in San Francisco on the new welfare rules for noncitizens. The "stormy" hearing lasted five and a half hours as Chicano and other groups vented their anger at the exclusions. Abe Tapia of the Mexican American

Political Association declared that "the regulations amounted to 'psychologi-cal genocide' against the people who live in fear of being deported." Speak-ers echoed Escalante's concerns about aged noncitizens getting caught in the welfare/immigration net. A representative of the Community Service Orga-nization talked about seniors who "have been here quite a few years—since immigration was not so strict. . . . It's a little unfair at this point to start asking for documentation." Japanese, Chinese, and Filipino groups also participated in the hearing and expressed concerns that the restrictions were "discrimina-tory toward the Asian and Latin communities."[11]

By merging demands for welfare rights, racial justice, and protection for immigrants, speakers at the San Francisco hearing signaled a new direction for activism, one that was exemplified by Escalante's Chicana Welfare Rights Organization. Activists now insisted that immigrant rights were inseparable from more familiar civil rights causes. They recognized how racism under-pinned xenophobia and how much attacks on immigrants were rooted in anti-Mexican sentiment that also affected US citizens. And, although they did discuss how welfare restrictions would hurt green card holders and long-term residents, speakers at the hearing explicitly included undocumented immigrants as a group deserving of public assistance and protection from deportation.

Welfare rights activism in the late 1960s and early 1970s, as Cybelle Fox has argued, along with Supreme Court decisions expanding the right to wel-fare for US citizens, led to a backlash from the federal government. Follow-ing Governor Reagan's example, Congress and federal agencies began adding "status restrictions" to all the major welfare programs, including Medicare, Medicaid, and Aid to Families with Dependent Children. By the mid-1970s, undocumented immigrants were officially banned from all federal welfare and health benefits.[12] Few undocumented people had ever used these pro-grams. In 1975 the US Department of Labor surveyed "a sample of persons who had been apprehended by INS" and "found that 77% contributed to Social Security and 73% paid federal income taxes. Only 0.5% received welfare benefits, 1.3% used food stamps and 3.9% had received one or more weeks of unemployment benefits; 7.5% had children attending public schools." Still, the official exclusion sent the message that the government was not only cutting welfare costs, but also taking steps against undocumented immigration.[13]

Local activists failed to stop the new California restrictions on welfare to immigrants. Fears of deportation had been a factor in Mexican-origin and Spanish-speaking residents' reluctance to seek health services since the 1920s, but the 1971 restrictions reportedly led to even more widespread avoidance of the health system and loss of health care access. In a 1973 investigation by the *Los Angeles Times*, doctors at the Los Angeles County–USC Medical Center said that few Mexican and Mexican American residents came to the public hospital "because so many barrio residents are afraid to come to the medical center or refuse to disclose the identity of . . . relatives." The director of the hospital's bilingual unit worried that "there's a hell of a lot of people out there who are sick but won't come here." And the director of the Los Angeles Department of Health Services said that "90 percent of the medical center's patients are admitted as emergency patients because so many refuse to seek care until they collapse."[14]

Although the state's attempt to deter undocumented residents from seeking services appeared to be working, local governments continued to claim that undocumented health costs were creating a massive burden on their budgets.

The Debate over Undocumented Health Costs: Los Angeles as Flashpoint

By drastically cutting state contributions, Governor Reagan's 1971 welfare reforms forced more costs onto California's counties, which were legally responsible for local health services to the poor. The Medi-Cal reductions led to lost revenues for county hospitals and clinics and an increase in patients without health coverage. Some counties closed their public hospitals and reduced other health services. The pain was especially severe in Los Angeles County, which was tasked with serving tens of thousands of poor residents. Despite cutting back on services, in the ten years following welfare reform Los Angeles County's health care costs increased eightfold.[15]

In Los Angeles, an elected Board of Supervisors governed the county's public health facilities, including its gigantic public hospital (County–USC). In 1976, a conservative supervisor named Pete Schabarum released a statement accusing the county of "providing $10.8 million in health services to illegals."[16] Schabarum was a former pro football player originally appointed to the board by Reagan and reelected to four additional terms. Like Reagan, Schabarum utilized anti-immigrant rhetoric and policy in pursuit of fiscally conservative austerity objectives (and vice versa).

Other members of the Board of Supervisors were skeptical of Schabarum's claims. There was no reliable mechanism for keeping track of how many undocumented people used the county's clinics and hospital, which (unlike Medi-Cal) did not require patients to report their immigration status. In addition, many of the costs cited by Schabarum may have been offset by patient payments (most county health services were sliding scale, not free) or other types of reimbursement. One board staff member remarked that undocumented people paid taxes and that it was unlikely they posed much of a burden on health services since they generally avoided them "because they fear detection and deportation."[17]

The Board of Supervisors decided to respond to Schabarum's complaint by convening an internal task force to study the "Treatment of Non-resident Aliens." In a memo on the task force's findings, Los Angeles County health director Liston A. Witherill again pointed out that immigrant patients who used health services generally paid sliding-scale fees and weren't getting it for free. And he pushed back against Schabarum even harder by arguing that county care for the undocumented might be required by law. According to California state statutes, counties were obligated to protect the public health, and this included "legal requirements of providing essential services to patients for the welfare and safety of the public." In addition, "There may be a risk of liability, both to the [Health] Department and its individual physicians, if non-residents turned away for lack of an 'emergency' later suffer disability or death for lack of treatment." Finally, Weatherill mentioned that he had received a telegram from a civil rights organization that "warned of possible court action if the Department of Health Services initiates non-resident alien screening procedures."[18]

This dispute at the Board of Supervisors indicates that the inclusion of undocumented patients in county health services had been uncontroversial—or at least not much discussed—until Schabarum chose to scapegoat immigrants for rising health costs. Soon Schabarum was joined in his efforts by the Pacific Legal Foundation, a nonprofit started by members of Reagan's welfare reform brain trust. Its lawyers wrote to the Board of Supervisors demanding an investigation into county funds being used for the "illegal purpose" of "providing nonemergency health care services for illegal aliens."[19]

These accusations forced some Los Angeles County leaders to begin finding explicit justifications for including people in health care regardless of immigration status. Their efforts were backed by similar work that Chicano and other activists were already doing. This included legal justifications. When a county attorney attempted to argue that immigrants could be excluded on nonresidency grounds, the National Health Law Program, a welfare rights organization, retorted that counties had full legal authority to provide care to the undocumented, based in past practice, California statutes, and constitutional law (including *Memorial v. Maricopa*), and also that inclusion fit with "contemporary moral standards" recognizing that "all persons have access to necessary health care."[20]

Immigration opponents and fiscal conservatives realized they needed a different approach to exclude the undocumented. In 1979, Los Angeles chief administrative officer Harry Hufford, with Schabarum's support, pushed for a new rule that would require all uninsured patients to apply for Medi-Cal before receiving care at a county hospital or clinic. Since the Medi-Cal application process included verifying citizenship or immigration status (the new Alien Status Verification Form), this measure would clearly deter undocumented immigrants from seeking care. Wary of a potential backlash from activists, Hufford described the proposal as a fiscal measure, solely intended to bring more revenue to the county through Medi-Cal.[21]

For the first time, Los Angeles officials were forced to join rights groups in publicly defending immigrant inclusion. Supervisor Edmund Edelman, a progressive who represented heavily Mexican parts of East Los Angeles, attacked Hufford's proposal as a "back door attempt to deny care." Labor unions, the Los Angeles County Bar Association, and even the local branch of the Red Cross spoke out against the measure. "Because this can result in deportation," opponents argued, "the undocumented will fear the entire [application] procedure and will defer badly-needed health care rather than risk exposure to INS." Despite the protests, a newly elected county board with a conservative majority implemented the new policy in 1980.[22]

But the Medi-Cal application requirement did not stand. The following year, the County Health Alliance, a Los Angeles antipoverty coalition, brought a lawsuit against the Board of Supervisors on the grounds that "the county has a duty to provide health care for all residents." Requiring a Medi-Cal application, the coalition argued, would "keep thousands of frightened illegal immigrants away from county hospitals and health centers," which could "endanger the health of all residents and could cost more in the long run." A judge immediately issued an injunction blocking the policy.[23]

The injunction infuriated Schabarum, who vowed, "This is not the end of it."[24] For the next several years, the conservative supervisor continued to pressure Los Angeles County to exclude undocumented nonemergency patients. He was not successful, but he and his opponents did find an area of consensus. Both conservatives and liberals agreed that any actual costs of health care for immigrants should be paid by the federal government. As the Los Angeles Board of Supervisors put it, Washington, DC, was responsible because "the financial consequences of undocumented aliens on local government stem from federally controlled immigration policy and practice."[25]

Federal Reimbursement for Undocumented Hospital Care: Immigration Policy as Health Policy

Starting in the mid-1970s, local politicians in California and the Southwest began to call for federal funding to reimburse care for undocumented immigrants. In June of 1977, Florida congressman Paul D. Rogers convened a hearing in the US House of Representatives on a set of bills that proposed federal reimbursement for "medical treatment of illegal aliens." While this idea seemingly contradicted official US government policies of exclusion, the proposals were framed not as a benefit to immigrants, but as support to hospitals and local governments. This emphasis was reflected in Rogers's opening statement warning that, if the US continued to turn a blind eye to the increase in undocumented immigration, "I fear that illegal aliens may place an ever-increasing burden on our health care delivery system which would impair the scope and quality of health care for our own citizens."[26]

The funding bills' primary sponsor was Bernie Sisk, a Democratic congressman representing part of California's Central Valley, home to a large population of farmworkers. Sisk testified that he first became concerned about the "alien" health care issue in 1972 when an undocumented resident in his district crashed his car and was rushed to the hospital with devastating injuries, including a crushed chest and kidney failure. The driver had no insurance and no money. His two-week hospitalization, before he was transferred to the university hospital at Stanford, cost Merced County $30,000 and threatened to "wipe out the entire medical budget for the year," according to Sisk. He told the hearing that Merced was spending $150,000 per year, and nearby Fresno County over $1 million, on emergency care for undocumented immigrants, adding, "To me the issue is whether local communities, who have no responsibility for maintaining the integrity of our borders, should continue to bear the burden of providing essential medical care to aliens whom the Federal Government maintains have no right to be in this country in the first place."[27]

Other California representatives echoed Sisk's complaints. Lionel Van-Deerlin talked about a private hospital in his district near San Diego "which just in the first five months of this calendar year has laid out $95,000 for taking care of illegals who are accident victims or women about to deliver babies. No hospital is going to turn down someone who needs emergency care, or who is about to deliver a child," he asserted, but "Why should local citizens be stuck with the tab when the national Government fails to meet its larger obligation to keep illegals out?"[28] "Being but a few miles above our international border with Mexico, San Diego has become a major way station in this underground railroad of illegal aliens," Rep. Bob Wilson added. "To the local taxpayer, the money he or she pays is already high. But to pay an additional sum to support such aliens through community health care facilities is to add an onerous burden to our citizens, especially those in our border cities."[29]

Congressmen from other states bordering Mexico chimed in. Rep. Morris Udall of Arizona told the hearing that a survey of hospitals in his state concluded that "emergency treatment of indigent Mexican nationals resulted in a loss of $1,750,000 in uncollected fees in 1976 alone." Texas congressman E. de la Garza said that hospitals in the border cities of Harlingen, McAllen, and Brownsville saw five thousand "illegal aliens" in their emergency rooms in that same year.[30]

Some congressmen proposed that the US Public Health Service (PHS) should reimburse hospitals for all this immigrant emergency care. They argued that PHS already paid for medical care for immigrants detained by federal authorities, so the agency should also be responsible for similar costs incurred by private hospitals. But Public Health Service officials countered that medical costs were only within their jurisdiction when an "alien" was actually in their custody. When asked who then was responsible for non-detained immigrants' health costs, PHS representatives could provide no satisfactory answer. Instead, they repeatedly referred to the upcoming immigration reform proposal from President Jimmy Carter. In essence, federal officials were telling Congress to wait for an immigration reform—that would never come, at least not during the Carter administration—to solve a health care cost problem.

The proposed funding bills went nowhere. According to San Diego health official Nancy Plaxico, a major reason for Washington's lack of interest was that "care for undocumented aliens . . . is perceived as a California–New York–Texas problem." In addition, powerful members of Congress, especially Senator Ted Kennedy, whose support was essential for health care measures, had no interest in "bailing out" California when that state was engaged, under Governor Reagan, in massively cutting taxes for its own residents.[31]

It is striking how speakers at the 1977 hearing discussed immigrant medical costs almost solely in fiscal rather than public health or humanitarian terms. There was no testimony from immigrant rights or civil rights organizations, nor from any immigrants or migrants themselves. And in an era before immigrant rights became a platform of the national Democratic Party, Democrats' anti-immigrant language was indistinguishable from that of their Republican counterparts. Democratic representative George E. Danielson's description of the "virtual flood of illegal aliens" in his district as "an issue which has grown from a fiscal annoyance . . . to something close to a fiscal catastrophe"[32] could have come from a member of either party. Politicians on both sides of the aisle engaged in the rhetoric of a health care cost crisis meeting an immigration crisis.

The attempt to secure federal reimbursement for undocumented health services failed, but the 1977 hearing was notable for other reasons. It was evident that reliable statistics on the extent of immigrant medical costs were nonexistent.[33] The figures presented to illustrate the undocumented "burden" were all anecdotes, estimates, or guesses. Hospitals and their congressional supporters had trouble justifying their calls for government reimbursement when they lacked accurate information about what costs would be covered. An immigration policy—demanding citizenship information from patients— would be required for reimbursement based on immigration status to be feasible. Still, the lack of accurate statistics did not prevent hospitals and members of Congress from continuing to demand, with increasing success over the next three decades, federal reimbursement for immigrants' emergency care (see chapter 7). But local governments' attempts to blame immigrants for their health costs would not go unchallenged.

"Illegal Aliens That Eat Up All Our Funds"

On April 15, 1979, fifteen-year-old George Olmos was rushed to San Diego Community Hospital with an accidental gunshot wound to his head. The California hospital did not have a neurosurgeon on call, so doctors phoned University Hospital, San Diego's county-supported premier trauma center, to request a transfer. A University Hospital physician asked if Olmos "was a Mexican citizen." Since Olmos was unconscious, the answer was unknown. University Hospital refused to accept him. The teenager eventually received surgery at another hospital, and he survived to tell authorities that not only was he a US citizen, but he had actually been born at University Hospital.[34]

This case added to the evidence for Chicano rights groups' contention that scrutiny of immigration status would lead to generalized discrimination against Spanish-speaking and Mexican-origin patients seeking lifesaving medical care. San Diego civil rights organizations filed complaints with HEW and the US Department of Justice charging the county with de facto racial discrimination. University Hospital received a warning from the state, but no sanctions were imposed.[35]

University Hospital tried to justify its actions by insisting that the refusal to accept Olmos was financial, not racial. The hospital director explained that "the county's policy of refusing to pay for hospital costs of transferred patients has made it necessary that we ascertain financial status before some transfers are completed." But the equation of undocumented Mexicans with hospital cost burdens was clearly a factor. The University Hospital physician who rejected the transfer allegedly said, "We are tired of being the dumping ground for illegal aliens that eat up all our funds."[36] San Diego County had recently filed a lawsuit against the federal government demanding $1.8 million in reimbursement for "medical care to undocumented aliens."[37] The suit was dismissed on technical grounds, but San Diego medical providers had clearly been hearing the message that "aliens" were to blame for the cost crisis.

There was no doubt that San Diego medical facilities saw a significant number of undocumented people with emergency conditions. The county shared a border with Mexico and was also facing growing overall costs for care of the indigent (people who did not qualify for Medi-Cal but still could not afford hospital costs). San Diego's decision to seek reimbursement for treating immigrants was financially strategic; there were no other sources to increase funding for indigent care, whether from the state or the federal government. The county also made reasonable efforts to quantify the amount it was spending on such care, using surveys of hospitals' own cost estimates when making its claim for reimbursement.[38] But they were still estimates, and the undocumented financial burden on medical facilities remained primarily a rhetorical tool: a tool to demand more funding, to express anger at immigrants, and to deny care.

It was also used by politicians to further their careers. On May 12, 1986, San Diego County supervisor Susan Golding held a press conference announcing her new plan to demand federal reimbursement for the costs of undocumented immigration. Golding, a Republican, stated that "we are being invaded by illegal aliens. . . . Last month, 72,000 illegal immigrants were apprehended by the Border Patrol in San Diego. For every one who is apprehended, as many as 10 may get through." The costs of this "invasion," according to Golding, threatened to "bankrupt county government." She presented a symbolic invoice for $23.27 million to Washington, DC, for "criminal justice, health and social service" costs related to immigration.[39]

Her claims were immediately challenged. San Diego's Committee on Chicano Rights (CCR), led by a tireless organizer named Herman Baca, demanded an "immediate apology and retraction" from Golding. Especially damaging were Golding's claims of a high crime rate among immigrants. The CCR declared that such claims—which were false—fomented "possible violence by bigots and racists against persons of Mexican ancestry."[40] At a rally and press conference on June 10, CCR was joined by numerous other Chicano rights organizations in denouncing Golding. Even the California Republican Hispanic Assembly declared, "In one stroke she [Golding] has destroyed every effort of the national Republican party to bring Hispanics into the GOP fold."[41] Even the San Diego County Sheriff's Department refuted Golding's claims about immigrant crime, and the supervisor quickly had to apologize (saying "My staff made a mistake.")[42]

On June 17, Golding came out with a proposal that dropped the crime accusations but doubled down on hospital costs. She repeated her earlier claim that "since 1980, the County of San Diego has spent more than $16 million on emergency health care for illegal immigrants." She backed away from the anti-immigrant rhetoric of her first proposal, stating that "there is no question that health services must be humanely provided to all who are in need" and that "it should also be obvious that our ability to supply services has been diminished for reasons other than the impact of illegal immigrants." She acknowledged that the county budget was suffering due to cutbacks in revenue sharing from the federal government. (Golding did not mention that the budget slashing from Washington was due to the economic policies of now-president Ronald Reagan.)[43]

In her original statement, Golding had admitted that when it came to how much hospitals and clinics were spending on care for the undocumented, "only rough estimates have been made so far" and that "there is presently no tracking system in place."[44] Her new proposal suggested various ways to more accurately measure immigration's impact on local budgets, such as a creating a "confidential" system for hospitals to record patients' immigration status. The impact of the CCR protests was evident, as Golding promised she would assure "a substantial representation of Hispanic interests" in these efforts.[45]

Many of the people objecting to Golding's first statement had referred to studies that showed that immigrants actually paid far more in taxes than they ever used in public services. Golding incorporated this information into her new proposal. She acknowledged the accuracy of the studies (one of which had been performed by San Diego County), but then noted that most of the taxes paid by immigrants went to the federal government, not the county. She then made a new proposal: "I believe that some of the tax revenues paid by undocumented workers should be returned to the communities that must bear the costs of providing needed services."[46]

Chicano movement leader Herman Baca celebrated how Golding had been forced to retract her comments on high crime rates among immigrants and gloried in the "complete defeat of her prior and absurd racist proposal. . . . She has to publicly admit that she knew nothing about the immigration issue and she still doesn't know anything." But Baca was still deeply concerned about the supervisor's focus on hospital use by immigrants. Golding may have "aired a different writer to clean-up her racist intents, but the racist intents of denying the undocumented Mexican worker county services, and scape-goating him for every problem that confronts the county is still present in her newest proposal." Her suggestion to recoup part of the taxes of undocu-mented workers further incensed Baca: he described it as an attempt to "use the Mexican worker's tax dollar on the one hand, and [on] the other hand [an] effort to eliminate this person. . . . Golding wants to represent their money but not their rights."[47]

Although her tax proposal never went anywhere, and she had had to admit that she had basically lied about immigrant crime rates, Golding's political career soared. In 1992 she was elected mayor of San Diego, running as a "progressive Republican." Her attempts to scapegoat the undocumented foreshadowed the rise of an anti-immigrant politics in California focused on public spending that would culminate in the battle over Proposition 187 in the 1990s. California activists' fight to defend immigrants' rights to life, work, and health was just beginning.

A New Labor Movement of Undocumented Workers, and a Clinic

Following a disastrous citrus strike in Yuma, Arizona, in 1974–75, Cesar Chavez decided to give up on that state. It was said that one hundred thousand farmworkers in Arizona, whose 370-mile border with Mexico was less patrolled than California's, were undocumented. Chavez's United Farm Workers had tried to keep migrants from Mexico out of the citrus fields with intimidation and violence, but the strategy to drive a wedge between citizen and noncitizen workers simply weakened the farmworkers' movement and helped lead to the strike's failure.[48]

In Maricopa County, Arizona, where the majority of farmworkers were undocumented, a handful of former UFW organizers rejected Chavez's approach. In 1977, they started the Maricopa County Organizing Project (MCOP). MCOP organizers focused on the conditions of gross exploitation suffered by undocumented Arizona farmworkers. Employers depended on migrants' fear of deportation to impose near-total control over their labor. They did not provide housing, and workers had to sleep in the fields under the citrus trees. There were no sanitary facilities, and the laborers were not given medical care; according to MCOP organizers, "any worker injured on the job was given liquor as a remedy or sent back to Mexico."[49]

As historian Ana Raquel Minian explains, the Maricopa County Organizing Project engaged in a unique, transnational organizing strategy. They identified the home towns of migrant citrus workers and traveled to Mexico in the off season to talk to them about how to improve their wages and working conditions in the north. When the 1977 harvest season began and the workers crossed the border back into Arizona, they were ready to take action.[50]

Thanks to this advance organizing, MCOP managed to run several work stoppages at citrus grower Goldmar, Inc. (owned by a relative of Republican politician Barry Goldwater), with a momentous result: the first labor contract

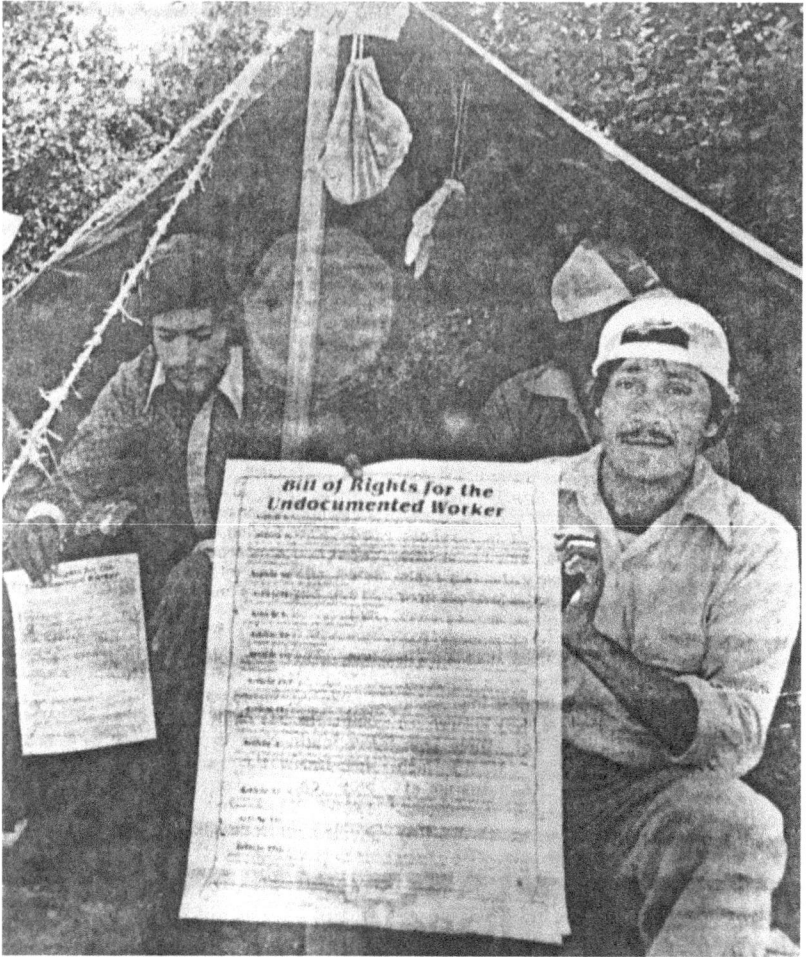

FIGURE 5.1. Striking Mexican citrus workers with an undocumented workers' bill of rights distributed by the Arizona Farm Workers Union, Bodine Ranch, Phoenix, Arizona. Photo by Lars Jones, *State Press* (Tempe, AZ), October 28, 1980. Maricopa County Organizing Project (MCOP) Records, Chicano/a Research Collection, Arizona State University Library.

in the United States signed with openly undocumented workers.[51] The MCOP then announced the creation of the Arizona Farm Workers Union (AFWU), an independent union not affiliated with the UFW. The AFWU held its first Constitutional Convention at the end of 1979. The new union pledged to "change the conditions" that farmworkers suffered in Arizona, including "lack of medical care and . . . decent housing," and declared that it would "seek full human, civil, and constitutional protection" for undocumented laborers.[52]

The AFWU went on to negotiate several contracts on ranches with large numbers of undocumented workers. These contracts included a medical plan similar to the United Farm Workers' RFK Plan (except that it used private insurance companies),[53] and also an innovative feature: they required employers to contribute ten cents per worker hour to a Farmworker Economic Development Fund in some of the workers' communities of origin in Mexico. Instead of attacking the exploitation of these workers by demanding their deportation, as the UFW had done, the Arizona union argued that only improved conditions in Mexico could address the long-term problem of undocumented migration.[54]

The MCOP/AFWU was led by a remarkable organizer, Guadalupe Sánchez, who had previously been an undocumented farmworker himself, and was also a member of the UFW before it left Arizona.[55] Sánchez vigorously argued that undocumented workers deserved to be unionized. In 1979 he wrote directly to Cesar Chavez, protesting the UFW's continuing efforts to turn workers over to the Border Patrol. "The undocumented workers have just recently started organizing themselves and have made great progress," Sánchez wrote. "They have sacrificed a great deal to accomplish what is considered an impossible task. . . . As long as the documented and undocumented workers are divided, the growers can use one group against the other." Chavez ignored Sánchez's pleas and ordered the AFWU to stop their organizing work. They refused his directive.[56]

Undocumented farmworkers deserved not only union protection on the job, according to Sánchez and the AFWU, but also a right to decent health care. In the antiunion environment of Arizona, services like medical care might be more sustainable, and do more to improve the conditions of farmworkers and their families over the long term, than union contracts that had to be constantly fought for and renegotiated. In 1979, MCOP applied for funding from the federal Rural Health Initiatives program to build a health center in Maricopa County. The application was successful, and the center, named Clínica Adelante, opened in 1980 in El Mirage, a farm town twenty-five miles northwest of Phoenix. It was staffed by a doctor and a dentist from the National Health Service Corps, a federal program that sent medical professionals to underserved communities.[57]

Like the UFW clinics, Clínica Adelante began as a more modest effort that enlisted volunteer physicians and nurses to provide care to union members. MCOP also brought attention to pesticide-related illnesses among farmworkers. But with so few union contracts, MCOP/AFWU could not count on employer fees to pay for a permanent facility like the UFW's Terronez Clinic. Instead, they pursued federal funding and worked to set up voluntary agreements with employers to contribute to the clinic's operations, charging growers twenty dollars per employee or family member each month.[58] Also like the UFW clinics, Clínica Adelante was not free to users; it used a sliding scale to charge patients for services. Unlike the UFW, the clinic accepted private insurance as well as federal funds.[59]

But the Arizona clinic's biggest difference from the UFW's programs was that it explicitly encouraged undocumented workers and their families to come for medical services. In a bilingual mass mailing sent to announce Clínica Adelante's opening, one bullet point appeared in Spanish only. It read, "¿Qué pasa si yo no tengo papeles? Nadie le preguntará si Ud. es ciudadano. Para nosotros es igual" (What happens if I don't have papers? No one will ask if you are a citizen. To us, it doesn't matter).[60]

By 1984, Clínica Adelante was growing increasingly popular and received only half of its funding from federal programs, with the remainder coming from patient fees and insurance. The *Arizona Republic* published a feature on the clinic that discussed the obstacles faced by undocumented workers who needed health care. It told the story of a woman working as a fruit picker who was fired when her pregnancy became visible. When "a patient from the clinic found her living in a garbage dump," she was taken to Clínica Adelante and found to be six months pregnant and undernourished. Her child was later born healthy. The article quoted Rita Goodman, a nurse practitioner at the clinic, saying proudly, "Many undocumented workers are afraid to go for help. They think they will be deported. We don't ask if they are a citizen or not. We are here to take care of them."[61]

Although other clinics had provided services regardless of legal status, Clínica Adelante set a new precedent for explicitly claiming a right to health care for the undocumented. As Ana Raquel Minian writes, the MCOP's work directly challenged "the notion that migrants' legal status rendered them ineligible for rights in the United States."[62] The Arizona organizers held the first US conference on undocumented workers rights, in Washington, DC, in 1978. In 1980, their efforts were celebrated at the First International Conference in Defense of the Full Rights of Undocumented Workers, held in Mexico City.

The conference was a major step in defining the rights of the undocumented, resolving: "It shall be the right of immigrant workers to health services, free and adequate medical attention, child-care and other services presently available to all United States Citizens. . . . Such right stems from their status of tax payers, workers and residents."[63] While this resolution was notable for including health care within the definition of rights, its authors disregarded the reality that "free and adequate medical attention" and other services were actually *not* available to all US citizens. In fact, the number of people in US with health insurance, after reaching its height in the mid-1970s, was declining, and both citizens and immigrants were very far from obtaining a right to health care.

Through the ER Door: Legal Action Leading to Unintended Rights to Care

In 1982, the US Supreme Court announced a momentous legal decision affecting the immigrant community. In *Plyler v. Doe*, the court ruled that undocumented children had the right to attend public schools. The lawsuit leading to this decision had come from both individual legal action and organized activism. It was brought by a group of undocumented parents in Texas who enlisted the support of civil rights attorneys from the Mexican American Legal Defense and Education Fund (MALDEF).[64]

Plyler v. Doe was a landmark decision in applying the Equal Protection Clause of the Fourteenth Amendment of the US Constitution to undocumented children's right to public education. But activists who hoped the ruling might apply to other arenas of American life for undocumented people faced disappointment. *Plyler* did not serve as precedent for later Supreme Court cases, and its purview has not even been expanded to include a right to public higher education, much less health care or other rights for the undocumented. The decision emphasized children's rights over those of immigrants, noting that schoolchildren were "innocent" of their parents' "crime" of undocumented migration. Given the vicious backlash in the subsequent decades, *Plyler v. Doe* was, in the words of legal scholar Michael A. Olivas, "the true high-water mark of immigrant rights in the United States."[65]

Legal action for health care rights took a more circuitous route in the 1970s and 1980s. Rather than emanating from the Supreme Court, limited rights for undocumented access to care originated in state-level court cases that were then, over an extended period of time, translated into congressional regulations buried in giant budget acts. This process went almost entirely unnoticed by the media and the general public. Quietly and unintentionally, by 1986 two new avenues to medical rights had been created for the undocumented: Emergency Medicaid and the right to hospital emergency care.

"Aliens"—a legal category that included both undocumented and other types of immigrants who did not have permanent resident status—had been banned from Medicaid coverage since 1973. In 1979, legal aid attorneys filed a class-action lawsuit on behalf of a New York woman named Lydia Lewis and other "aliens" who had been denied Medicaid due to their immigration or citizenship status. In its 1985 decision, the federal district court in New

York in *Lewis v. Gross* ruled that the alien restriction "violated the Medicaid statute." (This decision was made on technical grounds and did not affirm the plaintiff's contention that the ban was a violation of equal protection.)[66]

Because of *Lewis v. Gross*, the following year Congress decided to codify the Medicaid alienage restrictions by making them part of federal Medicaid law. In the new language adopted in 1986, Medicaid was amended to fully exclude aliens, but it specified a single exception: the federal government could contribute to state Medicaid programs "for medical assistance furnished to an alien . . . *for the treatment of an emergency medical condition*"(emphasis added).[67] This amendment to the Medicaid Act later became known as "Emergency Medicaid." Ironically, in officially banning "aliens" from Medicaid, Congress created a new, narrow type of access for immigrants: through the door of the hospital emergency room.

Because this change was part of the budget reconciliation process, which places strict limits on debate, there is no record of any discussion that occurred around the amendment. It seems likely that the Medicaid exception was included, not in order to create a new program for undocumented health coverage, but to align with another new law on emergency care recently passed by Congress. Following a drastic increase in instances of "patient dumping," in which private hospitals transferred severely sick or injured patients to public hospitals because they did not have health insurance, Congress had created the Emergency Medical Treatment and Active Labor Act (EMTALA) in another budget reconciliation earlier in 1986. EMTALA required all hospitals that have emergency departments to screen and stabilize anyone that came to their ER doors. Hospitals disobeying the requirement could be fined and be removed from the Medicare program, which was crucial to hospital funding.[68] The new law did not say anything about citizenship or immigration status; the right to emergency care applied to "any individual" who came to a hospital seeking such care.

As well as responding to patient dumping, EMTALA—which is still the only statutory right to medical treatment in the US—was the culmination of a set of state legal decisions in the 1970s that had gradually increased hospitals' obligations to provide emergency care. One of the most important of these cases, *Guerrero v. Copper Queen Hospital*, was brought on behalf of two children who were citizens of Mexico.

Teodoro and Marie Guerrero were a married couple who lived in Naco, Sonora, a town in Mexico that shared a border with its twin city of Naco, Arizona. Like many residents of this region, Teodoro and Marie crossed the border into the US daily as they drove to their jobs at a military base, about an hour from Naco.[69] While they worked, their two children went to their grandmother's house after school. In 1972, Saul Guerrero was five and Lourdes was fourteen years old. On a cold day in February, they were at their grandmother's when a stove exploded. Both children were badly burned.

Their parents rushed home from work as fast as they could. A doctor had dressed the children's burns, but there was no hospital on the Mexican side of the border, so the family piled into two cars to drive to the nearest emergency room, which was at Copper Queen Hospital in Bisbee, Arizona, only twenty minutes away. Border guards, accustomed to these medical emergencies, waved them through. But at the Copper Queen emergency room, a nurse refused to let the children enter. She took a look at them through the car window and told the parents to take them to the county hospital in Douglas, Arizona—another twenty-five minutes away. The nurse insisted that there were no beds available at Copper Queen.[70]

Cochise County Hospital in Douglas admitted Saul and Lourdes, and they both survived. But the parents were convinced that the children's pain would have been less, and their burns better treated, if they had been admitted to the first hospital. They found a lawyer and sued Copper Queen Hospital for medical negligence and malpractice. The case made it to the Arizona Supreme Court, which ruled in the Guerreros' favor. Arizona required hospitals to have emergency rooms, the court stated, and this implied that the state expected those emergency departments to provide care to everyone.[71]

Guerrero v. Copper Queen was an individual legal action, not a class action like *Lewis v. Gross*, and unlike in *Memorial v. Maricopa*, there was no activist doctor or attorney involved. Instead, it was a justice of the Arizona Supreme Court who ended up creating a new right to emergency care that included immigrants and migrants. The Guerreros had not alleged discrimination against noncitizens or even brought up the fact that they had crossed a border to seek emergency care for their children. But Justice Jack Hays decided, for unknown reasons, to add three crucial sentences to his decision. He wrote, "The appellants [Guerreros] are not residents of this state or county. Are they precluded from the benefits of the Arizona statutes and regulation on hospitals? *We think not*" (emphasis added).[72]

Hays's aside in the *Guerrero* decision went unnoticed at the time, but the case itself was one of a handful that created precedents for congressional action in the 1986 Emergency Medical Treatment and Active Labor Act. The text of EMTALA itself echoes the *Guerrero* decision, by making the treatment requirement applicable to any "hospital that has a hospital emergency department."[73] *Guerrero v. Copper Queen* is one of the most frequently cited cases on the law of emergency care, even appearing in an amicus brief that helped preserve the Affordable Care Act in 2012.[74] Like Henry Evaro in *Memorial v.*

Maricopa, the Guerreros were migrants who had been refused hospital care. Their legal actions ended up creating a right not just for migrants, but for everyone in the United States.

EMTALA was especially beneficial to public hospitals, which now had legal grounds to complain if private hospitals dumped patients at their doors. But it's difficult to fully celebrate the right to emergency care because of how it encapsulates the irrationality and contradictions of the US health system. It encourages the use of the most expensive type of medical care, and without other avenues of access, it contributed to transforming the emergency room into a primary care center for the poor. In addition, hospitals have numerous other means for turning away patients who cannot pay. Under EMTALA, they can transfer patients so long as they have been "stabilized," not treated.[75]

Still, the right to emergency care remains, alongside federally funded health centers, one of the two points of access in the US health system that are fully and legally available to anyone regardless of immigration status. There's no evidence that undocumented people began flooding emergency rooms after 1986—any increased pressure on ERs from this population was more likely due to changing immigration patterns, not to people taking advantage of the new law.[76] But private hospitals did begin blaming EMTALA for forcing them to provide vast amounts of uncompensated care to people without insurance—an argument that would be used to again demand more federal reimbursement to hospitals.

Reagan's Immigration Reform: Amnesty and Exclusion

In a televised debate between Ronald Reagan and George H. W. Bush in April 1980, both Republican presidential candidates expressed sympathy for undocumented immigrant children and approval of the *Plyler v. Doe* decision. Reagan even suggested providing Mexicans with work permits and allowing them to move back and forth across the border freely. But when pressed, Reagan declined to offer a specific proposal for immigration reform.[77] Reagan went on to win an electoral college landslide in 1980 and reelection in 1984. In 1986, he became the first president to sign immigration reform into law since Lyndon Johnson in 1965.

The legislation was the Immigration Reform and Control Act. IRCA, perhaps the most significant domestic policy achievement of the Reagan administration, heightened the contradictions of the US approach to immigration by imposing sanctions on employers who hired undocumented workers and increasing border enforcement, while at the same time creating an "amnesty" program for nearly three million undocumented residents.

The congressional negotiations that led to IRCA had lasted nearly fifteen years, spanning four presidential administrations. As historian Sarah Coleman has described, the final 1986 legislation took the form it did because of the large number of interest groups who weighed in, as well as political calculations by the Reagan administration. Reagan disliked employer sanctions because of his commitment to business deregulation, and in the final version the sanctions were watered down, voluntary, and nearly unenforceable.[78] The amnesty for unauthorized immigrants who had been in the country continuously since January 1 of 1982 was, surprisingly, one of the least controversial aspects of the bill. It was embraced by Latino rights groups as well as employers.

An aspect of the amnesty that conservatives disliked was the possibility of immigrants suddenly becoming eligible for welfare and social services.[79] To avoid this, Congress included a stipulation that public charge exclusions would apply to applicants for the amnesty program. In addition, people newly legalized under IRCA would have to undergo a five-year waiting period before becoming eligible for any type of government assistance "furnished . . . on the basis of financial need," including Medicaid.[80]

The legalization program did not constitute full "amnesty" for the undocumented. To meet the requirement of continuous residency since 1982 (with a shorter residency requirement for agricultural workers), applicants had to provide extensive documentation, such as pay stubs, driver's licenses, rent receipts, and doctor's bills, or provide a sworn affidavit. They had to undergo two medical exams performed by an INS-authorized doctor, and they had to pay for these exams themselves. There was also a fee of $185 per application.[81] These requirements put up immediate barriers for poor people who may have had spotty documentation of residency and never had access to private physicians. In addition, if they made it through the application process, the Medicaid waiting period ensured that poor immigrants would continue to live outside the borders of medical inclusion for another five years (actually a minimum of six and a half years, since there was a waiting period of eighteen months before being allowed to start the approval process for permanent residency).

Local immigrant rights advocates scrambled to help people legalize under IRCA and to find them medical care. The Coalition for Humane Immigrant Rights of Los Angeles warned potential applicants that people could be denied amnesty because they were poor. "If you have accepted welfare . . . wait to apply until you can support yourself," its pamphlet advised. "Do everything to be self supporting," and "prove you can get along without public cash assistance." Although public medical care, such as county clinics and hospitals, did not count as "public cash assistance" under public charge rules, advocates worried that people would be deterred from seeking medical care out of fear that their amnesty application would be denied. They also worked to identify sources of care for people waiting under the five-year Medicaid ban. Immigrants in this limbo could still be eligible for aid to the aged, blind, and disabled, for prenatal care, and for emergency treatment, but they needed to be informed of these rights.[82]

In the end, 2.7 million undocumented immigrants qualified for and received amnesty under IRCA. The legalization program, which from today's perspective seems almost unthinkably generous, had a flip side: increased enforcement and militarization on the US-Mexico border. IRCA's increased funding for the Border Patrol appeased restrictionists and sent a Cold War message about US strength and its ability to "control our own borders"—a ubiquitous phrase that made Mexican workers sound like foreign invaders.[83]

But IRCA failed to curb undocumented immigration. People continued to arrive without permission, and since repeated crossings became more dangerous due to the hardened border, more of them, and their families, remained in the US permanently. By government estimates, the undocumented population in the US grew by about 350,000 annually throughout the subsequent decade.[84] By 1993, about half of the country's undocumented population lived in California.

Exclusion By Law: The Battle over Proposition 187

In 1994, California anti-immigrant activists placed a measure on the state ballot to ban undocumented people from access to public education and nonemergency public health care. The battle over Proposition 187 captured the attention of the entire country as local debates over immigrants' rights swept onto the national stage.

Proposition 187, also known as the "Save Our State" initiative, was the brainchild of a group of restrictionists and fiscal conservatives from Orange County and other suburban areas of California. They included former INS and Border Patrol officials, Republican politicians, businesspeople, and local conservative activists. Their philosophy was embodied in the preamble language of their proposition:

> The People of California find and declare as follows:
>
> That they have suffered and are suffering economic hardship caused by the presence of illegal aliens in this state.
>
> That they have suffered and are suffering personal injury and damage caused by the criminal conduct of aliens in this state.

That they have the right to the protection of their government from any person or persons entering the country unlawfully.[85]

"Aliens'" use of health services and public education, according to organizers, was causing economic injury to California's taxpayers. Proposition 187
intended to deny all government-funded public services to undocumented
immigrants, increase penalties for people using false documents, mandate
cooperation between law enforcement and immigration officials, and require
"all public entities" to "verify the immigration status of anyone attempting to
use their services."[86]

The drafters of the measure specifically wanted to challenge *Plyler v. Doe*.
Proposition 187 would require schools to report not only the immigration
status of children, but also of their parents, and to expel children suspected of
being in the country illegally. But they did not attempt to go after EMTALA.
The health care provisions of 187 were harsh, banning all publicly funded care
to undocumented immigrants, including preventive and prenatal care, but
excepted "emergency medical care as required by federal law."[87]

Governor Pete Wilson, whose reelection campaign had relied on adver-
tisements intended to stoke fears of an immigrant invasion, threw his support
behind Proposition 187. With the measure placed on the ballot in June 1994
for the November election, opponents only had a few months to organize.
They faced a huge challenge; polls indicated strong support for the proposition among the white voters who made up the vast majority of the California
electorate, despite their shrinking percentage of the population.

A coalition formed to oppose Proposition 187, called Taxpayers against
187. In addition to Latino rights groups like MALDEF and LULAC, the Taxpayers against 187 coalition included organizations that had previously not
been involved in immigrant rights battles, including the AFL-CIO and the
California Medical Association, and several powerful Democratic politicians.
As political scientist Daniel HoSang has shown, Taxpayers against 187 decided
to appeal to the white electorate by taking a restrictionist and fiscally conservative stance. They conceded that undocumented immigration was a major
threat to California. Instead of defending immigrants against the falsehoods
propagated by restrictionists, the coalition argued that the proposition would
make "a bad situation worse" because it would fail to restrict undocumented
immigration and would end up costing taxpayers more.[88]

Ending health services to immigrants was a bad idea, according to the
coalition, not because it would hurt immigrant individuals and families, but
because it would hurt "mainstream" Californians. A Taxpayers against 187
pamphlet argued that, by forbidding immunizations and medical exams to

the undocumented, Proposition 187 "threatens everyone's health." It quoted health official Dr. Thomas Peters saying that "in one fell swoop, the carefully-crafted disease control system in California would be destroyed . . . it is not just someone else's health that would be threatened, it's yours." Immigrants "handle the food supply," the pamphlet went on, so denying them vaccines and health care could "spread costly and preventable communicable diseases across California."[89]

Proposition 187 opponents made fiscal as well as public health–related arguments. Rather than arguing that immigrants provided a net economic benefit to the state, as activists had done in the earlier Los Angeles and San Diego battles, the Taxpayers against 187 coalition chose to focus on how the proposition would further increase health costs. For example, the state stood to lose billions in federal funding, including for medical research, because 187 would violate federal privacy laws. Eliminating prenatal care for immigrants meant that their babies would end up costing the state Medi-Cal program more money. The "failure to treat and control serious contagious diseases, such as tuberculosis, among illegal immigrants," the *San Francisco Chronicle* noted, would "increase future costs to treat the disease in the general population." And requiring additional bureaucracies for hospitals and doctors to verify immigration status would add to the "escalating costs of publicly-funded health services."[90]

Another argument against Proposition 187 that did not center immigrant rights was based in traditional medical ethics. Requiring health care practitioners to ask about and report patients' immigration status violated medical privacy and the doctor-patient relationship. Proposition 187 "would turn doctors and nurses into INS agents," and "every teacher, social worker and nurse, the very people whose work depends so much on trust, would become a government snoop," according to a Taxpayers against 187 pamphlet. Finally, "by requiring verification and premising denial on 'suspicion,'" Proposition 187 "could cause unnecessary, and potentially life-endangering, delays and denials of services to people entitled to medical care."[91]

California's immigrant rights movement had expanded since the mid-1980s due to IRCA and also to Reagan's Central America policies. Many activists from this movement saw Taxpayers against 187's approach as a capitulation to racism and a betrayal of vulnerable people. They formed another coalition called Californians United against Proposition 187. Jan Adams, a Californians United leader interviewed by HoSang, said the fight against 187 was the most emotional organizing campaign she had ever been involved in. She described meetings with undocumented parents who expressed "moral outrage" at the idea that their kids' right to go to school and to "be able to get health care" was being "put to a vote."[92]

Unlike the Taxpayers against 187, the Californians United approach had more in common with the anti–Proposition 187 street protests and spontaneous high school walkouts that erupted across the state shortly before the election. The marches included one in Los Angeles on October 16 that drew between seventy and one hundred thousand people and was the largest in the city's history.

Throughout California, protesters passionately defended immigrants and denounced the cruelty of taking away education and health care. They carried signs reading "187 = Racism," "No Racism, No Scapegoating," and "Stop Immigrant Bashing Now." Some signs called attention to the state's reliance on immigrant workers: "These Hands Care for Your Children" and "These Hands Pick Your Food."[93] High school students joining the walkouts declared that "Prop. 187 is like a death penalty," "We're fighting for our parents, our loved ones, everybody," and "We have our rights."[94] In opposing the initiative, protesters made an affirmative case that immigrants deserved rights. One speaker at an East Los Angeles meeting rallied the crowd by announcing, "California does not need Proposition 187; California needs human rights for all."[95]

But, on November 8, 1994, Proposition 187 passed with 59 percent of the vote. According to exit polls, 63 percent of whites voted in favor, and 77 percent of Latinos voted against the initiative.[96] But Latinos made up only 11 percent of registered voters in California, even though they were almost 30 percent of the state's population. MALDEF and multiple other organizations immediately filed lawsuits to halt implementation of the law. Soon judges issued restraining orders delaying 187's educational, social services, and health care provisions.[97]

While lawsuits put the proposition in limbo, health departments and immigrant advocates feared that patients would meanwhile be deterred from seeking care. On November 9, the day after the election, the California State Department of Health Services announced that "no changes in eligibility or procedure" would occur until the state issued regulations for implementing the law. The Asian Law Caucus alerted rights groups that the restraining orders meant that "teachers, medical staff, and social service providers cannot ask immigration status nor report such information." The City and County of San Francisco issued a notice that "the Department of Public Health is not enforcing Proposition 187 at this time" and urged patients in bold letters to "PLEASE ATTEND YOUR REGULARLY SCHEDULED CLINIC APPOINTMENTS."[98]

But fears that the overwhelming passage of Proposition 187 would keep people away from seeking medical care started to come true. On November 24, about two weeks after 187's victory, the *Los Angeles Times* reported that a thirteen-year-old Anaheim boy named Julio Cano died of acute leukemia that had gone untreated. Julio had gotten sick on Monday, November 13, but his undocumented parents hesitated to take him to the hospital, because they "had been denied nonemergency care before. With the passage of Proposition 187, they believed their immigration status would be challenged," and they were unaware that the law had not taken effect. His father waited until payday on Friday so he could get sixty dollars to take his son to a private clinic. The family left the clinic with antibiotics but not a diagnosis. Julio got worse and died at home the next day.[99]

When the *Times* spoke to some of the authors of Proposition 187 about Julio's case, they "inveighed against Latino activists for exploiting a tragic situation for political ends" (the parents had met with MALDEF and agreed to add Julio's story to the group's lawsuit against 187). "Save Our State" leader Ron Prince said people like Julio's family were "endangering the children by bringing them here illegally." Governor Pete Wilson was asked about the case during a TV interview on *Good Morning America*. He replied, "We get all kinds of stories of that sort, I suppose." Wilson said that American citizens were the ones being denied health care because of the burden placed on hospitals by undocumented people seeking emergency care.[100]

The *Los Angeles Times* interviewed Julio's undocumented parents and found that the family were no strangers to medical exclusion. "Even before the passage of 187 . . . a daughter had been denied care at a Garden Grove hospital once because her condition was not deemed an emergency, and the mother said she went to UC Irvine Medical Center seeking a free pregnancy test once and was denied." From the Canos' story, it seemed that their concern about seeking care after Proposition 187 was not just that they would be turned away, which would be nothing new, but also that their immigration status would be reported.[101]

Other reports emerged of the negative health effects of Proposition 187. Los Angeles County announced that their health facilities had experienced a 20 percent drop in prenatal care visits between September 1993 and September 1994, even before the law passed.[102] The National Immigration Forum, an immigrant rights group based in Washington, DC, began documenting additional evidence that Proposition 187 was deterring people from using needed medical services or leading them to be denied services. Along with Julio Cano's case, they reported on an "elderly woman" in San Francisco who "died of a brain hemorrhage . . . because she was too afraid of being deported if she sought treatment." Other examples included California pharmacies and dental clinics demanding immigration papers, hospitals that asked for papers even though that part of the law was on hold, a woman suffering a miscarriage who was rejected from a private hospital and told "We don't treat Hispanics here," and a doctor calling a patient and his relative "'f—ing wetbacks' and telling them to go back to Mexico."[103]

In March 1998, most of Proposition 187 was struck down by a US district court. The judge ruled that the initiative was unconstitutional on two grounds: it violated the exclusive authority of the federal government to regulate immigration, and its educational provisions contradicted the *Plyler v. Doe* ruling affirming undocumented children's right to public education.

Although the law was never implemented, the battle over Proposition 187 was a watershed for immigration politics in the US. In California, it actually strengthened immigrant rights and Latino activism. It pushed organizers to start emphasizing voter registration and to fight for increased Latino electoral power. Political analysts agree that Proposition 187 was the turning point that led to the erosion of Republican Party influence in the state.[104]

The fight to defeat Proposition 187 also led activist groups nationwide to explicitly defend the rights of immigrants. The slogan "Immigrant Rights Are Human Rights" was seen on signs at marches from San Francisco to New York.[105] Older civil rights organizations such as LULAC and the GI Forum completed their transformation from anti-immigration to fully embracing immigrant rights. The slogan of New Mexicans against Proposition 187 was "Somos Un Mismo Pueblo"—"We Are the Same People."[106]

Finally, the proposition's direct attack on access to health care forced medical providers to openly defend access for the undocumented. The California Medical Association, the California Nurses Association, the California Association of Hospital and Health Systems, and the California chapter of the American College of Emergency Physicians all made public pronouncements against 187. Although "don't ask, don't tell" policies among medical providers had been common and would continue, the battle over Proposition 187 led them to articulate health care as a universal right, regardless of citizenship.

At the same time, Proposition 187 emboldened the nationwide anti-immigrant movement, which began to push for similar measures in other states. Legislation to reduce welfare and health benefits to immigrants would be embraced by both the national Democratic and the Republican Parties.[107] Even refugees and legal immigrants, groups that had previously been seen as deserving of public assistance to help them adjust to their new lives in the US, would soon have their access to health care ripped away.

6

Violence against Health

Medical Care for Refugees: More Deserving?

For most of the twentieth century, the US treatment of refugees—people fleeing war and persecution—took place within the framework of racially charged immigration restriction. In the 1930s and 1940s, the United States notoriously and shamefully refused to accept most Jewish refugees from Hitler's Europe. Its treatment of "displaced persons" following World War II was scarcely more generous. The Displaced Persons Act of 1948 "allowed refugees to enter the U.S. within the constraints of the existing [racial] quota system" and required those admitted to find their own housing and a job that would not displace a US worker.[1]

In the Cold War, US refugee policy became a tool of rivalry with the Soviet Union. The Refugee Relief Act, signed by President Dwight D. Eisenhower in 1953, authorized two hundred thousand nonquota immigrant visas for "refugees and escapees from communist countries." (Chinese refugees received two thousand visas under this program, while the immigrant quota for China was 105.) Thousands of Hungarian refugees fleeing a Soviet crackdown in 1956–57 entered under a special parole issued by the attorney general, and Congress later authorized their legal permanent residency. In 1961 the US announced a similar parole for refugees from revolutionary Cuba. More than fifty-eight thousand Cubans were admitted in the first year under this policy.[2]

When they arrived in the US, refugees needed a place to settle and assistance finding housing and jobs. Most resettlement assistance was provided by individual sponsors, churches, and voluntary groups. But as the number of refugees increased throughout the Cold War, the government gradually got more involved. The 1953 Refugee Act provided $5 million in federal loans to public and private agencies that worked to resettle refugees "who lack resources to finance the expenses involved." It also specified that any resettlement assistance refugees received would not label them as public charges, further confirming refugees' special status.[3]

The first direct federal expenditures for refugee resettlement were authorized in the Migration and Refugee Assistance Act of 1962, which gave the president discretion to provide funds for both international refugee programs under the UN and for refugees settling in the US. The 1962 act specified that the president could allocate loans or grants to local governments and agencies to spend on health care, education, and employment training for newly arrived refugees.[4] Three days after the act was approved, the Kennedy administration opened a Cuban Refugee Center in Miami. Named "Freedom Tower," the center provided Cuban arrivals with free medical care, food, financial support, and relocation assistance. It sent the message that Cubans fleeing Kennedy's archenemy Fidel Castro would be warmly welcomed in the US.[5] In 1966 Congress underscored the message when it passed a law giving permanent residency to all Cuban refugees admitted under parole status.[6]

Starting in the mid-1970s, a similar welcome was accorded to people fleeing newly Communist nations in Southeast Asia (Indochina). The first wave of refugees from Vietnam consisted of 130,000 people, most of whom were supporters of the failed US war in the region, who arrived primarily in evacuations organized during and after the fall of Saigon. In 1975, Congress created a program to provide resettlement assistance to refugees from Vietnam, Cambodia, and Laos by adding $455 million to the funds already available to the president for these purposes. People admitted under the Indochina programs also received legal permanent residency by act of Congress in 1977.[7]

The United Nations defined refugees as people "unable or unwilling to return to their country of origin owing to a well-founded fear of being persecuted for reasons of race, religion, nationality, membership of a particular social group, or political opinion." But critics pointed out that the preferential treatment of refugees from Communist countries violated this norm by elevating political considerations above all others and by using refugee policy as a geopolitical weapon. Due to increased attention to human rights during the Carter administration, in 1980 Congress passed the Refugee Act, which adopted the UN definition and allowed Congress and the president to set an annual number of refugee admissions and to utilize humanitarian and other considerations besides politics.[8] The act also established a permanent Office of Refugee Resettlement within the Department of Health and Human Services to provide grants to states and organizations that assisted refugees.

The 1980 Refugee Act authorized funds for "emergency" medical expenditures to treat refugees who were judged to have conditions "affecting the public health." In addition, it empowered the federal government to cover 100 percent of the costs of financial and medical assistance received by refugees during their first three years in the country.[9] In total, the new law significantly increased federal support for refugee health and welfare. Federal responsibility for refugee welfare services could be justified to conservatives because refugees were admitted "as a matter of national policy."[10]

However, shortly after Ronald Reagan arrived in the White House, he began seeking cuts to refugee assistance to "encourage self sufficiency and find savings."[11] Previously Cold War heroes, refugees were now labeled, in Reagan's world view, welfare seekers. In addition, they were no longer primarily eastern European but Asian and Latin American, adding to their undesirability and stigmatization.

Indochinese arrivals were also stigmatized as carriers of disease, especially tuberculosis, which had nearly vanished in the US due to the use of antibiotics.[12] In addition to coming from impoverished and war-torn homelands, many Southeast Asian refugees had spent months or years in crowded refugee camps awaiting resettlement, exposing them to tuberculosis, hepatitis B, and intestinal parasites. Refugees underwent extensive screenings both before and after their arrival in the US. Many were also found to be suffering from mental health problems, particularly post-traumatic stress. Public health researchers pointed out that screenings were not enough; the conditions they were found to have were controllable with adequate health care and follow-up treatments.[13]

A large majority of Indochinese refugees were poor enough to be eligible for Medicaid after their federal assistance expired. Unlike undocumented immigrants and those legalized by IRCA, refugees were not barred from enrolling in Medicaid, nor subject to IRCA's five-year waiting period. Membership in Medicaid was highly valued—among Khmer refugees in one California study, it was "like gold."[14]

When refugees attempted to enter the job market, they faced the irrationality of the US health system when they learned they would lose their Medicaid. Many jobs did not provide private health coverage or did not cover family members. Advocates noted how this worked against the professed goal of refugees becoming "self sufficient." It also worked against public health goals. For example, the husband of a Hmong woman with hepatitis B refused to be tested because, as a restaurant worker without health coverage, he knew they could not afford treatment.[15]

The Reagan administration's cuts to refugee benefits signaled a swift move away from the more generous approach of the 1980 Refugee Act. It also reflected a more general backlash against refugees among the US media and public. Since 1975, when "the great majority of the first [Indochinese] refugees arriving [were] professionals, skilled and clerical workers and businessmen," the numbers of refugees had grown and their characteristics had shifted. The increasing numbers of Vietnamese and Cambodians fleeing their war-torn countries in the late 1970s were described as "boat people." They tended to be poorer and less educated than earlier refugees and had spent long periods of time in refugee camps before being resettled.[16]

Increasingly, refugees were spoken of in the same breath as undocumented immigrants. In a 1982 *Reader's Digest* article that was reprinted in newspapers across the country, Carl Rowan and David Mazie wrote of the "estimated 6 million illegal aliens and refugees [that] have surged into the United States" in the preceding five years, "taxing our social services, overloading school systems and competing for jobs." Wisconsin congressman James Sensenbrenner condemned "our open-door policy toward immigrants and refugees." Along with measures against illegal immigration, he proposed reducing the number of refugees admitted per year and giving Congress more power over refugee admissions.[17] Formerly valorized as representing anticommunism, refugees no longer seemed deserving of their relatively privileged status.

The refugees and immigrants who threatened to turn the "melting pot" into a "pressure cooker," Rowan and Mazie wrote, were "primarily from Indochina, Mexico, and Cuba."[18] Conservatives had previously welcomed Cubans fleeing Castro's regime, but as the characteristics of Cuban migrants changed, like the Indochinese, they were redefined as undesirable.

The catalyst in this transformation had been the Mariel Boatlift, named for the Cuban port where the migration initiated. Between April and October 1980, 125,000 Cubans arrived in Florida on private boats, encouraged to leave their country by Fidel Castro. Soon word spread that some of the migrants had been released from Cuban mental institutions and prisons. The Mariel Boatlift also included more Afro-Cubans and young people than previous waves of Cuban migration.[19] The "*Marielitos*" were crammed into tent cities in Miami, including one in the Orange Bowl Stadium. The INS detained tens of thousands of these migrants and flew them to temporary housing at military bases.[20]

The Carter administration faced a dilemma. If the Cubans were accepted as refugees, they would immediately become eligible for federal health and welfare assistance. There was also the matter of the migrants from Haiti who had been coming throughout the 1970s. Significant numbers of Haitians had been denied asylum and placed in detention, which had led to intense criticism of the administration for discriminating against Black refugees. Carter decided to address the problem by creating a "Cuban-Haitian Entrant" classification, which allowed some Haitians and the new Cubans to stay in the

United States and to become permanent residents after two years. "Entrants" would be eligible for medical services, supplemental income, and emergency assistance benefits, with the federal government covering 75 percent of the costs.[21]

This was an improvement for those Haitians who qualified, but it represented the end of the Cubans' broader entitlement. No longer would Cubans be granted blanket refugee status because of where they came from. Even so, Cubans admitted via the entrant program still had a far more privileged position than other Spanish-speaking refugees, whose numbers were also swelling.[22]

The Politics of Sanctuary

Following the Nicaraguan Revolution in 1979, the United States turned its attention to Central America as a Cold War battlefront. Although US military and economic intervention in the region was not new, in the 1980s it entrenched its support of brutal and unpopular dictatorships that imprisoned, tortured, and murdered their opponents. In El Salvador, church workers and students were targeted by right-wing death squads allied with the pro-American president. In Guatemala, the US-backed military displaced and massacred tens of thousands of Indigenous people. And in Nicaragua, the United States funded and trained "Contra" forces, exalted by Ronald Reagan as "freedom fighters," seeking to overthrow the Sandinista government.[23]

These violent upheavals led to desperate migrations. As María Cristina García writes, "The wars in Central America displaced millions of people and forced them to migrate internally and across borders." Many went to other countries in Central America, Mexico, and Canada. Between five hundred thousand and 750,000 refugees, the majority from El Salvador, ended up in the United States. But the Reagan administration refused to recognize them as refugees. Unlike Indochinese fleeing communism, Central Americans fleeing right-wing regimes were labeled economic migrants and thus illegal immigrants. To grant them asylum would be to admit that the governments they were fleeing were violating human rights and would thus force Congress to reconsider US support for the regimes in El Salvador and Guatemala.[24]

The hypocrisy of US refugee policy was challenged by activists who began to both criticize US interventions in Central America and to defend the refugees who faced being sent back to their dangerous homelands. Participants in the sanctuary movement, which was part of the wave of protest against Reagan's foreign policy in the 1980s, provided people arriving from Central America with transportation, shelter, food, and legal help.

At first these activities were clandestine, but in 1982 activists in Tucson, Arizona, openly announced that the Southside Presbyterian Church would serve as a sanctuary for Central American refugees. The movement spread around the country as churches, synagogues, college campuses, and even some cities declared themselves sanctuaries. Activists risked arrest for aiding migrants, and in 1985, the US Justice Department indicted eleven sanctuary volunteers for alien smuggling. The publicity generated by their trial only led more people to join the cause.[25]

Medical providers got caught up in the sanctuary movement. In Brownsville, Texas, during an influx of refugees from Nicaragua, someone left a sick baby on the doorstep of Su Clínica, the community health center. Clinic workers sent a medical team to where the refugees were camped and, according to Su Clínica director Paula Gomez, "helped them set up tents and began transporting people in our own cars from the camp to temporary medical headquarters we had set up in a nearby gym." While caring for the refugees, the clinic staff found out that "the FBI was following us" but "we didn't stop. It was our version of the underground railway," Gomez remembers.[26]

Wisconsin public health nurse Leonard Cizewski provided sanctuary activists with guidance on refugee health care. He wrote that the health problems common among Central American refugees, including intestinal parasites, malnutrition, and anemia, were "diseases of oppression and poverty" and products of "unjust and exploitive social systems." The governments they were fleeing had failed to provide clean drinking water or vaccinations. In addition, post-traumatic stress resulted from the "institutionalized violence" refugees had experienced. Cizewski recommended that sanctuary volunteers serve as translators and advocates for refugees who needed medical care. He noted that hospitals and public health departments generally did not screen for immigration status, but also advised "appropriate caution" to avoid exposing refugees to detection.[27]

Salvadorans, Guatemalans, and Hondurans were not eligible for federal assistance, Medicare, or Medicaid because the US government did not recognize them as refugees. Fear of deportation, language barriers, and lack of money prevented them from seeking other types of care. In some cities with growing populations of Central Americans, the sanctuary movement set up medical clinics specifically to aid them. Sanctuary activists, Central America solidarity groups, and health professionals partnered to open La Clínica del Pueblo in Washington, DC; the Oscar Romero Holistic Health Clinic in Brooklyn, New York; and the Clínica Msgr. Oscar A. Romero in Los Angeles (the last two named for the assassinated archbishop of San Salvador). Care at the clinics was provided by Central American medical professionals as well as local volunteers.[28] US doctors and nurses in the solidarity movement also organized study and aid trips to Nicaragua and raised funds to send medical supplies to war-torn regions.[29]

Throughout the 1980s, the US government continued to detain and deport Central Americans. Between 1983 and 1990, only 2.6 percent of Salvadoran and 1.8 percent of Guatemalan applicants received asylum (Nicaraguans, from a country with a socialist government, were more successful, at 25.2 percent).[30] However, the sanctuary movement did win some significant victories.

In 1990, the settlement of a class-action lawsuit known as *American Baptist Churches v. Thornburgh* overturned the asylum denials of more than 150,000 Salvadorans and Guatemalans.[31] That same year, Congress passed a Refugee Act that included a new program called Temporary Protected Status (TPS). TPS allowed people from countries designated as undergoing armed conflict or disaster to receive temporary work permits and remain in the US without being targeted for deportation. In the subsequent decades, close to two hundred thousand Salvadorans have been able to remain in the country due to TPS.[32] TPS designation can be renewed indefinitely but can also be revoked by the government, so those under its protections live in a constant state of uncertainty. Also, people in the TPS program are not eligible for permanent residency (unless otherwise qualified), or for any type of public assistance.[33]

Despite these limitations, the sanctuary movement was among the most successful US migrant rights movement of the twentieth century. In addition to forcing the courts and Congress to protect hundreds of thousands of asylum seekers, it led to a proliferation of organizations, including medical clinics, that continued to provide advocacy and services after the end of the Cold War. Sanctuary and solidarity activism demonstrated the connections between foreign and domestic politics, between immigration and refugee/asylum policies, and between refugees and undocumented immigrants. Finally, the movement transformed political language by making the word "sanctuary" synonymous with protection for undocumented people.

But the attack on the rights of refugees from the wars in Central America was just one aspect of the US war on migrants in the 1980s. The Reagan administration opened another front by using a global pandemic as an excuse to exclude, detain, and discriminate against immigrants.

Deporting a Disease: HIV/AIDS Exclusions

On May 5, 1987, over three million undocumented people in the US became eligible to apply for amnesty under the Immigration Reform and Control Act. Less than one month later, Congress added a new disease to the list of condi-

tions that made an alien excludable from the United States. The disease was
AIDS, which had been ravaging communities in the US since 1981, but was
not publicly discussed by President Ronald Reagan until 1987.[34]

Compared to the government's slowness in acknowledging the pandemic,
Congress's action to exclude HIV-positive immigrants was lightning fast.
Jesse Helms, the notoriously bigoted and homophobic US senator from North
Carolina, proposed the amendment, and the Senate passed it with a vote of
96–0 on June 3, 1987. The new exclusion represented a desire to "do something" about AIDS that would not (its supporters hoped) cause much debate
or controversy or cost any money.[35] It was, yet again, an example of using immigration policy to enact health policy—or rather, a policy to discriminate
based on a health condition.

This was not just an extension of the long-standing practice of excluding
immigrants who carried certain contagious diseases. The new policy imposed
exclusion, and potential deportation, on people who simply tested positive for
HIV, whether or not they had developed symptoms of AIDS (which could take
many years). Testing positive could expose migrants to severe discrimination
and stigma, whether in the US or in their home countries. In addition, there
was no evidence that exclusion would control the spread of AIDS, and the
World Health Organization had advised against screening travelers for HIV
because of the minimal effectiveness of such a policy.[36] Disregarding both
the ineffectiveness and the discriminatory effect of HIV exclusions, the US
also announced that applicants for the IRCA amnesty already living in the
country had to take an HIV test.

The HIV alien exclusion and testing requirements coincided with the
eruption of activism around the AIDS pandemic. ACT UP (AIDS Coalition to Unleash Power), the stunningly effective grassroots organization that
would transform public health and help speed progress against the disease,
held its first meetings in New York City in the spring of 1987. When gay rights
activists in Los Angeles started their own chapter of ACT UP a few months
later, their very first public action was against the HIV testing requirement for
immigrants and applicants for IRCA amnesty.

The new organization called a protest at INS headquarters in downtown
Los Angeles on December 23, 1987. They announced that "ACT UP L.A. is
profoundly concerned with the mandatory HIV antibody testing regulation" for immigration and amnesty applicants. They called the requirement a
"human rights violation" that would lead to deportations, family separations,
and violations of confidentiality and would discourage people from applying
for amnesty.[37]

The seventy-five people who showed up to protest in front of the INS,

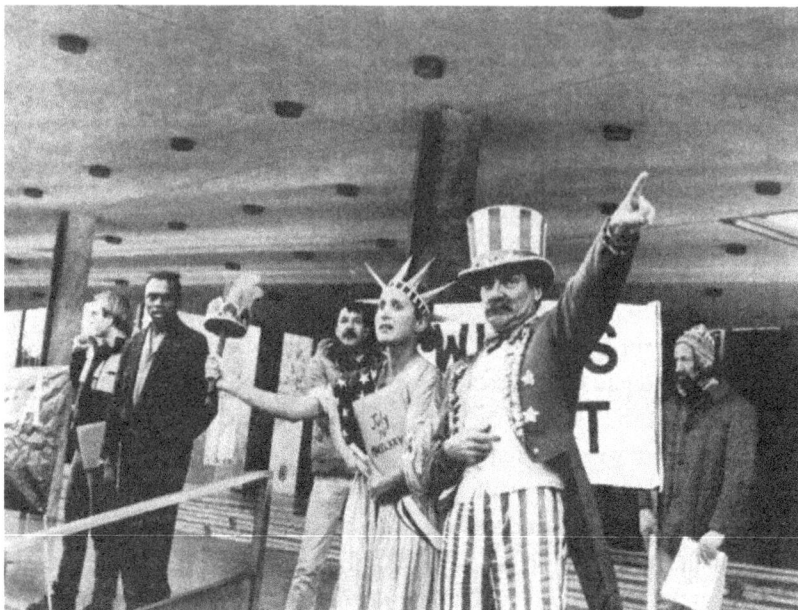

FIGURE 6.1. ACT UP Los Angeles members perform street theater to protest the Immigration and Naturalization Service's HIV testing requirement, December 23, 1987. Photo by Sandy Dwyer, *News* (West Hollywood, CA), January 8, 1988, 18. ONE Archives at the USC Libraries.

and the press, were treated to a theatrical performance. An ACT UP member dressed as the Statue of Liberty stepped in front of the crowd. She began to welcome immigrants "in a variety of languages." Then a costumed Uncle Sam interrupted, "informing her she must take the HIV antibody test." Her result was positive, and Uncle Sam told the Statue of Liberty to leave the country. The players then led the crowd in chanting "Who's Next?"[38]

In focusing on the exclusion and testing policy, ACT UP Los Angeles found common cause between gay rights and migrant rights. Both communities were already subject to stigma, neglect, and discrimination that was exacerbated by panic about AIDS. Activists feared that mandatory testing could lead to quarantines of any targeted group. In addition, ACT UP's passionate defense of migrants reflected its growing commitment to fighting racism, reinforced by the influence and leadership of Black and Latino activists in both the Los Angeles and New York organizations.[39]

ACT UP Los Angeles continued protests targeting the immigration ban. In March of 1988, they joined the immigrant rights group La Resistencia to picket in front of the Mardi Gras Motel in Inglewood, which the INS had converted to a privately run detention center housing Central American refugees. ACT UP member Larry Day told the protesters, "We are here to demand justice for our immigrant brothers and sisters" and called for coalitions between immigrant and AIDS rights organizations. At a "Shut Down the INS National Phone Zap" in 1990, ACT UP organized people to inundate the immigration service with faxes and phone calls demanding the end of the exclusion policy.[40]

ACT UP emphasized that the ban on HIV-positive immigrants affected not just those seeking entrance to the country, but also those who had been here for many years.[41] Longtime residents who were eligible for the IRCA amnesty had to undergo HIV testing before being approved. In San Francisco, immigrant rights attorneys created an HIV Task Force to assist applicants for amnesty who were struggling with the consequences of HIV testing. When one Mexican-born woman was informed that she tested positive, she "became very depressed." Her husband and lawyers from the task force encouraged her to retest, and that result was negative. Yet the positive results had already been sent to the INS and nearly caused her to give up pursuing legalization. "Task Force members have heard of at least ten seropositive (HIV-positive) persons who were eligible for legalization but did not apply because they believed they would be denied outright," attorneys reported. There were also several cases of men who tested positive for HIV being told by their INS-appointed doctors that they actually had AIDS. One Guatemalan man was so distraught at this inaccurate news that he attempted suicide.[42]

The California Department of Health Services warned that amnesty applicants who did test positive, or who already knew they had HIV, would "remain in the United States in an illegal underground status" or be forced or choose to leave the country, "at a time when they most need proper medical guidance and assistance." There was a process for HIV-positive applicants to receive a waiver of exclusion, but "the process was long, the standards were strict, and advocates worried [that] most did not know about it." According to an INS spokesman, "From the small number of waiver requests coming in, we can assume that the majority of people testing positive decided not to pursue their legalization applications."[43]

While amnesty applicants faded back into the shadows, the ban on HIV-positive people entering the US became a target of high-publicity protests. In 1989, Dutch activist Hans Paul Verhoff, who had AIDS, was denied entry to US to attend a conference in San Francisco. In response, activists announced a boycott and protests of the Sixth International AIDS Conference in San Francisco the following year, due to what ACT UP called the "heinous travel and immigration ban." In 1992, international protests over the US AIDS exclusion forced the conference to be moved from Boston to Amsterdam. Spanish immigrant Tomás Fabregas announced his HIV-positive status and said he would travel home from the Amsterdam conference to test the travel ban. The Hollywood star Elizabeth Taylor and other celebrities joined Fabregas at his press conference, and he returned to the US "without incident."[44]

The HIV/AIDS movement argued that the travel exclusion was connected to other health care and immigration injustices. A 1991 ACT UP Los Angeles pamphlet stated that the ban was part of the "sordid history" of "allowing ignorance and prejudice to dictate the treatment of non-citizen visitors, workers and immigrants." The immigration and exclusion bans were "bad medicine" both because they failed to stem the spread of disease (AIDS was not transmitted through casual contact) and because they prevented HIV-positive people from seeking care. ACT UP Los Angeles called for universal health care and condemned the unequal US health system: "We believe that people with AIDS will never receive decent, humane treatment from a society that stands by silently while immigrant women are forced to give birth in the hallways of over-crowded, under-funded public hospitals."[45]

By insisting that prejudice and inequality exacerbated the spread of HIV/AIDS, ACT UP contributed to a shift in the global response to the pandemic. By the late 1980s, international health agencies, including the World Health Organization and the Red Cross, were condemning travel and immigration bans as both unjust and ineffective. Following the WHO's adoption of a non-discrimination policy in 1987, all the countries that had them dropped HIV travel restrictions—except the United States.[46]

AIDS activists condemned testing requirements and immigration bans as a slippery slope to quarantine and the loss of civil and human rights. In the case of one group—Haitians—they were proved correct.

Detain and Quarantine: The Haitians' Ordeal

People from the Caribbean nation of Haiti had faced discrimination in US immigration and refugee policy long before the AIDS crisis. Haiti's undemocratic governments served the United States as allies against Cuba, so people fleeing those regimes were not welcomed on political grounds, the way Cubans or Indochinese were. And as people of African descent, Haitians' Blackness also singled them out as "undesirable" migrants.[47]

A wave of Haitian migration began in 1972, with people fleeing torture and imprisonment under the brutal rule of Jean-Claude "Baby Doc" Duvalier, heir to the US support of his father "Papa Doc." The United States issued a blanket denial of asylum for Haitian refugees from the regime. This meant that all Haitians seeking asylum were placed under deportation orders. However, they still were entitled to the limited due process required under official deportation procedures, leaving them in limbo awaiting their asylum hearings, often for years. Many Haitian asylum applicants were placed in detention in the US. Those who were released were not eligible for work permits or any kind of welfare, so they had to rely on local charities to survive.[48]

As Congress discussed how to deal with the new influx of Mariel Cubans in 1980, the plight of Haitians already in the US came to public attention. Walter E. Fountroy, Washington, DC's nonvoting representative and member of the Congressional Black Caucus, condemned the "shameful" treatment of Haitians, which he called not just political but racial, noting that "any other boat people are welcome here." Haitians, Fountroy said, "have been languishing and starving in southern Florida for 8 years without any sort of humanitarian assistance from the Federal government." In comparison to other refugees, Haitians got "no work permits. No medical care. No assistance in terms of food and survival. . . . That treatment is unprecedented." Fountroy was especially incensed by the detention of Haitians: "I do not know of any [other national group of] aliens that have been imprisoned upon arrival here. That seems to us to be particularly discriminatory."[49]

Pressure from civil rights groups, the Congressional Black Caucus, and Haitian migrants themselves helped persuade President Carter to create the Cuban-Haitian Entrant Program in order to demonstrate that the two groups were being treated more or less equally. Neither group received official refugee designation or protection from deportation, but their new entrant status did allow Haitians who arrived before October 10, 1980, to eventually apply for permanent residency. Even that protection was short-lived, as the new Reagan administration soon reverted to treating Haitians differently, imposing a policy of "interdiction" that allowed the US to intercept vessels carrying Haitians and rapidly repatriate the passengers. In addition, the administration announced that all Haitians who did reach the US would be put in detention, without the possibility of bond.[50]

Then, another rationalization for discrimination worsened the plight of Haitian refugees. Starting in 1982, Haitians were stigmatized as AIDS carriers. That year, the US Centers for Disease Control designated "4 H's" as the high-risk groups for HIV: homosexuals, hemophiliacs, heroin users—and Haitians. Although the CDC admitted by 1985 that people from Haiti should no longer be considered a risk group, they remained excluded from giving blood. In New York City in 1990, tens of thousands of Haitian Americans, migrants, and their supporters protested the continuing ban. Marchers carried signs reading "We're proud of our blood" and "Let's fight AIDS, not nationality."[51]

In 1991, a violent coup in Haiti overthrew the democratically elected leader Jean-Bertrande Aristide, and more refugees headed to the US. Thirty-

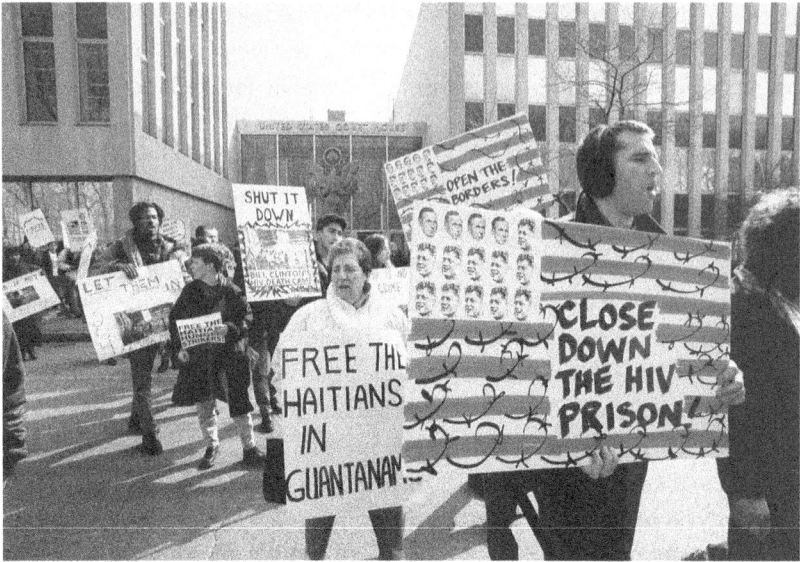

FIGURE 6.2. Original caption: "Members of ACT UP join residents of New York's Haitian community to demonstrate outside the Brooklyn Federal Courthouse, March 8, 1993. The two groups are protesting the continued lock up of AIDS-infected Haitian refugees in Guantanamo Bay." AP Photo/Andrew Savulich. Courtesy Associated Press.

seven thousand Haitians were interdicted in a single year. Not wanting to bring them to the mainland, the US government detained them at sea and then began to forcibly repatriate them, until stopped by a judicial order. To get around the legal restrictions and protests by refugee rights groups, the George H. W. Bush administration decided to move all detained Haitians to the US military base at Guantánamo, Cuba. There they were held under military guard. The government announced that it would begin evaluating asylum claims at Guantánamo without giving the Haitians a right to legal representation. Under this policy, a majority of the claimants were repatriated to Haiti.[52]

Detained Haitians at Guantánamo who passed the asylum screening were given a set of medical tests. If they tested positive for tuberculosis or HIV, they were separated into a different area of the camp and held behind barbed wire. They were barred from entry to the US due to their HIV status, and Guantánamo became a quarantine prison for three hundred Haitian refugees.

They were held in terrible conditions, with overflowing portable toilets, spoiled food, and little protection from the elements. The refugees organized and went on a hunger strike. On the mainland, ACT UP also engaged in vigorous protests against the detention of Haitians. Human rights attorneys filed a lawsuit that temporarily closed the facility, but soon Guantánamo reopened to detain still more Haitians and Cubans.[53]

Detention and Health Activism

By the time Guantánamo was targeted by protests, detention had already become an increasingly central part of the US immigration regime. The practice of detaining Haitian refugees in the 1970s and Cubans in 1980 had paved the way for the Reagan administration to expand the system of immigration detention centers. Detainees were previously held mostly in jails, prisons, and temporary facilities around the country, but in 1985 Congress authorized funds to construct a permanent immigration detention facility in Louisiana and also to begin outsourcing detention to private companies.[54]

As hundreds of thousands of Central American migrants were apprehended and placed in custody in the 1980s, conditions in detention facilities came to the attention of sanctuary groups and human rights attorneys. The El Centro detention facility near the Mexican border in Imperial County, California, which opened in 1945, had previously held almost exclusively Mexican migrants and became the target of protests by Chicano activists in the 1970s. The protests had focused especially on El Centro's "inadequate medical care," which, according to a *Los Angeles Times* exposé, consisted solely of a single first-aid kit. By the early 1980s, large numbers of Salvadoran men were being sent to this facility to await deportation (women were held in a separate facility in the town of El Centro). The detention center became extremely overcrowded, and a 1981 congressional report found filthy conditions, inadequate shelter from the blistering heat, and no medical care; a man with an apparent bullet wound was given only aspirin. El Centro was supposed to function as a temporary holding facility, but some men had been there for nearly two years.[55]

Since so many Salvadorans and Guatemalans were being sent to El Centro, the facility became a focus of the sanctuary movement. In 1982, volunteers from the National Council of Churches of Christ began visiting prisoners held there, and the American Friends Service Committee (AFSC), a Quaker activist group, set up an office nearby.[56] Sanctuary workers saw detention as another facet of the Reagan administration's mistreatment of Central American refugees. Working alongside and sometimes led by the prisoners themselves, they began to expose the injustices of the detention system, including medical neglect and abuse.

On May 27, 1985, around three hundred detained migrants at El Centro began a hunger strike. Half were Salvadorans, but there were also strikers from Asia, Europe, Canada, and the South Pacific. They demanded an end to the overcrowding, to being forced to stand outside in the heat or cold for most of the day, and to the denial of access to legal representation. The hunger strikers also focused on the medical conditions in the facility. They reported that "there is only one doctor to treat 400–500 men. Aspirin is the only medication dispensed, regardless of medical complaint, and no doctor is available on weekends."[57]

The crackdown against the hunger strike came swiftly. Fifty protesters were deported immediately, and some of the inmates' elected leaders were transferred to other facilities. After a week, border patrol agents in full riot gear entered the detention center and brutally beat some of the remaining strikers. Although their demands were not met, the protesters were released on bonds paid by sanctuary activists.[58]

Medical neglect was a problem not just at El Centro, but at detention facilities around the country. A 1990 AFSC report described overcrowding and "unacceptable conditions of detention" at centers in New Mexico, Texas, and Florida. "A common complaint was the lack of medical attention for detainees. . . . All reported poor sanitary conditions." At a detention center in South Texas, migrant women "complained of lack of hygiene, and of not being allowed to bathe and change uniforms more often than every eight to twenty days. . . . Eight women complained of a lack of medical attention." There was a waiting list of up to two weeks to see a doctor. One pregnant woman had a high fever and bleeding, and "by the time she received medical attention, she had already miscarried."[59] Another report on detention centers found, among other problems, widespread "unhygienic conditions, poor or absent medical care, [and] the inappropriate use of medication, including sedatives."[60] Medical abuse and neglect would continue to be among the chief targets of protests against the many injustices of immigrant detention.

The 1992 presidential campaign of Arkansas governor Bill Clinton gave hope to AIDS activists and opponents of immigration detention. Clinton promised to end the policy of detaining and deporting Haitians and also spoke of lifting the ban on HIV-positive immigrants and travelers. But soon after he won the election, Clinton reversed his positions. It took a judge's order, not presidential action, to release the Guantánamo detainees in 1993. However, the Clinton administration reopened Guantánamo as a processing center for refugees the following year and continued to force Haitians to return home.[61] The HIV immigration exclusion would not be repealed until 2009.

Clinton's hardline stance on Haitian detention was only the first of his many actions to appease anti-immigrant forces. His NAFTA free trade policy supported the free movement of products, but cracked down on the movement of people. In 1994 Clinton's Border Patrol initiated Operation Gatekeeper, which "hardened" the California-Mexico border and pushed migrants toward more dangerous crossings to the east. In 1995 Clinton asked Congress for $1 billion to "fight illegal immigration" and to expand his administration's "get-tough policy on the border."[62]

The electoral victory of Proposition 187 in California, as well as Republican gains in the 1994 midterm elections, pushed Clinton even further to the right on immigration. In his 1995 State of the Union address, he announced that "all Americans, not only in the States most heavily affected but in every place in this country, are rightly disturbed by the large numbers of illegal aliens entering our country. The jobs they hold might otherwise be held by citizens or legal immigrants. The public services they use impose burdens on our taxpayers."[63] Clinton's remarks indicated that federal policy would embrace Proposition 187's linkage of immigration and welfare costs. It was not only the undocumented who would suffer as a result.

"Reforming" Welfare, Punishing Immigrants

In 1996, Clinton signed into law the landmark welfare reform drafted by the Republican Congress, known as the Personal Responsibility and Work Opportunity Reconciliation Act (PRWORA). PRWORA achieved Clinton's promise to "end welfare as we know it." It "eliminated welfare as an entitlement, imposed time limits on public assistance, mandated that welfare beneficiaries work, and substantially increased state authority in administering welfare programs."[64] The legislation also placed new restrictions on legal immigrants' ability to access welfare by making new legal residents ineligible for federally funded benefits for five years.

The new restrictions on legal immigrant welfare had a dual purpose: to cut welfare budgets and to appease the perceived public appetite for anti-immigrant measures. The law's sponsors claimed that the five-year waiting period for legal immigrants would save taxpayers billions of dollars—nearly half of the $54 billion in savings promised by the total welfare reform bill. And Republican representative Rick Santorum, one of the bill's main architects, announced that "immigrants should come to America for opportunity . . . not welfare."[65]

In addition, according to historian Sarah Coleman, White House pollsters reported that the idea of restricting legal immigrants' access to welfare was popular among the independent and swing voters that Clinton coveted. Following the Republican takeover of Congress in the 1994 midterm elections,

Clinton was desperate for a victory on the welfare reform he had promised. He signed PRWORA, but tried to have his cake and eat it too by publicly criticizing the provisions targeting legal immigrants as too harsh.[66]

Some prominent Democrats were shocked that legal immigrants had been targeted in the welfare reform. San Francisco mayor Willie Brown wrote, "Tens of thousands of legal immigrants who have worked hard and paid billions of dollars in taxes, who have raised families, started businesses and created jobs would be disqualified from vital safety net services." Brown said that costs of providing health care would shift from the federal government to states and counties and "all hospitals would be responsible for providing emergency care to immigrants who lose access to cost-effective preventive care."[67]

Immigrant rights groups also condemned the new restrictions. The Latino Coalition for a Healthy California announced, "This welfare reform legislation has now become a new force in attacking immigrant communities across the U.S." The National Latina Health Organization argued that removing benefits from legal immigrants would exacerbate the poverty that was already high among this group. They pointed out that "in California, poverty rates among immigrants are higher than average, however, they utilize fewer public benefits than average. . . . Proponents of welfare reform should be concerned with how to reach out to these populations so that they may gain access to social services rather than instituting policies that will even further alienate them."[68]

The passage of another Clinton-era law, the Illegal Immigration Reform and Immigrant Responsibility Act of 1996, exacerbated legal immigrants' fears of accessing welfare. This act focused primarily on expediting deportations and further militarizing the border, but it also strengthened the ability of the US to exclude immigrants or deny them legal residency based on "public charge" criteria. The new emphasis on public charge exclusions had a chilling effect on legal immigrants' willingness to seek needed medical care.

In the aftermath of welfare reform, Lisa Sun-Hee Park, an anthropologist, conducted interviews with nearly two hundred California low-income immigrant women, welfare caseworkers, and immigrant advocates. Her informants spoke of the ways that fear of being labeled a public charge deterred dangerously sick or injured people from obtaining health care. Examples included legal immigrants who refused to call an ambulance despite having a heart attack; waited more than thirty days to go to the emergency room with severe burns (this patient ended up dying from infection); and refused surgery for uterine cancer. Many pregnant women avoided prenatal care, and "a number of patients . . . had limbs amputated due to untreated gestational diabetes." Emergency medical care was supposed to be exempt from public charge consideration, but caseworkers struggled to convince immigrant patients that they would be safe if they went to the emergency room. As researcher Lynn Fujiwara put it, hearing about the welfare reform and public charge laws left low-income immigrants "confused, panicked, and in despair. . . . The power of the anti-immigrant discourse proved lethal in itself."⁶⁹

One of the most tragic results of welfare reform was its effect on poor elderly immigrants. Many low-income immigrants had been in the US for decades but had never naturalized due to language or other barriers. The poorest of these senior citizens had been eligible for SSI (Supplemental Security Income), a federal program that provided a small amount of cash support. But in addition to the five-year welfare ban for new immigrants, PRWORA ended food stamps and SSI for all immigrants who had not become citizens.

Seventy-five-year-old Ignacio Muñoz of Stockton, California, had been a farmworker for three decades and received legal status in the IRCA amnesty. He was on SSI, disabled, and had no family. When he heard that his benefits would be cut off, Muñoz shot himself. This seems like a shocking and isolated incident, but in fact immigrant suicides due to welfare reform were reported across the country. In Miami, an elderly Cuban man died after jumping off a building. He was just one several Cubans who committed suicide after hearing they would lose their old-age benefits. Among Southeast Asian refugees, elders' fear of becoming a burden on their families was overwhelming. In Fresno, California, a Hmong man took his own life because he believed his Medicaid benefits would be terminated. An eighty-five-year-old Laotian grandfather in rural Wisconsin hanged himself after he learned of the SSI cutoff.⁷⁰

Undocumented immigrants were already ineligible for federal benefits, but the 1996 welfare reform further codified their exclusion. Section 401(a) of PRWORA prohibited "non-qualified aliens" from receiving "any Federal public benefit." The only exceptions were Emergency Medicaid, disaster relief, and public health services like immunizations or treatment of communicable diseases. States could provide their own benefits to undocumented people, but only by passing new laws.

In California, welfare reform provided an opportunity for Governor Pete Wilson to once again go after undocumented immigrants' health care. Immediately after PRWORA passed, Wilson terminated California's prenatal care program that had been open to undocumented women. Surprisingly, the same judge who had struck down Proposition 187 allowed the prenatal care program to end. In her words, PRWORA meant that "Congress has decided the states should deny health benefits to illegal aliens."⁷¹

Several counties in Texas had long provided care to undocumented people through their public hospitals. In July of 2000, state attorney general John

Cornyn announced that "public hospitals in Texas may not provide free or discounted preventive care to undocumented immigrants," basing his opinion on the 1996 welfare reform law. He warned hospitals that they stood to lose federal funds for offering the services. An organization called the Young Conservatives of Texas then stepped in and began to file complaints against counties that continued to provide care to immigrants. They persuaded the district attorney in Houston to launch a *criminal* investigation of the Harris County Hospital District. The Young Conservatives' leader Mark Levin, a third-year law student at the University of Texas, claimed that it was "an abuse of power for hospital districts . . . to continue to illegally force taxpayers to underwrite free health care for every citizen of another country who illegally crosses the border." Levin went so far as to warn that Texas was on the road to becoming "Mexico's Nursing Home."[72]

Texas medical practitioners defended the provision of nonemergency care to undocumented immigrants. Dr. Jeff Stark at Ben Taub Hospital in Houston said Cornyn's ban was a violation of the Hippocratic oath. Dr. Ron Anderson of Dallas's Parkland Health and Hospital System, which delivered more babies than any hospital in the state, called the attack on prenatal care "mindless and mean-spirited." He told a reporter that "a woman who delivers without prenatal care is six times more likely to deliver a baby who requires costly intensive care treatment upon birth." Hospital administrators pointed out that "forcing people to emergency rooms for minor illnesses like flu or chicken pox, prenatal care or serious diseases that needed early intervention is costly public policy." Hospitals in Dallas, Houston, and San Antonio announced that they would continue providing care. However, prenatal services for undocumented immigrants were discontinued in Fort Worth and in Montgomery and Nueces Counties.[73]

Thanks to the outcry from health providers and immigrant rights groups, and press coverage that was mostly critical of the health care ban, in 2003 the Texas Senate approved a bill that would allow counties and local governments to provide preventive care regardless of immigration status. This put Texas in compliance with PRWORA, which allowed states to offer nonemergency care to the undocumented only if they passed new laws. For John Cornyn, who won a US Senate seat in 2002, the negative reaction to his ruling was apparently transformative. He said that "he had 'only been doing his job'" when he issued the opinion against preventive care. Cornyn even announced that he supported federal legislation to allow preventive care for undocumented immigrants because "lack of access is neither humane nor compassionate nor cost effective."[74]

Some anti-immigrant groups continued to defend bans on preventive care.

Jack Martin of the Federation for American Immigration Reform (FAIR) said that "poor aliens, who are facing medical problems . . . should not be allowed to become a burden on the U.S. taxpayer." Preventive care for the undocumented was *not* "a public health issue," Martin continued; "We think it is an immigration law issue."[75] And in 2001 the US Court of Appeals ruled in *Lewis v. Thompson* that the federal exclusion of undocumented immigrants from prenatal care was not a violation of equal protection.[76] But the outcome of the Texas controversy seemed to indicate that, even among some anti-immigrant politicians, public health concerns could be an entering wedge to more inclusive policies. Even for conservatives like Cornyn, denying prenatal care could be a bridge too far.

Prenatal care proved to be an opening to limited rights to access in the states. Some of the harshness of PRWORA was mitigated by a new program created by Congress in 1997: the State Children's Health Insurance Program (SCHIP). SCHIP provided federal matching funds for states that sought to expand health coverage to children in families who did not qualify for Medicaid. Some states began to allow SCHIP enrollment for undocumented pregnant women through a mechanism known as the "unborn child option." Since their children would be citizens, the mothers received a temporary right to coverage by extension. By 2014, sixteen states had elected to provide coverage to undocumented pregnant women through their SCHIP programs.[77] Immigrant rights advocates pointed out the irony of unborn and newborn children being granted rights that their parents were denied.[78]

SCHIP is one of a patchwork of methods that have allowed immigrants some access to nonemergency health care despite the federal limitations. In addition to prenatal care, states could opt to use their own funds to provide medical coverage to children who were otherwise not eligible for Medicaid or SCHIP. By 2002, twenty-two states and the District of Columbia had elected to create such programs, which mostly covered legal immigrant children who were affected by the five-year PRWORA ban. Undocumented children were included only in Massachusetts, Rhode Island, and Washington, DC. While committing state funds to these programs could be expensive, those states who had them balanced that concern with the high cost of emergency care these children would otherwise incur. Also, states that filled PWRORA gaps tended to be those with more generous welfare programs already, no matter their political climate around immigration.[79]

In the rest of the states, Emergency Medicaid was the only type of coverage available to undocumented immigrants and to legal immigrants under the five-year ban. PRWORA did not ban any immigrants from two federal nutrition programs, school lunches and the WIC (Women, Infants, and Chil-

dren) program, and all immigrants continued to be eligible for care in federally funded clinics, but clinics were far-flung and had long waiting lists. In
California, which had 30 percent of the country's immigrant population, six
counties had no federally qualified health center at all.[80]

Despite a few avenues for access, welfare reform continued to have a negative effect on immigrants' ability and willingness to seek health services. Even
though Medicaid was exempted from public charge definitions in 1999, legal
immigrants continued to fear that use of Medicaid and other health services
would leave them vulnerable to deportation. A study conducted in Texas
found that up to 30 percent of legal immigrants had "voluntarily withdrawn"
from Medicaid in the two years after the passage of PRWORA. Both legal and
undocumented immigrants avoided nonrestricted services like free clinics
and WIC programs because they saw any government program as potentially
dangerous. Local health practitioners and immunization clinics reported a
drop in services to immigrants following highly publicized Border Patrol and
INS raids in Houston, Fort Worth, and El Paso.[81] The two Clinton-era policies of increased border enforcement and harsh welfare restrictions worked
together to damage access to health care for immigrants and their families.

A Right to Health Coverage: New Labor Activism

As Clinton and Congress tore the safety nets away from immigrants and
refugees, activist groups began to focus more of their demands on migrants'
access to health care. The immigrant rights movement also became more involved in health politics due to the increased nationwide attention to the topic
during and after Clinton's attempt to overhaul the nation's health care system
in 1993–94. For the first time, Latino rights groups had been invited to participate in discussions of national health reform. Although the reform effort
failed, activists emerged with a clearer idea of how the lack of universal health
insurance hurt immigrants and communities of color. Because it proposed to
exclude the undocumented, the Clinton health reform attempt led to explicit
defenses of undocumented people's right to basic health care from groups like
the American Nurses' Association, the American Public Health Association,
and the American Civil Liberties Union.[82]

Also in the 1990s, more labor unions began to openly organize undocumented workers. The battles of the "new labor movement" reflected how the
US had transformed from a manufacturing to a service economy. If the labor movement was to have a future, it required organizing industries like
hotels and restaurants, health care, and cleaning services. And "new" labor

organizing focused not just on wages but also on benefits, including health coverage.

Many workers who formed the backbone of the new economy were undocumented immigrants. By the mid-1980s, only 25 percent of undocumented workers were farm laborers.[83] Millions of others worked in construction, hotels, restaurants, and factories; cleaned homes, hospitals, and offices; and cared for children and the elderly. These were mostly low-wage jobs, often paid under the table, leaving workers without benefits or access to social security.

The decline of US manufacturing in the 1980s led to the loss of many unionized jobs. As the service sector expanded, employers fought to reduce the influence of labor unions in service industries too. For example, large office buildings began outsourcing their janitorial work to subcontractors. In California, office building janitors had previously had strong unions, and the switch to subcontracting not only destroyed unions, but also greatly eroded working conditions. In Silicon Valley, unionized janitors had been paid ten dollars an hour, plus benefits, including health insurance. Janitors hired from subcontractors "were paid an average of $5.50 an hour and received no health insurance or other benefits."[84]

Unionized jobs had been held by Black and white citizen workers, but the subcontracted workforce was overwhelmingly immigrant, many of them undocumented. US labor unions believed that immigrants, especially the undocumented, were difficult if not impossible to organize, but they were proven wrong. The "Justice for Janitors" organizing campaign of the Service Employees International Union (SEIU) began to win major victories thanks to the enthusiastic participation of undocumented immigrant workers, mostly from Mexico and Central America.

SEIU had a long history of organizing janitors, hospital workers, and other service workers. It created Justice for Janitors in 1988 to revitalize unionization in an industry where it was under threat. When the campaign launched in Los Angeles, they engaged in highly visible tactics, including large protests in front of buildings that used nonunionized janitors. At a typical Justice for Janitors event, the mostly Latino immigrant workers chanted slogans in Spanish, including "Con unión, hay protección" (With a union, there is protection).[85]

In 1990, Los Angeles janitors won a union contract with one of the largest cleaning contractors in the city. According to scholar Ruth Milkman, "This was the triumphal conclusion of a two-year organizing drive that brought SEIU's janitorial membership in the city to 8,000, up from 1,800 five years earlier—the largest private-sector union victory involving Latino immigrants since the UFW campaigns of the early 1970s." Organizers realized that it did not take much convincing for immigrant workers to participate in organizing drives. This was due to several factors, including workers' familiarity with unions and political work in their home countries, their strong social and family networks, and their lived experiences of injustice. In addition, many workers refused see their deportability as an obstacle to workplace activism.[86] Immigrant workers also strongly valued benefits to protect their families, especially health insurance.

In the United States, the only affluent nation without universal coverage, health insurance is closely tied to employment. But from its peak in the 1970s, job-based health insurance had plummeted. By 1991, nearly 35 percent of Americans were uninsured, the highest number since before the passage of Medicare and Medicaid.[87] For undocumented immigrant workers, with public insurance foreclosed and private care unaffordable, unionization was a crucial path to health security.

Justice for Janitors continued to rack up victories in Los Angeles, so that by 1991, 90 percent of downtown office buildings were being "cleaned by unionized workers." SEIU's settlement with the giant contractor Bradford Building Services included health coverage not just for the newly unionized workers, but also for their families. Dependent health insurance was extremely important to immigrant workers who had come to the US and worked long hours to provide a better life to their children. Cleaning worker Sonia Garcia, for example, got involved in the union because "as a single mother, [she] became interested in how janitors could win family health insurance." Garcia eventually became the union representative for her workplace and encouraged other family members to work for the union.[88]

Undocumented organizing also blossomed in the garment industry, which in Los Angeles relied almost entirely on immigrant workers. The majority of Los Angeles's 150,000 Latino and Asian garment workers were women, and many were mothers. Garment labor was heavily subcontracted and highly exploitative, with many workers paid less than minimum wage. In addition, "Medical insurance is virtually non-existent for the worker herself, and out of question for her family." The wealthy manufacturer instead "forces his workers to rely on the impoverished L.A. County health system."[89] In one nationally publicized incident in 1995, when investigators raided several garment workshops in El Monte, a city in Los Angeles County, they found migrants from Thailand in conditions that resembled not just sweatshops, but involuntary servitude.[90]

The garment industry was targeted for unionization by UNITE, which had formed out of the merger of the International Ladies' Garment Workers' Union and the Amalgamated Clothing and Textile Workers' Union. Their campaign had some minor successes, but faced even more daunting obstacles than the janitors, especially when major garment manufacturers began moving their operations to Mexico. When health insurance via unionization was elusive, immigrant workers turned to other forms of organizing and provision for health care access. For example, the Oakland, California, organization Asian Immigrant Women Advocates (AIWA), which provided health and safety trainings to women in the Silicon Valley electronics industry, started a health clinic for garment workers that was reminiscent of the ILGWU's clinic in New York City. The clinic, along with AIWA's innovative Peer Health Promoter Network, involved immigrant women in reporting and organizing around safety violations and pervasive health problems, such as repetitive stress injuries, in the garment industry.[91]

Throughout the 1990s, union organizing and worker activism also spread in the highly immigrant-dominated restaurant, hotel, and home health care sectors. An indication of the movement's impact came in 1996 when Miguel Contreras was elected president of the powerful Los Angeles Federation of Labor. Contreras had started working in the grape fields with his migrant worker parents at age five. He joined the UFW at seventeen and became a lead organizer. In the 1980s he organized service workers in the Hotel and Restaurant Employees Union. Contreras was the first person of color to head the labor federation, and his ascension signaled the newly central role of Latino, immigrant, and service workers in the labor movement. And in 2000, the AFL-CIO, the nation's largest labor federation, announced its support for amnesty for undocumented workers and for ending employer sanctions.[92]

Deaths of the Invisible

In New York City, on September 7, 2001, Sekou Siby played a game of soccer with his friends from work. Siby was from Ivory Coast, and his fellow players were immigrants from several countries in Latin America. As the game ended, his friend Moises Rivas asked Siby to trade shifts that coming Tuesday. On September 11, Rivas went to work at the Windows on the World restaurant, at the top of the World Trade Center. Everyone who played soccer that day except Siby and one other friend perished when the Twin Towers fell.[93]

Seventy-three workers at the Windows on the World restaurant died in the terrorist attacks on September 11, 2001. Many of them were undocumented immigrants. In the aftermath of the attacks, which killed 2,750 people in New York, it became obvious how much the city's economy depended on undocumented workers. They labored primarily as "cooks, dishwashers, waiters, delivery persons, maids, and child care workers." In addition to the immi-grants who died on that day, whose number will never be known, hundreds who survived lost their livelihoods because their workplaces were destroyed.[94]

Immigrant rights organizations worked around the clock to help families and survivors apply for aid. The INS promised not to arrest undocumented victims of 9/11, but many survivors could not provide the work documenta-tion required to receive financial help. Families of the dead also lacked the paperwork needed to receive compensation payments for the loss of their loved ones, who may have been the primary support of their relatives either in the US or their home country.[95] Their problem "reflected a common situation for undocumented immigrants who are paid 'under the table': the inability to provide what seems like simple proof of their existence."[96]

Some of the undocumented workers lost that day did have official recog-nition of their existence: they were members of the Hotel and Restaurant Em-ployees Union at the Windows on the World restaurant. Union membership automatically qualified survivors or family members for disaster assistance. Unions also provided grief counseling and temporary continuation of health insurance.

The loss of health insurance proved to be a serious consequence of 9/11. Union insurance was temporary, and many restaurant workers who died out-side of the Twin Towers were not unionized. New York City chefs and restau-rant owners formed an aid organization, Windows of Hope, to raise money for restaurant workers and survivors affected by the disaster. After hearing from family members that "in addition to financial assistance, they needed health insurance . . . [and that] the large number of dependent children of those lost on 9/11 made lack of insurance a real worry for surviving parents," Windows of Hope pledged to pay for health insurance for victims' family members for five years.[97]

While some were able to provide sufficient paperwork for government compensation, most undocumented victims and family members had to rely on charity, return to their home countries, or scrape by without assistance. Despite the outpouring of generosity and concern following 9/11, New York State did not allow undocumented people to access the temporary Disaster Relief Medicaid program. And many remained as invisible in death as they had been in life. The immigrant rights organization Tepeyac, which worked closely with undocumented survivors and families, concluded that "an ex-tensive search of the number and identities of undocumented workers who were lost in the World Trade Center and its vicinity . . . was never carried out or even seriously attempted." This also meant that many US-born children of those killed never received compensation for the loss of a parent.[98]

Retaliation for the 9/11 attacks led to decades of war in the Middle East and the creation of new generations of refugees. For many refugees, migrants, and immigrants, safety and health in the US continued to be elusive. From experiencing violence in their homelands, they might go on to suffer physical attacks by border officials, abuse, medical neglect, and exposure to disease in detention, the denial or withdrawal of access to health care, and danger and even death in their workplaces. In the face of this violence against health, and the relentless reinforcement of their invisibility, immigrant communities would continue to fight, refusing to give up on their American dreams of health, safety, and well-being.

Undocumented, Uninsured, Unafraid

In 2003, a terrible medical accident occurred at Duke University Medical Center in Durham, North Carolina. A seventeen-year-old girl who had been waiting three years for a heart-lung transplant was accidentally given organs of the wrong blood type, and her body rejected them. Almost immediately, Duke located another set of organs and transplanted them into the patient to try and rectify its mistake. But the young woman, whose name was Jesica Santillan, died shortly after her second operation.

Members of the local community, who had supported Jesica and her mother since they arrived from Mexico three years earlier, reacted with grief and horror. Jesica had been diagnosed with a fatal condition at age twelve, and only a tricky and rare heart-lung transplant could save her. No such procedure was available in Mexico, so her mother Magdalena hired a *coyote* to help her and Jesica cross the border. They had heard that Duke Medical Center was the best place in the world for the type of transplant Jesica needed, so they headed to North Carolina. After they arrived, Duke placed the sick girl on the transplant waiting list. Local residents who heard of the Santillans' plight arranged for her mother to get a job and ran a successful campaign to raise the $500,000 Duke required for the transplant. No one anticipated that the procedure meant to save the young woman's life would end up killing her.

But the media soon turned away from the tragedy of the shocking medical mistake to focus on another aspect of the case: Jesica and her mother were undocumented Mexican migrants. How was it possible that an "illegal alien" had received not just one, but two sets of organs, when many US citizens remained on transplant waiting lists? The press revealed that the United Network for Organ Sharing (UNOS), the organization governing US transplant protocols, allowed up to 5 percent of available organs to go to foreign nationals. UNOS pointed out that in practice, probably less than 1 percent of organs went to undocumented immigrants, since payment for the prohibitively expensive procedures was still required. Jesica's case was very unusual because of the community funds raised for her; in addition, Duke accepted Jesica for the transplant because her mother had health insurance through her job at a local college.[1]

Even as Jesica Santillan briefly clung to life, her story led to a backlash of invective against immigrants that focused on the issue of health care utilization. Debates over immigrant health burdens on the taxpayer took a new turn, as undocumented people were now accused of literally stealing lifesaving treatments from US citizens. A Raleigh woman said she would take herself off the organ donor list so that her organs would not go to "illegals." In a letter to the editor, a New York man asked, "Why were Jesica Santillan and her mother, illegal aliens from Mexico, even at Duke University and not in an INS holding cell?" An anti-immigrant blogger posted, "if Jesica recovers from the second heart-lung transplant, will any federal immigration authority have the guts to enforce the law and send her and her family back to Mexico?"[2] (These last two comments, typical of many, were an indication of how militarized enforcement, detention, and deportation had come to be seen as normal and expected functions of the US immigration system.)

Very few undocumented immigrants received organ transplants, as UNOS pointed out. Emergency Medicaid did not cover transplants or aftercare. Sometimes immigrants who could not get a hospital to provide a transplant went back to their home countries to die. When migrants did get transplants, it might only be after community protests against their exclusion. In Chicago in 2001, Children's Memorial Hospital denied a liver transplant to eleven-year-old Ana Esparza, but an outcry from community members led to her being transferred to a Florida hospital that agreed to do the procedure. The following year, Cleveland Clinic turned down a Guatemalan undocumented woman who also needed a liver transplant. When local political leaders and Latino community groups intervened on her behalf, the clinic agreed to put her on the waiting list. She died before she could receive the operation.[3] Journalists also reported that not only did undocumented people rarely get transplants; they donated about twice as many organs as they received, and Latinos in North Carolina pledged to donate their organs after death more often than non-Latinos did.[4]

The anger over Duke's decision to provide organ transplants to Jesica Santillan reflected anxiety over two seemingly intractable problems in the US: undocumented immigration and the inaccessibility and expense of health care. Immigrant health care utilization lay at the intersection of both.

Some hospitals faced severe financial problems due to the number of un-insured people coming to their doors. Because of the emergency room access stipulated by EMTALA, it was illegal to turn them away. Hospitals that pro-vided a significant amount of unreimbursed care to uninsured people were es-pecially subject to escalating costs, and some closed down. It was time, again, to blame immigrants. The same blogger who wanted the Santillan family sent "back to Mexico" wrote that "the costs of illegal alien health care are crippling hospitals across the country" and "dozens of hospitals" along the US-Mexico border "have either closed their doors or face bankruptcy because of losses caused by uncompensated care given to illegal immigrants."[5] Hospitals' losses and closures were due to many factors, one of the most important being re-ductions in federal payments to hospitals.[6] As they had done since the 1970s, hospital leaders looked to undocumented immigrant utilization as a way to argue for increased federal funding.

Hospital Reimbursement Redux: A Disproportionate Share of the Blame

In 2000, the Arizona College of Emergency Physicians reported that the state's "emergency healthcare system is in imminent danger of collapse" and "cur-rent resources supporting emergency care are inadequate to meet the needs of all patients at all times." They cited several hospital closures, high levels of uninsurance in Arizona (28 percent), and the use of emergency rooms by immigrants as contributing to the crisis. Among the solutions the emergency physicians proposed was "separate Federal funding for immigrant and illegal alien healthcare."[7]

Arizona was already notable for its fiercely localistic and conservative health politics—the state hadn't even adopted a Medicaid program until 1983, nearly two decades after it became eligible, resisting the program for primar-ily ideological reasons—and a combative approach to immigration.[8] Starting in the late 1990s, Arizona became even more of a hotspot for anti-immigrant politics as a new border wall in California pushed thousands more migrants to cross from Mexico to the US via the harsh Arizona desert. Medical provid-ers argued that they unfairly bore the brunt of the surge in undocumented pa-tients, due to both lax federal immigration enforcement and the burdensome federal mandate of EMTALA. The Arizona Hospital Association agreed with the College of Emergency Physicians that "increasing numbers of undocu-mented aliens are presenting in Arizona hospital emergency departments."[9]

In seeking greater federal responsibility for immigrants' emergency care, Arizona hospitals argued for a redistribution of existing funds known as Dis-proportionate Share Hospital payments (DSH). DSH funds had been added to the Medicaid and Medicare programs incrementally by Congress (in 1981 and 1985, respectively) to provide additional payments to hospitals, particularly in urban areas, that served a "disproportionate" share of poor and uninsured patients. DSH resources were not initially intended to support services to the undocumented, but hospital officials in Arizona and other border states increasingly asked that the payments be redirected to hospitals treating large numbers of immigrants in their emergency rooms.[10]

Although Arizona hospitals were already receiving millions in DSH funds (they got $81 million from just the Medicaid portion of DSH in 2000),[11] hospital lobbyists continued to press for more federal support specifically for the treatment of undocumented patients. They found a sympathetic ear in Arizona senator Jon Kyl, a conservative Republican who twice introduced legislation for additional emergency care funding for Arizona and other states with large immigrant populations. He succeeded on the third attempt, in 2003, when President George W. Bush signed the Medicare Prescription Drug, Improvement, and Modernization Act (Medicare Part D).

Into this law, Bush's signal domestic legislation and the only change to Medicare's coverage provisions in its history, Congress quietly tucked Kyl's Section 1011, authorizing $250 million a year in hospital reimbursements to states based on their proportion of the estimated undocumented population. A slightly higher proportion of the funds would go to six states with the largest number of immigrants apprehended by the INS. This ballpark formula based on apprehensions was yet another indication that there were no statistics measuring the actual extent of hospital utilization by the undocumented. It so happened that the state with the highest number of apprehensions, and thus the greatest allocation of funding, was Kyl's home state of Arizona. This was a particularly glaring example of an immigration policy (aggressive border enforcement) underpinning a health care policy (the allocation of federal hospital dollars to states engaging in aggressive enforcement).[12]

Not all border state politicians jumped on the federal funding bandwagon. Some saw the funding as unfairly supporting undocumented immigration. Representative Dana Rohrabacher of Orange County, California, who like Kyl was a conservative Republican, called the appropriations for undocumented emergency care "a travesty." "At this time when we cannot afford the money to pay for prescription drugs for our seniors," he told Congress, "we are going to be spending $1 billion to treat people who have come here illegally." Rohrabacher added, "We all remember Jesica Santillan. She was an illegal alien who died after receiving not one, but two, heart and lung transplants in North Carolina. . . . There are American citizens who desperately need organs, and they are being knocked out of line by a family who broke the law to come here."[13] Rohrabacher proposed an amendment that would require hospitals to report undocumented patients to immigration authorities.

His proposal was immediately attacked by congressional Democrats, whose response reflected liberals' shift toward a politics more sympathetic to immigrants. Representative Linda Sánchez of California announced that "using our health care system as a subagency of the Immigration Service is a ludicrous idea." Texas's Sheila Jackson-Lee quoted the American Medical Association: "by requiring physicians to report patients and perhaps withhold necessary care, this bill would in effect require physicians to violate their Hippocratic Oath."[14] Rohrabacher's proposal was defeated. For the next four years, hospitals in the states selected for Section 1011 quietly received $250 million annually to offset emergency treatment of undocumented immigrants.[15]

This episode perfectly captured policymakers' opportunistic manipulation of the immigration/health policy nexus. Arizona's Kyl won funding for cash-strapped hospitals in his state by invoking the federal government's failure to slow the influx of undocumented people. Rohrabacher then tried to enlist hospitals as agents in federal efforts to catch and deport undocumented immigrants. Although he did not invent the idea of medical facilities playing this role, Rohrabacher's proposal went further in attempting to attach an immigration reporting requirement to federal health care funding. In doing so, he was clearly inspired by his own state's Proposition 187, which had tried to do the same a decade earlier for state- and locally funded medical services.

In 2004, the federal Government Accountability Office (GAO) attempted to study the actual costs to hospitals of undocumented immigrants. Its report concluded that, due to the lack of accurate statistics or reporting, the "GAO could not determine the effect of undocumented aliens on hospitals' uncompensated care costs."[16]

But among academic researchers, a consensus was emerging that contradicted the persistent notion that undocumented patients were a burden on hospitals and health care. Over several decades, investigators had looked for evidence to understand immigrants' relationship to the health system, and to evaluate whether migrants paid more in taxes than they utilized in medical services. One of the earliest of these studies, "Health Care for California's Undocumented Mexican Immigrants," was published around 1980 by a researcher at the University of California, San Diego. It admitted to a paucity of data but concluded that "some evidence to date suggests that unrecovered funds for medical service is outweighed significantly by immigrant tax contributions." Texas researchers came to a similar conclusion in 1984: "Undocumented aliens in Texas contribute more revenue to the state than the cost to the state to provide them with public services." As advocates continually pointed out, undocumented people did not generally seek free health care; the nonemergency care they did receive was not free, and in the Texas study, most found a way to pay their bills, usually in installment payments. However, a few catastrophic high-cost cases in which undocumented patients could not pay were publicized in the newspapers, contributing to the idea that they posed a medical cost burden.[17]

Starting in the 1980s, the anthropologist Leo R. Chavez published a series of landmark studies on migrants' use of health care. In a 1982 article, Chavez described hospitals' and governments' attempts to shift responsibility for services to the undocumented as "a game of pass the buck." His 1992 book, *Shadowed Lives*, which was based on his years of fieldwork with undocumented migrant communities in Southern California, included examples of migrant workers who were reluctant to seek health care, even for life-threatening illnesses and injuries, due to both their fear of detection and lack of insurance or money. Many workers, Chavez writes, "either take their health problems back to Mexico or simply suffer with them."[18] In another study, Chavez and coauthors concluded from interviews with Mexican and Central American migrants in Texas and California that, while emergency rooms were "an important source of care" for those without health insurance, there was "little evidence that hospital services, including emergency rooms, were overutilized by undocumented interviewees."[19]

Over the next twenty years, health services researchers continued to find that undocumented people minimized their use of medical care. In 2012, the Commonwealth Fund, a nonpartisan health care think tank, completed a report that summarized dozens of studies that had been made of undocumented health care utilization in the past two decades, along with new research. It concluded that "this population uses fewer health services of all types, including emergency services, when compared to U.S.-born and legally-residing immigrant groups . . . we estimate that unauthorized immigrants are significantly less likely than naturalized citizens and U.S.-born citizens to visit the emergency department."[20] Another study found that "non-citizens were less likely to use ED [emergency department] services (8.7%) compared to naturalized immigrants (10.6%) and U.S.-born Americans (14.7%)." In addition, there was no correlation between the number of undocumented immigrants in a state and the amount of uncompensated care provided by hospitals.[21] Too many uninsured people were using emergency rooms for basic health care, but they were primarily US citizens, not migrants.

By identifying immigrants as the cause of high costs, hospital lobbyists and state and federal politicians sought a scapegoat for the US health care crisis while continuing to avoid addressing the system's fundamental dysfunc-tions. They also obscured the reality, evidenced by multiple research studies and by lived experience, that undocumented immigrants' encounters with US health care were characterized not by overutilization, but by exclusion, fear, and even punishment.

When Hospitals Deport

On August 3, 2008, the front page of the *New York Times* featured a story titled "Deported, by U.S. Hospitals." Reporter Deborah Sontag wrote about the case of Luis Alberto Jiménez, a young Guatemalan immigrant, who was working as a gardener in Florida in 2000 when he became the victim of a horrific accident with a drunk driver. His injuries were devastating; he was severely brain damaged and unable to care for himself. The hospital that treated him, Martin Memorial, looked in vain for a rehabilitation center that would take Jiménez. Finally, after several years and $1.5 million in costs, Martin Memo-rial Hospital "leased an air ambulance for $30,000 and 'forcibly returned him to his home country'"—to a tiny town in the mountains where no medical care was available.[22]

Sontag reported that the practice of hospital deportation, which she also described as "international patient dumping," occurred frequently all over the country. Sometimes patients requested to be transferred home, but many of these deportations were involuntary. The article listed dozens of examples, including one hospital in Phoenix that deported ninety-six patients in a single year and another that tried to deport a citizen baby of immigrant parents. Ac-cording to Sister Margaret McBride, an administrator at the Phoenix hospital, "We don't require consent from the family" to remove patients to another country. Legal as well as undocumented immigrants were subject to hospital deportation. And since the deportations were conducted by private entities, not the government, patients were not provided with due process.[23]

Emergency Medicaid, the only form of reimbursement available for the care of uninsured undocumented immigrants or indigent legal immigrants in their first five years in the country, does not cover the costs of long-term care. DSH funds, at least according to hospitals, were insufficient to keep indi-gent patients for long periods of time. Sontag reported on a private company, MexCare, that was founded in 2001 solely to provide deportation transport for hospital patients. MexCare advertised itself as "an alternative choice for the care of unfunded Latin nationals" that promised "significant saving to U.S. hospitals."[24]

In 2012, researchers from Seton Hall Law School and New York Lawyers for the Public Interest released a report concluding that medical deportation was "widespread but barely publicized." They found over six hundred cases in the US over a five-year period.[25] Hospitals viewed medical deportation as a cost control measure. "The federal government, the states, everybody says they're not paying for the undocumented," said the CEO of the Iowa Health System, one of whose hospitals had deported two comatose Mexican men by private jet.[26] Medical deportation is an immigration procedure that serves the health care policy goal of cost savings.

Medical deportations were nothing new. They had been happening since the mid-nineteenth century, and especially during the 1930s, when hospitals turned over patients to the immigration authorities for becoming public charges. But earlier hospital deportations had been primarily measures of immigration enforcement, rather than of cost control for individual hospitals. They took place not primarily with the justification of saving money, but because in the era before EMTALA, undocumented status sufficed as a reason for expelling a patient, even with a severe emergency condition. For example, in the late 1970s, a public hospital in Texas "transferred two illegal aliens back to Mexico and both died two days later at a hospital in Nuevo Laredo."[27] In 1978 University Hospital in San Diego refused to accept the transfer of a severely burned patient because she was undocumented. The hospital that attempted the transfer put her in an ambulance and sent her across the border to a hospital in Tijuana.[28]

Attempts to stop medical deportations were rare, because hospitals often conducted these activities in secrecy. Occasionally, families might sue the hospital, or local governments, activists, or foreign consuls might protest. In the San Diego case of the burned woman, the California State Department of Health Services reported the transferring hospital for violating the state's emergency (pre-EMTALA) treatment law, leading to an investigation by a grand jury. In Phoenix in 2008, a Honduran woman went into a coma during childbirth. She was in the country legally with Temporary Protected Status, but the hospital tried to have her shipped back to Honduras. Her family hired a lawyer, and the attempted deportation was stopped when she came out of the coma.[29]

In August of 2010, Quelino Ojeda Jiménez, an undocumented migrant from Mexico, was working on the roof of a building in Chicago when he slipped and fell to the ground twenty feet below. The fall was so severe that it left him paralyzed and on a ventilator at Advocate Christ Hospital. There he remained for nearly four months. But right before Christmas, "hospital staff disconnected him from equipment and rolled him away on a gurney as one of his caregivers pleaded for them to stop." Ojeda was then "loaded onto an air ambulance and flown to Oaxaca, capital of the Mexican state where he was born."[30]

Before his deportation, as Ojeda lay in the hospital, members of the local Mexican community had rallied around him and created an informal support network for the injured man, who was otherwise alone in Chicago. One of these caregivers was by his side and tried to stop the medical deportation as Ojeda was strapped into the gurney and wheeled away. It was due to the existence of this network that Ojeda's case was publicized and appeared on the front page of the *Chicago Tribune*. Community members rallied further support from civil rights and disability rights groups and from the Mexican Consulate in Chicago, but the attention only came after Ojeda's removal had already taken place. A little over a year later, Ojeda died at the General Hospital of Juchitán in Mexico of pneumonia and sepsis. He was twenty-one years old.[31]

Hospitals also engage in encouraging undocumented patients to accept voluntary repatriation, at great risk to their health. In 2009, Grady Hospital, a large public hospital in Atlanta, Georgia, shut down its free dialysis clinic as part of a budget-cutting effort. The clinic served many indigent people with end-stage kidney disease, and its patients included dozens of undocumented immigrants. Even though the clinic had been a lifeline for people who would otherwise die without treatment, dialysis was not considered an emergency measure covered by EMTALA, so it was provided at the discretion of the hospital. Most of Grady's citizen patients were covered by Medicare and easily found treatment at other dialysis centers in town. But for its undocumented immigrant patients, Grady offered something different: three months of treatment at a private clinic, and then airfare to their home countries.[32]

Faced with a stark choice between a slow death in the US without dialysis and a return to homes of origin with inadequate medical care, the immigrant kidney patients, mostly from Mexico and Central America, decided to find a lawyer. Their attorney, Lindsay R. Jones, filed a class-action suit against Grady Memorial Hospital, but it was dismissed. The judge was "unpersuaded . . . that patients have a constitutional right to the sought-after relief."[33]

It was true that in the United States, no one could claim a constitutional right to dialysis. But, instead of giving up, Jones decided to try a new strategy: defining the denial of lifesaving care as a violation of international human rights. He reported the case of the Grady patients to the Inter-American Commission, the human rights arm of the Organization of American States (a Western Hemisphere alliance akin to a regional version of the United Nations).

The Inter-American Commission normally focused on exposing human rights abuses in Latin American countries. It did issue "Precautionary Measures"—requests for urgent state action on human rights violations—

aimed at the US, but these were primarily for cases of prisoners on death row.[34] The organization had never before gotten involved in US health care rights, but in 2010, the Inter-American Commission announced a precautionary measure on behalf of "31 Undocumented Immigrants Residing in Atlanta, Georgia, United States whose dialysis treatments at Grady Memorial Hospital were scheduled to be terminated on February 3, 2010." The US government needed to take urgent action, according to the commission, not only because "the lives and the health of the 31 persons are at grave risk," but also because the hospital's decision had a "disproportionate impact" on immigrants who were ineligible for other forms of care due to their undocumented status. The commission's statement also implied that, by only offering repatriation and not long-term treatment, the hospital was coercing patients to leave the country.[35]

The Inter-American Commission has no concrete power in the United States, and the Grady patients' lawyers were under no illusions that it did. Attorney Jones explained that "we want to make this an international human rights issue," and that even though the commission might not have the power of enforcement, they had a "political stick."[36] And this strategy worked. The publicity it generated forced Grady Memorial to find alternate dialysis care for nearly forty undocumented patients.[37] In this case at least, US espousal of international human rights was put to the test by shining a spotlight on the abuse and neglect of immigrants by the American health care system.

But some of the patients had taken the self-deportation deal. Grady officials had argued that "a Mexican citizen has a much better chance of finding long-term government assistance from the Mexican government than they do in Georgia." MexCare, the transportation company that repatriated them, offered to cover one year of Mexican health insurance for the patients, but failed to disclose that the insurance program did not cover dialysis. A later study found that "of the ten to thirteen patients who relocated, many faced difficulty obtaining dialysis after the transition period and two died."[38]

Despite the Grady patients' partial victory, and continuing reports showing that both voluntary and involuntary medical deportations are widespread and can result in death, no attempt has been made to regulate these practices or to develop a formal reporting mechanism for medical repatriation. Unless family or local activists get involved, hospital deportations take place privately, without the participation of local or federal government. Air ambulance services like MexCare for repatriating (voluntarily) and deporting (involuntarily) patients have become a booming business.[39]

A 2021 report on medical deportation emphasized that, even though the practice is not conducted by US immigration authorities, "hospitals are able to rely on the government's role in terrorizing immigrant communities with the threat of deportation to swiftly conduct involuntary transportations or coerce patients into consenting to their transportation." Like undocumented immigrants' underutilization of medical services, dangerous medical deportations and repatriations are yet another health consequence of the fear of immigration enforcement.[40]

The Health Effects of Immigration Status and Immigration Enforcement

Some researchers have offered one possible explanation for immigrants' low utilization of health care: they may simply be healthier as a group.[41] But there is also ample evidence that the experience of migration, of living in the US as an undocumented immigrant, and exposure to immigrant enforcement all have measurable, negative effects on health. Being an immigrant can exacerbate the need for health care, making it even more injurious when care is not accessible or is denied.

For undocumented people, the act of migration itself is dangerous to their health and even their lives. Having to cross the border clandestinely exposes migrants to violence, drowning, accidents, dehydration, and deadly heat. After they arrive, undocumented people face exclusion from welfare programs and from nonemergency medical care. They often work in hazardous, low-wage occupations without health insurance benefits. In her 2000 study of immigrant families in Houston and San Diego, researcher Shawn Malia Kanaiaupuni found that "legal status is key to health status." Even citizen children, if one or both parents were undocumented, were at higher risk of poor health outcomes than children of legal immigrants.[42]

In addition, undocumented status affects health due to the stress of living in a country with a harsh regime of immigration enforcement. The fear of deportation, Leo R. Chavez writes, "can be just as devastating as deportation itself, leading to self-monitoring behavior such as avoiding medical appointments, not seeking help from police, or staying at home and avoiding 'dangerous' public spaces, even going to the grocery store."[43] A 2019 international meta-analysis found that the more severe the restriction policy a country has, the worse the health outcomes for migrants.[44]

Immigration enforcement has negative effects on both mental and physical health. Children who constantly think about the possibility of their parents' deportation experience "clinical levels of separation anxiety." In interviews conducted by researcher Luis H. Zayas, children of undocumented parents talked of recurrent nightmares of chase, capture, and families torn apart. They suffered persistent feelings of fear, guilt, and shame, all of which can lead to depression and other psychological disorders.[45]

Immigration enforcement in the US became even harsher after 2001. The "hardening" of the border had begun in the 1980s and intensified in the 1990s, and then policy changes in response to the 9/11 attacks implemented militarized immigration policing throughout the US. In 2002, the INS was absorbed into the Department of Homeland Security, and federal immigration functions divided between Customs and Border Protection, Citizenship and Immigration Services, and Immigration and Customs Enforcement (ICE). As public health scholar William Lopez writes, "following the events of 9/11, federal immigration law transformed from a means of labor control to a tool of maintaining national security and managing terrorism," and "the focus of immigration enforcement . . . shifted from the border to the interior of the United States."[46]

Lopez's powerful account of the aftermath of a 2013 immigration raid in rural Michigan shows how enforcement in the interior had far-reaching health effects. After raiding a workshop where many undocumented men worked, ICE and a local SWAT team conducted a "no-knock" raid on an apartment housing mothers, teenagers, and small children. Armed and armored agents broke down the door, stormed in, and forced everyone, including the children, to the floor at gunpoint. All the men at the workshop, as well as an eighteen-year-old at the apartment, were arrested and deported. Their family members were left behind to pick up the pieces. The women and children who underwent the apartment raid suffered shock, post-traumatic stress syndrome, and thoughts of suicide. The emotional trauma had physical effects: after experiencing the raid, a young mother with a three-month-old baby was no longer able to nurse her child. She explained that her milk "didn't work anymore." As Lopez writes, the physical trauma of the raid "increased the reach of ICE . . . into the women's futures" and those of their children.[47] Other scholars have found a correlation between immigration raids in a community and the negative health outcome of lower infant birth weights.[48]

Witness and Protest against the Health Violence of Immigration Enforcement

The harmful health effects of immigrant policing had been recognized by civil and human rights groups for decades. In the 1970s, some rights organizations began to document and protest abuses against migrants by the US Border Patrol and other immigration agencies. Many of the rights violations involved the denial of medical care.

In 1979, San Diego's Committee on Chicano Rights, along with the United California Mexican-American Association and the Legal Aid Society of San

Diego, filed a petition with the US Department of Justice alleging "violations of human, civil, and constitutional rights perpetrated by the Immigration and Naturalization Service, U.S. Border Patrol and U.S. Customs Service against persons of Mexican and Latin ancestry." In addition to numerous examples of Border Patrol violence and harassment, the petition detailed the case of a sick baby, a US citizen, who died after being refused entry at the border. The baby's mother was an undocumented Salvadoran who had taken a bus for three days to get her child to San Diego for treatment. She got some citizen friends to drive to Tijuana and pick up the baby. When they tried to cross back into the US, a woman border patrol officer exclaimed that the child was "dehydrated and starving!" but refused to accept their documentation, saying, "We can't let sympathy get to our jobs" and "I'm sorry but we cannot let the baby go through." One of the women ran back into Tijuana and flagged down a policeman who took her and the baby to Tijuana General Hospital, where he died.[49]

The San Diego activists' "Petition for Congressional Investigation" also reported the case of a four-year-old Mexican child who had received heart surgery at a San Diego hospital. When his aunt tried to bring him back for follow-up treatment, showing officials a letter from the child's doctor, they were denied entry, and placed in an INS waiting room. "The child died during the wait in the waiting room while INS personnel ignored the aunt's pleas for help." In these cases, the petition accused the Border Patrol of rights violations including "Arbitrary Refusal to allow a U.S. citizen to pass [when in] urgent need of medical treatment." It also alleged that officials failed to inform border crossers of the possibility of humanitarian parole, which could allow temporary entry in the case of a dire medical condition.[50]

The American Friends Service Committee (AFSC), a Quaker organization focused on nonviolence, had begun its US-Mexico Border Program in 1977 to advocate for the human rights of migrants. In 1987 they started the Immigration Law Enforcement Monitoring Project to keep track of cases of abuses reported by migrants, legal residents, and US citizens. Between 1989 and 1991, the AFSC project documented 1,274 cases of Border Patrol violations, including rapes, sexual abuse, beatings, and shootings.[51]

In cases documented by the AFSC and Americas Watch, another human rights organization, it is evident that this abuse often had a medical component. Officially, INS policy required "proper and timely medical attention" to injured suspects.[52] However, there were numerous cases of agents denying or delaying medical attention to migrants they had beaten or shot. Border Patrol Agent Michael Elmer "shot an unarmed man in the back" and, instead of seeking emergency care for him, dragged him behind a tree trunk where he died. Doctors estimated that the man may have lived with medical attention. Another "suspect" was beaten in the stomach by officers and then repeatedly begged to see a doctor, which officers refused for many hours. Finally, he was taken to Chula Vista hospital, where he was operated on for a damaged pancreas.[53]

Additional cases of medical care delay and denial were included in a report for a 1993 congressional hearing on Border Patrol violence. In Nogales, Arizona, when a Mexican man refused to stop for the Border Patrol, the agents attacked him and his leg was broken. In detention, they confiscated his asthma inhaler, and he "suffered an asthma attack that caused loss of consciousness." Agents took him to the hospital but brought him back to detention without the X-rays recommended by the doctor. He finally got an X-ray confirming the leg fracture only after returning to Mexico. A man's finger was severed when agents dragged him off the fence at San Ysidro while he was trying to flee. His finger landed on the Mexican side. He was detained face down on the ground for an hour, "begging for medical attention." The agents kept telling him to go to Mexico for treatment. When they took him to a hospital after the hour's delay, his hand was already badly infected.[54]

Civil rights groups were also concerned about how border enforcement affected longtime Mexican residents and US citizens. They documented numerous cases of citizens being picked up or harassed by border officials solely because they appeared to be Mexican.[55] In the cities and towns along the US-Mexico border, fear of the Border Patrol affected everyone of Mexican descent. A Mexican American community group in the border community of McAllen, Texas, described "a history of depredations visited upon our populace by the INS. . . . For example: A pregnant mother of two was questioned so intensely and incessantly at the border that she fainted dead away. One man was put through a full body cavity search. . . . Another woman was strip searched because she came across the border into Texas with $200 cash in her purse—at holiday time! . . . A woman was separated from her children." All of these incidents involved US citizens or legal residents.[56]

In 1989, a hospital in McAllen decided to exploit residents' fear of immigration enforcement as a way to save money. When administrators purchased new uniforms for the hospital's security guards, they chose outfits that were dark green, with gold badges and holsters for walkie-talkies—virtually identical to the outfits worn by officers of the Border Patrol. The choice was no coincidence. According to the local newspaper, "The man who sold McAllen Medical Center their badges says administration specifically requested uniforms that look like those of the Border Patrol."[57]

Word about the uniforms quickly spread through the community. One

McAllen woman, a US citizen, said she was "shocked and scared when she saw the hospital's uniform. 'We all know that they (INS) will just pick up anybody and take us, even if we have papers.'"[58] A discussion of the hospital's policies on talk radio led to "a collective expression of concern and outrage." The Latino community interpreted "the manner in which MMC dresses its security guards" as "unswervingly directed toward us." A doctor at the hospital told the local paper that "they're basically trying to scare off the Mexicans."[59]

Apparently with some success. While McAllen Medical Center was one of the largest providers of indigent care in Texas, legal aid attorneys provided statistics showing that Hispanic people's utilization of MMC's emergency room was significantly lower than at other safety net hospitals in the region. MALDEF, the Mexican American Legal Defense and Education Fund, filed a federal civil rights complaint to demand an end to the hospital's practice of using Border Patrol uniforms to deter patients.[60] "Similar complaints have proven successful" according to a Texas Rural Legal Aid attorney. "One to a Brownsville hospital brought down a sign that had advised patients that 'We cooperate with the Border Patrol.' Another prevented a Yuma, Ariz., hospital from insisting patients show them immigration papers, and displaying a 'we cooperate' sign."[61]

Activists focused on how border enforcement in hospitals was not just an immigration issue, but also a civil rights issue. Immigration enforcement had become synonymous with racial profiling and affected the health of US citizens as well as migrants. And once more, hospitals were attempting to pass the buck on health care costs to the immigration system. But the burden on emergency rooms in Texas border cities was primarily caused by an overall shortage of primary care and a lack of doctors who were willing to take Medicaid.[62] These hospitals fully understood that immigration enforcement was a deterrent to health seeking, and chose a route of intimidation that may have temporarily led to a reduced patient load, but failed to address the main reasons that they were losing money.

Direct Action in the Desert

Another type of border activism consisted of providing direct support to migrants who were under threat of harm by immigration enforcement. In 2004, sanctuary movement activists in Arizona founded the organization No More Deaths. "As the increased militarization of the border has intentionally pushed people into more and more remote and difficult terrain," they explained, "even more people are at risk." No More Deaths likened the border to a war zone, with many innocent victims: "The Department of Homeland

Security's militarized approach to border security has led to massive civilian casualties."[63] Between 1998 and 2018, at least 7,500 people died attempting border crossings.[64]

The Arizona activists began their work in the desert simply by leaving supplies of water in places migrants might find them. They publicized the tragically high number of migrants whose bodies were found in the desert. No More Deaths also worked to document the abuse of border crossers by immigration officials, which continued to include the denial of medical care. Doctors, nurses, and paramedics volunteered their services, some hiking deep into the desert to locate migrants in need of emergency first aid. If asked by the Border Patrol "What are you doing here?" No More Deaths volunteers were advised to respond, "I am here because I want to do everything I can to end suffering and death in the desert."[65]

In response to the increasing numbers of injuries and deaths in desert crossings, the Border Patrol expanded its own medical aid unit, called Borstar (Border Patrol Search Trauma and Rescue Unit). Even so, activists continued to find repeated instances of immigration authorities refusing their obligations to provide medical help to apprehended migrants. Some No More Deaths volunteers worked in Mexico to treat migrants who had been held in short-term US custody and then returned across the border. One first-aid worker reported, "I have witnessed and/or treated dozens of injuries including sprained ankles, injured arms and hands, lacerations, severely blistered feet, sunburns and dehydration among returned migrants who had received no medical care of any kind while in U.S. custody."[66]

While the danger of border crossings worsened, it did not prove a deterrent to continued undocumented migration. Between 2000 and 2006, undocumented immigration increased by 23 percent, and the number of undocumented people living in the United States approached eleven million.[67] In addition to the continuing economic crisis in Mexico and other parts of Latin America, border enforcement itself ensured that significant numbers of people who would otherwise have returned to their home countries were virtually trapped in the United States. By discouraging recrossing and reentry, the militarized border also created incentives for the migration of families, and of unaccompanied minors who had no other choice for a reunion with a parent or other loved ones in the US.

While immigrant rights activists denounced the humanitarian crisis at the border, anti-immigrant groups railed against what they described as an intensified "alien invasion." "Minutemen" groups sprang up in Arizona and patrolled border areas, sometimes armed, confronting migrants and even asking US citizens for their papers. The Minutemen invoked the heightened fears of terrorism after 9/11 and warned that millions of people "from all over the world" were "breaking into the country" and threatening American society generally, including the education and health care systems. Said one Minuteman volunteer, "I'd like to see my brother get a wheel chair lift rather than an illegal alien get a free education."[68] If the provision of public services in the US was a zero-sum game, groups like the Minutemen wanted to take immigrants out of the equation. It was an old argument—but this time immigrants fought back as never before.

"Today, They'll Understand": A Mass Movement for Immigrant Rights

On March 10, 2006, over 250,000 people marched in Chicago in support of immigrant rights. It was the largest protest in the city's history. Asked why he joined the march, Alex Garcia, who had taken the train in from Joliet with his coworkers, told the *Chicago Tribune*, "Most people don't realize how much work we do, but it's part of their daily lives. We are putting up all the buildings and cooking all the food. Today, they'll understand."[69]

The movement spread throughout the country. By May, somewhere between 3.7 and five million people had taken to the streets peacefully to demand recognition of immigrants' contributions and their rights to life and dignity—the largest immigrant rights protests in history, anywhere.[70]

The protests were triggered by a bill that passed the US House of Representatives in December of 2005. HR 4437—known as the Sensenbrenner bill for one of its Republican sponsors, James Sensenbrenner of Wisconsin— intended to criminalize undocumented residency and make immigrants subject to arrest by local police. It proposed to make illegal border crossing a felony and to provide substantial funds for additional border enforcement and fencing. Its provisions against immigrant smuggling potentially made humanitarian assistance to undocumented migrants, such as provided by sanctuary activists and groups like No More Deaths, a crime. Although the bill did not mention health care, one of Sensenbrenner's arguments on its behalf was that reducing the number of immigrants in the country would help US citizens because, as he told a group of his constituents, "most of these workers do not have health insurance" so "Americans end up paying higher health care premiums."[71]

Following the huge protests, the Sensenbrenner bill died in the Senate. But the mass immigrant rights movement did not see any additional immediate victories. A law supported by President George W. Bush to pour more funds into border enforcement (the "Secure Fence Act") passed. A bipartisan proposal in Congress to provide a path to citizenship to undocumented residents, known as the DREAM Act (first introduced by Senators Orrin Hatch, a Republican, and Dick Durbin, a Democrat, in 2001), again met with defeat. Intensified raids and deportations would continue under both the Bush and Obama administrations.

But the 2006 movement was still a substantial step forward for immigrant rights. Political scientists Kim Voss and Irene Bloemraad note that, in addition to the massive numbers, the protests "were remarkable in another way: they focused on, and were in substantial part animated by, people without citizenship in the political system they challenged."[72] The marches were fully and openly led by, not just on behalf of, undocumented people. Young undocumented workers, college students, and even high school students began to emerge as leaders who refused to remain "in the shadows" and who fought to create change despite their inability to vote or run for office. In doing so, they expanded the meaning of democracy and political participation.

The election of Barack Obama to the presidency in 2008 brought hope but also frustration to the immigrant rights movement. Obama's campaign promises included ending the Iraq war and bringing the economy back from financial crisis, and he also vowed to seek a pathway to citizenship for undocumented residents. At the same time, he used "strengthen border security" and "crack down on employers" language. In his inaugural address on January 21, 2009, Obama did not mention immigration.[73] During his first year in office, he focused on a major health care reform—but his proposal couldn't avoid getting entangled in the politics of immigration.

"You Lie!": A New Kind of Exclusion

Obama was determined to sign a comprehensive health care overhaul into law. But when legislators held "town hall" meetings across the country in the summer of 2009 to discuss health reform proposals, they were met with a wave of protests from antitax, anti-Obama Tea Party activists. Many who attended the town halls were conservatives who wanted to register their opposition to "socialized medicine." Misinformation, including the idea that reform would create "death panels" to withhold care from the elderly, and the falsehood that Obama was not a US citizen, fueled the anger at these meetings.[74]

One of the most common accusations hurled during the town halls was that the plan would "give free health care to illegal immigrants." Obama's opponents repeated the long-standing falsehood that people migrated to the US to get easy access to health and welfare benefits. A leader of the antiimmigrant forces claimed that "the legislation amounts to a reward for illegal aliens and another power boost to the magnet that draws illegal aliens."[75]

When Obama went before Congress on September 9 to reassure the nation that the new health care law "would not apply to those who are here illegally," South Carolina representative Joe Wilson shouted out, on national television, "You lie!"

Among its many provisions, the Patient Protection and Affordable Care Act (ACA), which also became known as Obamacare, established insurance exchanges in which people could purchase private coverage and receive subsidies depending on their incomes. In the initial proposal, undocumented immigrants were barred from access to the subsidies, but would have been able to purchase unsubsidized insurance plans in the exchanges with their own money. However, when a new version was unveiled by the House on September 16, it stipulated that only citizens and legal residents could purchase *any* kind of insurance in the exchanges.[76]

The White House indicated support for the exclusion of undocumented immigrants from the bill. According to an Obama spokesperson, it was not a change of heart by the president, just a clarification of intent. But immigrant rights groups were furious. The executive director of LULAC said that Congressman Wilson "had acted like a buffoon," but "at the end of the day he sort of got his way."[77] Since most undocumented immigrants would not have been able to afford unsubsidized plans anyway, their exclusion was largely symbolic. But it was a symbolism that mattered, a capitulation to anti-immigrant politics that used the undocumented as pawns to achieve a legislative goal. It also reinforced the false idea that immigrants burdened the health care system. As a National Council of La Raza leader reminded the *New York Times*, "These folks are [already] not getting public benefits."[78]

After the ACA passed in 2010, health care providers and researchers continued to report on the ways that exclusion affected immigrants' health and that of their families. The requirement to demonstrate legal status in order to purchase ACA insurance added yet another deterrent to families with undocumented members.[79] Legal immigrants did benefit from Obamacare because they were allowed to purchase subsidized plans. An especially important change was that in states that expanded Medicaid with federal ACA funding, the five-year waiting period for legal immigrants to receive Medicaid was removed. However, since the Supreme Court overturned the ACA's mandatory Medicaid expansion, legal immigrants in states that elected not to expand their programs were still severely disadvantaged.[80]

One part of the Affordable Care Act would potentially increase access to care for the undocumented: the expansion of community health centers (CHCs). The 2010 act made the CHC program permanent and provided additional federal funding for the centers, which do not ask about immigration status. Between 2010 and 2018, the number of patients served by CHCs grew from 19.5 million to 28.4 million. However, CHCs have long waiting lists, provide limited services, and still do not exist in large swaths of the country, particularly rural areas.[81] The limited and flawed avenues of federally funded clinics and hospital emergency rooms continue to be the most common ways for immigrants to access medical care. As one study put it, Obama's landmark health reform left "the number of uninsured undocumented immigrants . . . virtually unchanged."[82]

DACA and Health Coverage

On March 10, 2010—two weeks before President Obama signed the ACA into law—the immigrant rights movement entered a new phase. Young undocumented people in Chicago held an event called "Coming Out of the Shadows." Under the banner "Undocumented and Unafraid," hundreds marched from Union Park on the Near West Side, chanting "Obama, escucha, estamos en la lucha" (Obama, listen, we are in the fight). After arriving at Federal Plaza downtown, eight undocumented young people took the stage in front of the iconic Alexander Calder *Flamingo* sculpture. Each speaker announced "I am undocumented" and shared their story. They had been born in Mexico, Central America, or Southeast Asia and had come to the US as babies, small children, or teenagers. Each denounced Congress's failure to pass the DREAM Act and the increase in deportations under Obama. They claimed the right to stop living in fear and demanded "Legalization Now!"[83]

These activists had decided to stop waiting for Congress to move on immigration reform and instead to pressure Obama to take executive action. Across the country, immigrant youth mobilized to gain the president's attention. They sat down in the middle of a street in Atlanta and used bullhorns to broadcast their undocumented status and their demands. They protested and heckled at events where Obama was speaking.[84] Their tactics worked. On June 15, 2012, the president announced that he was creating, by executive order, a program called Deferred Action for Childhood Arrivals, or DACA.

DACA allowed young people who had been brought to the US as children to apply for a temporary reprieve from the danger of deportation and to receive a work permit. Between 2012 and 2021, nearly nine hundred thousand immigrant youth participated in the program. Recipients must apply every two years to renew DACA, paying a hefty application fee of $495 each time. They must also be willing to disclose their names, addresses, and undocumented status to the federal government. The work permit and temporary relief from fear of deportation have been essential in helping many young people to come out the shadows. On the other hand, DACA recipients are still not eligible for welfare programs or federal student aid, and they were not given access to Affordable Care Act insurance.

Latinx and immigrant rights organizations praised DACA but expressed concern about the continued health insurance exclusion. The National Hispanic Leadership Agenda, a coalition of thirty-nine Latino and public health groups, wrote to Obama in 2014, asking him to make DACA recipients eligible for coverage under the ACA. They argued that executive action was "warranted in light of the chronic and severe lack of access to health care faced by the immigrant community, particularly Latino immigrants. . . . For DACA recipients in need of health care, the denial of affordable care and coverage undoubtedly leads to human suffering and diminished health."[85]

DACA provided further evidence of how immigration status can affect health status—this time in a positive way. Even with the ACA exclusion, DACA has helped improve health coverage for many undocumented youth. Work permits can provide more access to employer insurance and even the ability to purchase individual coverage. A 2018 study found that DACA led to an increase in recipients reporting that they had a usual source of medical care and made them less likely to defer care for financial reasons.[86] Just as immigrant enforcement damages health, relief from enforcement can enhance it.

Taking the Fight to the States (and Cities)

In the wake of the 2006 protests and the failure of the Sensenbrenner bill, anti-immigrant forces turned their attention back to state legislation. An Arizona law known as SB 1070, passed in 2010, required police to ask for immigration papers during any stop, arrest, or detention if they had "reasonable suspicion" that the person was undocumented. It also criminalized transporting, shielding, or harboring undocumented immigrants. Other states began discussing similar initiatives, which came to be known as "show me your papers" laws. Alabama's law, passed in 2011, was the harshest in the nation. In addition to a "show your papers" provision, it also required schools to report students' immigration status, barred undocumented students from public higher education, and made it a crime for landlords to rent to undocumented people and even for a citizen to transport undocumented immigrants in a car. The law was intended, according to its sponsor, to "attack . . . every aspect of an illegal alien's life."[87]

Even though the more draconian provisions of these state laws were struck down by the courts, their passage still had a negative effect on the health of immigrant and Latino residents. Researchers found that the Arizona law led to worsening mental health status among Latino youth in the state, including nonimmigrants. Young people reported anxiety about family separation, fear of racial profiling by the police, and increased thoughts of suicide. Numerous studies showed that in states that passed these harsh laws, immigrants' access to health care decreased, due not only to new restrictions but also to increased hostility or reluctance from providers, fear of immigration enforcement in health care settings, and worsened poverty.[88]

Just as immigration opponents turned to state action in the wake of federal inaction, so too did health rights activists. The exclusion of undocumented immigrants from the Affordable Care Act led to an upsurge of mobilizations to expand access to care on the local level. Although they did not achieve the national visibility of the 2006 demonstrations, local fights did lead to some concrete victories for immigrant health care access.

Some improvements in the states came from the top down. Congress's 2009 reauthorization of SCHIP (State Children's Health Insurance Program) included an option for states to cover certain categories of legal immigrants who had been excluded due to the five-year ban. In a classic example of US health care rationing (which refuses universalism by creating categories of inclusion and exclusion), states could make exceptions to immigrant exclusions and cover pregnant women, children, or both in their SCHIP or Medicaid programs. By 2020, thirty-five states opted to cover legal immigrant children, and twenty-five states covered legal immigrant pregnant women. While some of the states who chose the coverage expansions already had a history of committing some state funds to health coverage for poor legal immigrants, others were motivated by the offer of fresh federal matching funds.[89]

In the 2010s, immigrant rights groups began winning some other victories in the states, including allowing undocumented people to obtain drivers' licenses (eighteen states by 2022) and giving undocumented students access to in-state college tuition (twenty-two states by 2022). And after the undocumented were excluded from the Affordable Care Act, state-level immigrant rights activism began to focus on health care expansion. Thanks to pressure from young immigrants engaging in activism "out of the shadows," in 2012 both New York and California enacted legislation to allow low-income DACA recipients to enroll in their Medicaid programs, getting around federal regulations by only using state funds for this purpose. Also in California, a campaign by immigrants and allies led to the passage of a bill in 2015 extending the full benefits of its Medicaid program (Medi-Cal) to undocumented children. Excepting California, the states expanding immigrant health care were not the ones with the most undocumented residents; instead, coverage legislation tracked state Democratic Party dominance, local legislators committed to immigrant rights, and, especially, strong and vocal movements in defense of the undocumented.[90]

Health care expansion in the states also correlated with the presence of "sanctuary cities." Sanctuary cities began as part of the sanctuary movement of the 1980s, when dozens of localities declared themselves safe havens for Central American refugees. In the 2000s, the term came to mean cities and towns that officially limited the cooperation of local police and other public service providers with federal immigration authorities—the opposite of "show your papers." Some of the largest cities in the country, including Chicago, Los Angeles, Denver, and Philadelphia, have passed ordinances declaring themselves to be sanctuary cities, and even some states call themselves sanctuaries. On the other hand, in some parts of the country, sanctuary ordinances have been banned by conservative state legislatures.

Sanctuary cities can actively provide better access to health care for noncitizens. San Francisco's municipal health care programs for the indigent, Healthy Kids and Healthy San Francisco, are both open to undocumented immigrants. At San Francisco safety net hospitals and clinics, medical practitioners and staff actively work to counter immigrants' fears; for example, offering alternatives to the social security number for medical records and reassuring patients "it is safe here." Researchers found that undocumented Mexican immigrants with diabetes in two sanctuary cities, San Francisco and Chicago, were able to access care and reported outcomes that were similar to those of documented and US-born Mexican American patients.[91] Again, relieving the fear of immigration enforcement resulted in improvements to health.

Health Care Dreamers: Undocumented Medical Practitioners

The US health care system has long relied on immigrant nurses and doctors to address its shortage of medical providers. Special visa categories have allowed highly skilled professionals to move to the US temporarily or permanently, and the government has periodically created programs to bring in foreign nurses. Since the 1960s, for example, over 150,000 nurses from the Philippines have migrated to the US. The health system's dependency on doctors and nurses from overseas has been controversial because of the way it encourages "brain drain" of skilled talent from low-income countries. It also highlights

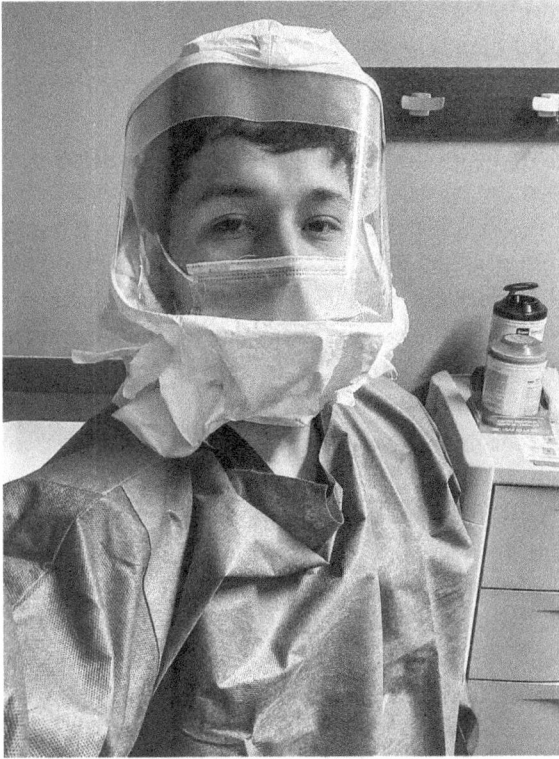

FIGURE 7.1. DACA recipient Jose Flores of DeKalb, Illinois, served as a traveling certified nursing assistant during the COVID-19 pandemic and was commended in Congress (see epilogue). He plans to start medical school in the fall of 2024. Photo courtesy of the Latino Oral History Project, Center for Latino and Latin American Studies, Northern Illinois University, and Jose Flores.

the failure of the US to train sufficient numbers of medical professionals to meet the needs of its population, especially its poor population.[92]

At the same time that the US has sought to import physicians and nurses, it has prevented immigrants already in the country from pursuing medical and other professional careers. PRWORA, the punitive 1996 welfare reform act, prohibits certain categories of immigrants from obtaining professional licenses unless states create enabling legislation. This includes immigrants with provisional status that allows them to obtain work permits, such as Temporary Protected Status and DACA.

The political activation of young undocumented people that led to the creation of DACA also produced a movement to extend professional licensing to DACA recipients. Many young immigrants who grew up and were educated in the United States had been turned away or discouraged from pursuing vocations in health care. Some had earned degrees in nursing or other health fields, paying their own way because they were not eligible for scholarships, but then were not able to practice their profession due to the licensure ban. Now, they demanded to be allowed to put their educations and passions to use.

Jiyarut "New" Latthivongskorn, the son of Thai restaurant workers, had been brought to the US as a young child. While majoring in biology at the University of California, Berkeley, he became involved in immigrant rights activism. "From personal experiences of having very little or no access to health care," he remembered, "I wanted to become a physician who would change policies and influence the status quo of how healthcare was delivered."[93] In 2012, Latthivongskorn and two other DACA recipients formed an organization they named Pre-Health Dreamers and began organizing peer support groups for undocumented students seeking medical careers. Their movement spread from California to campuses around the country. By 2019, there were nearly two hundred undocumented students enrolled in US medical schools, and ten states had passed laws that allowed DACA recipients to become licensed health care providers.[94]

State-level Medicaid expansions, sanctuary cities, and "DACA-mented" medical students represented local responses to health care exclusion. But exclusion and even targeting of the undocumented continued at the national level. The Obama administration did put forth some policies in response to immigrant rights activism: in addition to DACA, Obama announced a "Priority Enforcement Program" to focus deportations on those with criminal records and recent border crossers, rather than families and long-term residents. Even so, more than five million people were deported or removed during the Obama administration, leading immigrant rights groups to refer to him as "Deporter in Chief."[95]

But it was evident that activism for immigrant health rights was having an impact, at least on political rhetoric. During the 2016 US presidential primary campaign, Hillary Clinton announced that she was in favor of allowing undocumented immigrants to buy into Obamacare coverage with their own money, and presidential candidate Bernie Sanders indicated that his Medicare for All proposal would not exclude anyone based on citizenship. Such pronouncements would have been unimaginable just a few years earlier and would have been impossible without activist responses to the Obamacare exclusion that called attention to health care injustice against immigrants. However, this progress faced an existential threat when Donald Trump was elected president.

Trump Terror against Health

Trump had campaigned on an anti-immigrant and specifically anti-Mexican platform. He threatened to massively expand deportations and promised to build a wall along the entire southern border "and make Mexico pay for it." In his first two years in office, he enacted a ban on entrants from Muslim countries, rescinded DACA and Temporary Protected Status, and continued to describe migrants from poor countries as criminals and "animals." Although his administration did not end up implementing mass deportation, Trump's rhetoric and policies created an atmosphere of terror in immigrant communities.

The worsened climate under Trump hurt immigrant health and access to care in several ways. Undocumented people became even more reluctant to seek medical help. For example, a free clinic in Phoenix, Arizona, was usually triple-booked with immigrant patients, but after Trump took office, the clinic "felt its patients retreat. There were more missed appointments, fewer answered phone calls, and more patients checking in with anxiety attacks."[96] One study found that, in the three years following the start of Trump's presidential campaign in 2015, undocumented immigrants' completed primary care visits dropped by 43.3 percent for children and 34.5 percent for adults.[97]

Fear increased when immigrant enforcement under Trump began to target places that had previously been deemed off-limits or lower priorities for deportation. Under an Obama-era memorandum, ICE (Immigration and Customs Enforcement) and other enforcement agencies were supposed to steer clear of "sensitive locations" like churches, schools, courthouses, and hospitals. But on October 24, 2017, Border Patrol officers entered the Texas hospital room of ten-year-old Rosa María Hernández, who had cerebral palsy and was recovering from surgery, and detained her for deportation. After the ACLU filed a complaint, the child was reunited with her parents, but the case was not an isolated incident. That same year, undocumented parents seeking care for their seriously ill newborn in a Corpus Christi hospital were arrested by immigration agents. A Salvadoran asylum seeker was diagnosed with a brain tumor and underwent surgery at another Texas hospital, but then agents forcibly returned her to detention.[98] For undocumented patients, hospitals became spaces of potential terror.

On May 7, 2018, Trump's Department of Justice announced a "zero tolerance" policy for unauthorized migrants at the southern border. All undocumented border crossers, including asylum seekers not utilizing ports of entry, would be charged as criminals. When families were apprehended, the parents were jailed and the children taken to shelters across the country. Parents were not told where their children were being taken. The splitting of families was deliberate, a cruel attempt at deterrence. By the end of May, two thousand families had been separated—a number that would eventually rise to over six thousand. Advocates for migrants began reporting horrific incidents. Federal officials forcibly removed a baby from its breast-feeding mother. A father committed suicide in jail after his family was taken away. In a Texas warehouse, hundreds of children, including babies and toddlers, were held in cages made of wire fencing. Parents were deported back to their home countries without their children.[99]

The devastating effect of detention and family separation on physical and mental health was already well known. In 1979, officials of the World Health Organization had recommended that countries recognize the negative effect of family separation on "somatic (physical) and psychological" health when developing immigration policies. Even when families were kept together in detention, which was the policy under the Obama administration, studies found that the trauma of detention negatively affected children's brain development. In 2019, the United Nations high commissioner for human rights, Michelle Bachelet, condemned the US zero tolerance policy. Bachelet, a former pediatrician, said, "Detaining a child even for short periods under good conditions can have a serious impact on their health and development." In 2020, a report by Physicians for Human Rights (PHR) described family separation as "causing 'significant distress' and ongoing functional impairment." PHR concluded that the zero tolerance practices rose to the level of the international human rights violations of torture and enforced disappearance.[100]

Trump also set out to make life more difficult for *legal* immigrants and to reduce legal immigration. He especially sought to end the immigration of Muslims, Africans, and poor people. Several of his administration's initiatives on legal immigration focused on health. In a draft executive order leaked in the first days of his presidency, Trump demanded more rigorous enforcement of public charge rules to deny entry to low-income immigrants and expel legal immigrants who used public benefits. He wanted to broaden the criteria for being excluded as a public charge, adding the use of noncash benefits including housing assistance, food stamps, and Medicaid. Although the final rule was not issued until 2019, the persistent threat of a draconian redefinition of public charge enforcement led legal immigrants to drop out of health care programs that they were entitled to use and added green card applicants, asylum seekers, and people seeking naturalization and citizenship to the groups living under a climate of fear.[101] And for those who sought medical help despite the fear, Trump issued a rule to end the requirement that hospitals inform patients of their rights to language interpretation.[102]

The Trump administration's final public charge rule expanded how health and health care criteria would be weighed in excluding people from the country. Having "a medical condition that is likely to require extensive medical treatment" branded applicants as likely to become a public charge. In addition, being "older or younger than working age" and lacking private health coverage were added as negative factors. Applicants were more likely to be approved if they had higher incomes or private health insurance. This last requirement was further intensified when Trump released a proclamation suspending entry of immigrants unless they could provide proof of having private health insurance or the ability to pay for it. The title of the order repeated the familiar but long-discredited zero-sum calculation: "Suspension of Entry of Immigrants Who Will Financially Burden the United States Healthcare System, in Order to Protect the Availability of Healthcare Benefits for Americans."[103]

The cruelty of raids, detention, family separation, and attacks on immigrant health were intended to deter further migration and make life harder for those already in the United States. Such attempts at deterrence had always failed in the face of the many pressing reasons that people migrate, but there was another dimension to these actions: the targeting of groups that threatened white supremacy. Many of Trump's immigration policies were orchestrated by his adviser Stephen Miller, who openly expressed white nationalist beliefs, including the idea that immigration from poor countries would lead to the end of the US as a white nation.[104] Immigrant health and well-being posed not just an illusory fiscal burden, but a threat to white dominance.

The Trump administration's attacks on immigrants were met with vigorous protests. Immigrant rights supporters had to contend with setbacks to progress, such as the rescission of DACA, as well as new threats like the zero tolerance policy. But the movement also grew, especially as more people joined the outcry against family separation in 2018. Rallies and marches were held in communities around the nation, and a Facebook fundraiser asking for $1,500 to reunite a family ended up with $20 million in donations. Doctors, nurses, and medical students protested at detention centers and marched to the border to demand an end to family separations. A physician who flew from Washington, DC, to Texas to attend a protest explained, "As health professionals we must speak up about the toxic stress, the broken families, the long-term consequences of these actions."[105]

Immigrant health rights activism at the local level also intensified, and there were even some victories. In Philadelphia, family members and activists were able to stop the hospital deportation of an undocumented immigrant who was in a coma following a motorcycle accident. Their protests and publicity got him transferred to a long-term care facility instead. Local activists continued their work to expand access to health care for the undocumented. In 2017 Cook County, Illinois, created a program for all low-income residents who were ineligible for Medicaid, regardless of immigration status, which gave them access to hospitals and primary care. The program was the result of several years of organizing by immigrant rights groups. In June of 2019, California extended Medi-Cal coverage to everyone eligible under age twenty-six, becoming the first state to offer health insurance to adult undocumented people. And in 2020, Illinois became the first state to create a health care program for low-income undocumented seniors.[106]

In June 2019, in a nationally televised debate, the Democratic candidates for the presidency were asked for a show of hands if they supported providing health coverage for all undocumented immigrants. All ten of the candidates—including Joe Biden—raised their hands.[107] Coming almost exactly ten years after Democrats decided to exclude the undocumented from the Affordable Care Act, this represented nothing less than a sea change in mainstream attitudes toward immigrant health care. This change was brought about by the movement that had sparked in 2006, brought people out of the shadows in 2012, and refused to capitulate during the agony of the Trump years. But there were more horrors to come. During the COVID-19 pandemic, the nation's deep-seated inequities within its labor, health, and immigration systems intensified, with deadly consequences.

From Pandemic to Power

The global pandemic created carnage for immigrant and migrant communities. Immigrants made up a disproportionate number of the essential workers who were unable to shelter from COVID's assault. As a result, immigrant communities in the US had more deaths among working-age people than did the general population. Essential workers were also forced to bring the virus home to vulnerable family members. Both Trump and Biden used the pandemic as an excuse to close the border and put migrants at even greater risk.[1] But the devastation of COVID-19 also led to strengthened activism that targets the injustices of the US immigration/health nexus.

The pandemic hit immigrants especially hard, and undocumented people were further hurt by being excluded from the emergency unemployment insurance and federal stimulus payments that helped workers survive. Communities responded by building on old forms of mutual aid and developing new ones. Volunteers made cloth face masks. Soup kitchens and food distributions sprang up everywhere. Long-standing mutual aid organizations such as the Chinese Progressive Association in San Francisco offered modest cash payments to families in need. Groups that had been founded in the upsurge of undocumented rights organizing, like Movimiento Cosecha and Undocu-Black Network, started their own mutual aid funds and projects.[2] As in the nineteenth century, these activities were a response to neglect and abandonment by government. As a group of Chicago activists put it, "Mutual aid has long been a way for communities to survive hostile systems."[3]

In industries with many undocumented workers, the devastation of the pandemic required both mutual aid and organizing for workplace safety. Shutdowns led to the loss of many low-wage jobs for workers who did not have access to benefits. Among Spanish-speaking house cleaners, for example, less than a third received stimulus checks, and more than 90 percent did not receive unemployment pay. Mutual aid was one way to respond to this exclusion, and funds were established for laid-off workers in the restaurant, garment, and even domestic service industries. In "essential" sectors, workers were forced to continue laboring in conditions that exposed them to COVID. Health care workers, food production workers, and farmworkers engaged in strikes, walkouts, and informational picketing to demand adequate protective equipment, social distancing, and other protections.[4]

In US meatpacking plants, whose workers are almost all immigrants and people of color, fifty-nine thousand people were infected and more than 250 died in the first year of the pandemic. A congressional investigation found that employers had refused to implement more stringent safety measures and that the Trump administration had pushed back against local health department orders to close the plants.[5] Workers, families, and unions fought to bring attention to how workers were being exposed to the virus. In Greeley, Colorado, families held a rally, carrying signs with the names of their loved ones who had died. Several families of immigrant workers brought lawsuits against meatpacking employers. One worker's family sued an Iowa pork plant where several workers perished. At that plant, managers had made bets about how many workers would fall sick. A LULAC official in Iowa said, "We knew it was bad, but to have people in management positions look at our people as just pieces on a game board to play with, that is so inhumane."[6]

Another reason for the high rates of deaths among immigrant workers was that very few of them could afford to take time off work when they got sick. In the low-paid, immigrant-heavy service sector of the US economy, only about 20 percent of workers have access to paid sick days. Workers' inability to stay home exacerbated the danger of infection at workplaces. The lack of employer-sponsored health insurance in these same low-wage occupations also made it more difficult for immigrant workers to access care when they became infected.[7]

Immigrant workers in hospitals and other health facilities suffered a disproportionate share of deaths. Two-thirds of health workers who died of COVID in 2020 were people of color, and one-third were foreign born. A clear reason for the correlation between race, immigration status, and vulnerability to COVID among health workers was labor exploitation: "Lower-paid workers who handled everyday patient care, including nurses, support staff and nursing home employees, were far more likely to die in the pandemic than physicians were." One of the most disturbing statistics on immigrant health worker deaths was the high number of Philippine migrant and Filipino American nurses who perished—between 20 and 30 percent of all COVID deaths among nurses. The US had long relied on migrants from the Philippines to address health care worker shortages, and it seems that the combination of workplace conditions (many worked in the most dangerous settings such as nursing homes) and being an older age cohort made these nurses especially vulnerable. Like other essential workers, health workers have had to fight against indifferent and hostile employers and government to demand safer working conditions.[8]

Along with its workplace and health policies, US immigration policies made the pandemic worse for immigrants and migrants. Trump's repeated references to the "China virus" encouraged racist attacks on Asian Americans and immigrants. White nationalist Trump adviser Stephen Miller had been looking for a way to invoke Title 42, an obscure public health law that allows the government to prevent people from entering the country if they might spread disease. When COVID hit, the Trump administration almost immediately began using Title 42 to expel large numbers of migrants and to prevent people from entering, including asylum seekers. In 2020, 340,000 migrants were expelled under a health policy, Title 42, which had been converted into an immigration policy.[9]

In practice, Title 42 worked against public health. Most migrants were coming from countries with lower COVID rates than the United States. When people were detained under Title 42 to await expulsion, their risk of being exposed to coronavirus worsened because of the crowded conditions. Some migrants who were deported to their home countries ended up bringing the disease with them from their exposure in the US. If they were expelled into or forced to remain in Mexico, many migrants landed in overcrowded shelters or tent cities where it was a constant struggle to remain safe from infection.[10]

Health providers, public health experts, immigrant rights groups, and migrants themselves have protested the policies that forced people to get sick and violated the rights of immigrants and asylum seekers. The protests intensified after the Biden administration continued to use Title 42 to expel migrants, even as it declared the pandemic was mostly over. A letter to the US Centers for Disease Control signed by 1,300 medical and public health professionals asserted, "As public health experts have long objected, the Title 42 order lacks epidemiological evidence to justify banning the entrance of only migrants and asylum seekers at US borders." In May 2022, hundreds of migrants gathered near the port of entry in Nogales, Mexico, holding signs saying "500 Days Waiting" and "Title 42 is Racist." A woman who was fleeing violence in southern Mexico told a reporter at the protest, "We are not a virus. . . . We are just desperate." Antiracist activists point out that the Biden administration used Title 42 especially forcefully against Haitian asylum seekers.[11]

Yet in the US coronavirus response, there were some avenues of inclusion. In 2020, Congress did not exclude noncitizens from free COVID testing programs, and even Trump said "yes we will test that person," referring to undocumented immigrants.[12] When it came to the vaccine rollout in 2021, Biden's Department of Homeland Security announced that "it is a moral and public health imperative to ensure that all individuals residing in the United States have access to the vaccine" and "DHS encourages all individuals, regardless of immigration status, to receive the COVID-19 vaccine once eligible under local distribution guidelines."[13]

Encouragement could only go so far, especially in the context of the severe immigration enforcement that had amplified fears of accessing health services. Despite officially open access (until the end of the public health emergency in 2023), many factors still worked against immigrants' ability to obtain the lifesaving vaccines. Florida initially announced that proof of residency would be required to receive the vaccine. Some states prioritized vaccinating the elderly before essential workers, which doubly disadvantaged immigrant workers, who tended to be younger as a population.[14] Although there was much concern about vaccine hesitancy among minority communities, some studies found that immigrants were more eager to get vaccinated than the general population. Lower levels of vaccine uptake by immigrants early in the pandemic were due less to hesitancy than to lack of supply, barriers to access such as location of vaccine distribution sites and the need for internet access to make appointments, the inability to miss work, and fears of having to provide identification.[15]

With a dose of activism, vaccine uptake among immigrants could be spectacularly successful. In Alabama, by June of 2021 close to 90 percent of Vietnamese Americans and immigrants had been vaccinated, compared to only 34 percent of all people in the state. This was in great part due to the work of an immigrant rights organization, Boat People SOS, that blanketed the community with vaccine information and worked to counter rumors and disinformation. In Chicago, community organizers successfully pressured the city to concentrate vaccine distribution on the neighborhoods hardest hit by COVID. When a community health center in the Gage Park neighborhood partnered with activist organizations to open a vaccine clinic in February 2021, the demand was overwhelming. Within a few months, Chicago's Latinx neighborhoods, which started out with the lowest levels of vaccine uptake, became the most vaccinated in the city. "After so much obliviousness by leaders all over, we feel like we are being seen right now," sixty-three-year-old Antonia Quiñones, who received the vaccine after a push by community activists in the Little Village neighborhood, told the *Chicago Tribune* in Spanish, "but it was after demanding and fighting for this, we made this happen for ourselves."[16]

As immigrants protected their own communities, they also made vital contributions to fighting the pandemic and helping countless others. On farms, in food production, in grocery stores, restaurants, and warehouses, and in many other roles, immigrants risked their health, and many lost their lives, to keep the economy going and feed the population. In hospitals and nursing homes, immigrant nurses, physicians, and aides assisted patients who were sick and dying of COVID, going beyond their medical roles to provide language interpretation and to communicate with terrified families. Those seeking further evidence that immigrants helped save lives in the pandemic could even point to the immigrant scientists who invented the N95 face mask and led the quest for COVID vaccines.[17]

The enormous contributions of immigrants during the pandemic have led to calls for rewarding the undocumented with a path to legal status. As one rights group put it, "Their sacrifices have kept America going through the pandemic. It's time to provide legal certainty to those on the frontlines." A poll taken during 2020 showed 73 percent support for providing a path to citizenship for undocumented essential workers.[18] In December 2022, Illinois senator Dick Durbin took to the floor of the US Senate to renew his call for such a path for DACA recipients. Durbin had made this kind of speech over one hundred times, and this time he focused on one young man's contributions during the pandemic. Jose Flores had been brought to the country from Mexico when he was eleven months old. As a child in DeKalb, Illinois, he served as an interpreter for his family during medical appointments, and "his passion for healthcare bloomed." Blocked from premedical studies due to financial barriers, Jose trained as a certified nursing assistant. When the pandemic hit, "Jose was deployed across the country to meet urgent health-care needs. . . . His work took him far from home," Durbin recounted, "which meant that he was unable to be by his grandfather's side when his grandfather passed away from COVID. It was one of the many sacrifices Jose made to pursue his passion for serving our nation."[19]

Yet immigrant workers' sacrifices were nothing new, and the rewards were never given. The proposed HEROES bill in 2020 would have given stimulus checks and temporary relief from deportation to essential undocumented workers, but Trump declared it "dead on arrival" and it failed to pass the Senate.[20] Under Biden, DACA has been reinstated in limited form, and in May 2024, in a notable victory for health rights, he announced that DACA recipients would become eligible for the Affordable Care Act. However, Congress continues to fail to make progress on the DREAM Act or other meaningful immigration reform. The path to citizenship and, for the non-DACA eligible, protection from the brutality of immigration enforcement, are as out of reach as they were before the pandemic.

The notion of rewarding essential workers for their contributions during the pandemic also reinforces some troubling assumptions, namely, that we "primarily value immigrant lives when they are sacrificed."[21] It should not take a pandemic for the US to recognize how its prosperity and comfort is dependent on migrant and immigrant labor. The pandemic intensified their "sacrifices," but it was business as usual that the economy's reliance on immigrant workers led not only to their exploitation, but to their sicknesses and deaths. An emphasis on reward for sacrifice also contradicts the human rights principle that people should deserve or receive rights based on their humanity, not their economic contributions. Rather than rewards for continuing exploitation, we should be asking what justice might look like.

One way to start would be to recognize that the injustices of the US health care system are not just visited on immigrants. As the pandemic again brought starkly to light, health care access in the United States is precarious for everyone. The exclusion of immigrants reflects and reinforces the many other types of health care exclusion that Americans experience every day, including exclusions based on race, geographic location, income, insurance coverage, occupation, workplace, and age. Structural inequalities that lead to poor health outcomes affect both immigrants and citizens. The US is still the only wealthy nation that allows a substantial portion of its population to go without health insurance, and is the only such nation that does not require paid sick leave for workers. These policy choices made the pandemic worse and contributed to the country's devastatingly high number of deaths from COVID.[22] Addressing the ways that the health care system hurts immigrants also requires addressing how it hurts everyone.

Similarly, action to improve immigrant health and access to care is good for everyone. This book has described numerous examples of ways that fights to expand health rights for immigrants and migrants created modest but meaningful improvements in the system as a whole and made inroads toward greater inclusion for citizens as well as noncitizens. Ethnic hospitals were the first to admit chronic and contagious patients. Settlement house nursing services demonstrated the effectiveness of preventive and follow-up care. Immigrant labor organizing generated improvements in workplace health and safety. The fight for bracero rights led to the Migrant Health Act. Lawsuits brought by and on behalf of migrants expanded rights to informed consent (*Madrigal v. Quilligan*), the right to travel (*Memorial v. Maricopa*), and the right to emergency care (*Guerrero v. Copper Queen*). Activism on behalf of

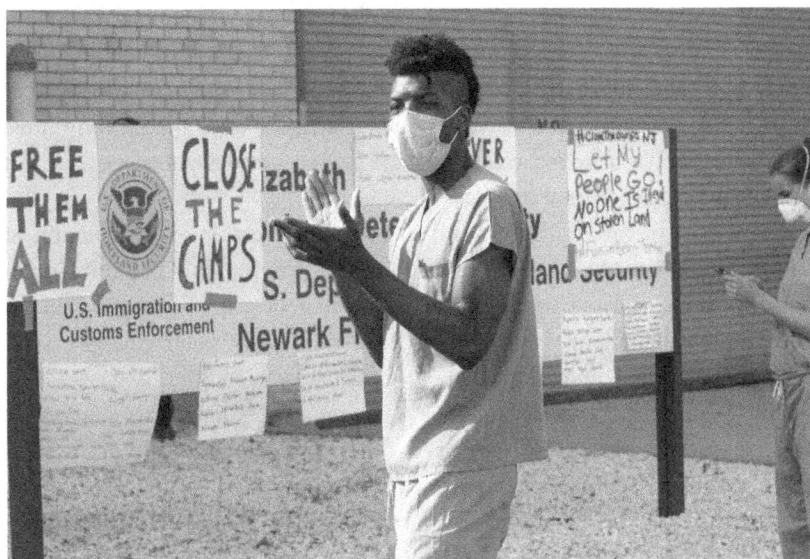

FIGURE 8.1. Health care workers' demonstration at the Elizabeth, New Jersey, Contract Detention Facility for US Immigration and Customs Enforcement early in the pandemic. This action was part of a nationwide protest calling attention to dangerous conditions at immigrant detention centers across the country. May 16, 2020. Rickyflores.com, photo courtesy Ricky Flores.

language and provider diversity pushed hospitals to better serve and represent their communities. Clinics offering access to the undocumented put forth the idea of noncategorical community health services open to all.

The fight for immigrant health shows that borders are incompatible with health for all. I mean this both literally and figuratively. Numerous examples throughout this book show the literal devastation to health wrought by the political border. The border's tangible effects on health and mortality include deaths in the desert, drowning in rivers, pesticide baths, exposure to infectious disease, border patrol violence, medical neglect, family separation, and exploitive labor conditions. Internally, the categorization of people as foreigner, immigrant, undocumented, noncitizen, recent arrival, and so on, dictates their ability to obtain needed health care. Figurative borders also permeate the US health system, which separates everyone into categories of entitlement or exclusion that determine their access to care and their ability to thrive and survive.[23]

To improve health for all, a politics of care needs to replace the politics of borders. "Care" requires "recognizing and embracing our interdependencies."[24] That means ending the invisibility and exploitation of all essential workers, both citizen and noncitizen, and of all the caregivers, paid and unpaid, upon whom economies and families depend. It means prioritizing policies and government spending that support caregiving, protect the most vulnerable, and improve health for all. It also means recognizing the role of US foreign, economic, and environmental policies in creating the conditions that force people to migrate and become refugees and asylum seekers, and taking steps to repair that damage.

A politics of care undermines the separateness created by the fiction of borders. This is necessary not just for human thriving, but also for human survival. If we continue to place borders above people, we will not be able to meet the great challenges of our time. Pandemics and climate change do not recognize national boundaries.

If this amount of transformation seems impossible, the history told in this book opens our eyes to the possible. Profound change can begin at the local level. Mutual aid, clinics, and sanctuaries put the politics of care into practice. Community actions have reunited families and even shut down detention centers.[25] Immigrant health rights activism shows that people who are supposed to be powerless can lead the way to a more democratic and caring society for all.

Acknowledgments

Thank you to everyone who helped make *Borders of Care* possible. Years ago, Alice Kessler-Harris taught me that immigrant workers helped create the American welfare state. Alan Derickson, Alan Kraut, and David Rosner, pioneering historians of immigrant and worker health, have provided continual and generous encouragement. Keith Wailoo's invitation to contribute to the project *A Death Retold* gave me my first opportunity to write about the health rights of the undocumented, which led to this book.

Researching and writing *Borders of Care* involved branching out into disciplines beyond my comfort zone, giving me the great privilege to learn from amazing scholars in migration and Latinx studies. I have mentioned as many as possible in the book's text and endnotes and would also like to express special gratitude for the work of Natalia Molina, Leo R. Chavez, John Mckiernan-González, Mae Ngai, Cybelle Fox, Carl Lindskoog, Chantel Rodríguez, and Michael Aguirre.

I am grateful for feedback on my research from audiences at Texas State University, Johns Hopkins University, Yale University, Boston College, the London School of Hygiene and Tropical Medicine, University College London, the World History Association, the Newberry Library Borderlands and Latina/o Studies Seminar, Loyola Stritch School of Medicine, NIU History Department Brown Bag Seminar, the American Association for the History of Nursing, the NIU Center for Latino and Latin American Studies, and the Latino Medical Student Association. For their efforts in hosting these talks I thank John McKiernan-González, Ahmed Ragab, Jeremy Greene, John Harley Warner, Naomi Rogers, Martin Summers, Stephen Colbrook, Ivón Padilla-Rodríguez, Emiliano Aguilar, María Eugenia López-García, Xócitl Bada, Mark Kuczewski, Brigid Lusk, Christina Abreu, Alex Mold, and Tammy

Proctor. Thank you to Samuel Roberts, Anne Pollock, Deborah Levine, Mical Raz, and David Courtwright, for entrusting me with the 2023 Garrison Lecture of the American Association for the History of Medicine.

I benefited from working on collaborative projects and publications led by Alex Mold, Laura Madokoro, Patti Lenard, Martin Halliwell, Sophie Jones, Ryan Essex, and Maggie Rivas Rodriguez. Teresa Ortiz Gómez, Esteban Rodríguez-Ocaña, Matt Murphy, and faculty and students at the Andalucian School of Public Health made my time in Granada, Spain, a transformative one. I was given a unique opportunity to develop many of the themes in *Borders of Care* by serving as guest curator for a National Library of Medicine "Outside/In" exhibition on immigrant health history, using photographs and archival materials from the library's collections. I am grateful to Patricia Tuohy, Jiwon Kim, and Erika Mills of the NLM Exhibition Program for their guidance and enthusiasm.

Many archivists and librarians helped with this project. I thank the staff of the Chicano/a Research Collection, Arizona State University; the Center for Southwest Research, University of New Mexico; the Walter Reuther Archives, Wayne State University; the Immigration History Research Center and Social Welfare Archives, University of Minnesota; the University of California, Santa Barbara; California State University, Los Angeles; Stanford University; and of all the other libraries and archives I cite in the book. When libraries were closed to the public during the pandemic, archivists and staff at the University of California, Los Angeles; San Diego State University; Stanford University; and California State University, Northridge worked hard to provide me with hundreds of pages of scanned materials.

Funding for my research travel was provided by Northern Illinois University's Division of Research and Innovation Partnerships, Center for Latino and Latin American Studies, and Department of History, led by Jerry Blazey, Christina Abreu, and Valerie Garver, respectively. I also benefited from two NIU sabbaticals. NIU's Office of Student Engagement and Experiential Learning and the College of Liberal Arts and Sciences provided stipends for the undergraduate student researchers who worked with me. Our union, the United Faculty Alliance of Northern Illinois University, successfully fought for research funds in our collective bargaining agreements. I thank Kristin Huffine, former acting director of the Center for Latino and Latin American Studies, for starting NIU's Latino Oral History Project and for encouraging me to teach Latino history. Valerie Garver deserves additional thanks for being the most supportive, compassionate, and effective department chair anyone could ever wish for.

I learned so much from the student researchers who contributed to this project: Betsania Salgado, Laura Vivaldo Cholula, Sandra Puebla, Stephanie Salazar, Ainsley Galvez, and Jackie Barranco. Working with the students of NIU's Dream Action changed my life, and Dra. Sandy López, NIU's director of Undocumented Student Services, is a constant inspiration. Dr. Mark Kuczewski welcomed visits from our aspiring physicians and nurses to Loyola Stritch School of Medicine. The amazing Jose Flores kindly allowed me to share his story and photo.

For reading and commenting on chapters, I am grateful to Tammy Proctor, Colleen O'Neill, Sarah Blue, Claire Barnes, Jennifer Nelson, Sean Farrell, Taylor Atkins, Kathy Bean, and Naomi Rogers. Any remaining errors are mine alone. Dana Yarak, the best writer I know, patiently read every line and hopefully helped me improve my prose. I also thank Dana for his work with Al Otro Lado supporting asylum seekers in Tijuana, and for conducting many of the oral history interviews with health care workers we used for our article "*La Primera Línea*: Latina/o Frontline Health Workers during COVID-19's First Wave."

Erika Mills and Casey Yarak provided essential help with images and photos. Thank you to Karen Darling and Fabiola Enríquez Flores of the University of Chicago Press for their guidance and expertise. I am so fortunate to be able to work with Karen on not just one, but two books! Mark Reschke provided meticulous copyediting. The anonymous reviewers of the proposal and manuscript provided eloquent commentary and excellent suggestions.

For their generous and steadfast support and kindness, and for always cheering me on, I thank Jessica Adler, Ted Brown, Martin Gorsky, Nic John Ramos, Susan Reverby, and Nancy Tomes.

Archives Consulted

Abbreviations following collection names are used in the endnotes.

ACT UP NY Historical Archive (online)
Arizona Historical Society, Tucson
    Medicine and Health Care Delivery in Southern Arizona Oral History Project
Arizona State Library, Phoenix
    Debi Wells Series, Papers of Governor Jane Dee Hull
Arizona State University, Tempe, Hayden Library
    Alianza Hispano Americana Papers (Alianza Papers)
    Maricopa County Organizing Project Records (MCOP Records)
Bracero History Archive (online)
California State Polytechnic University Pomona, Special Collections
    Douglas Adair United Farm Workers Collection
California State University, Los Angeles, Special Collections
    Gloria Arellanes Papers
California State University, Northridge, Special Collections and Archives
    MELA (Madre del Este de Los Angeles) Collection
Chicago History Museum, Chicago
    Mary McDowell Papers
Guantánamo Public Memory Project (online)
Huntington Library, San Marino, CA
    Edmund D. Edelman Papers
    Gloria Molina Papers
New York Public Library, New York
    Lillian Wald Papers
San Diego State University, Special Collections
    Enriqueta Chavez Papers

Grace Molina de Pick Papers

Samuel Hayakawa Papers

San Francisco Public Library

San Francisco Department of Public Health AIDS Office Records

San Francisco State University Archives

San Francisco Pride at Work Records

Stanford University Special Collections, Palo Alto, CA

Anne Loftis Papers

Centro de Acción Social Autónomo Papers

James Vizzard Papers

Mexican American Legal Defense and Educational Fund Records (MALDEF
Records)

Texas A&M University, Corpus Christi

Hector P. García Papers

University of California, Berkeley, Bancroft Library

National Council on Agricultural Life and Labor Records

Paul Taylor Papers

University of California, Los Angeles, Chicano Studies Research Center

Grace Montañez Davis Papers

Ron Lopez Papers

University of California, Los Angeles, Special Collections

Edward Roybal Papers

University of California, San Diego Library

Farmworkers Movement Documentation Project (FMDP) (online)

University of California, San Diego, Special Collections and Archives

American Friends Service Committee US-Mexico Border Program Records
(AFSC Papers)

Ben Yellen Papers

Herman Baca Papers

University of California, Santa Barbara, Special Collections

Alicia Escalante Papers

Comisión Feminil Mexicana Nacional Collection

Ricardo Cruz/Catolicos por la Raza Papers

University of Illinois, Chicago, Daley Library

Immigrants' Protective League Papers

University of Iowa, Iowa Women's Archives

Muscatine Migrant Committee Records

University of Minnesota, Minneapolis, Immigration History Research Center
Archives (IHRC)

Immigration and Refugee Services of America Collection

James V. Donnaruma Papers

University of Minnesota, Minneapolis, Social Welfare Archives

Henry Street Collection

University of New Mexico Center for Southwest Research, Albuquerque
    La Cooperación del Pueblo de Tierra Amarilla Collection
    Eduardo Hernandez-Chavez Papers
    Frank I. Sanchez Papers
University of Southern California, Los Angeles, ONE Gay and Lesbian Archives
    ACT UP/Los Angeles Records
University of Texas at Austin, Benson Library
    José Angel Gutiérrez Papers
Wayne State University, Walter Reuther Library, Detroit, MI
    Florida Christian Migrant Ministry Records
    Marion Moses M.D. Papers
    UFW Administration Files
    UFW-Arizona State Office Collection
    UFW Information and Research Files
Wisconsin Historical Society, Madison
    Chicago Religious Task Force on Central America Records
World Health Organization Archives, Geneva, Switzerland
    M5-372-4 Co-ordination with United Nations on the Protection of Social and
        Human Rights of Migrant Workers

Notes

Introduction

1. Kaiser Family Foundation, "Key Facts on Health Coverage of Immigrants," September 17, 2023, https://www.kff.org/racial-equity-and-health-policy/fact-sheet/key-facts-on-health-coverage-of-immigrants/; Hastings Center, "Undocumented Immigrants and Health Care Access in the United States," https://undocumented.thehastingscenter.org/issuebrief/health-care-use/.

2. "Health Insurance Coverage in the United States: 2020," U.S. Census Bureau, September 14, 2021, https://www.census.gov/library/publications/2021/demo/p60-274.html.

3. On the inequities and injustices of the US health care system, see, e.g., Luke Messac, *Your Money or Your Life: Debt Collection in American Medicine* (New York: Oxford University Press, 2023); Anne Pollock, *Sickening: Anti-Black Racism and Health Disparities in the United States* (Minneapolis: University of Minnesota Press, 2021); Elizabeth Rosenthal, *An American Sickness: How Healthcare Became Big Business and How You Can Take It Back* (New York: Penguin Press, 2017); Beatrix Hoffman, *Health Care for Some: Rights and Rationing in the United States since 1930* (Chicago: University of Chicago Press, 2012).

4. E.g., Claire Klobucista, "U.S. Life Expectancy Is in Decline. Why Aren't Other Countries Suffering the Same Problem?," Council on Foreign Relations, In Brief, September 8, 2022, https://www.cfr.org/in-brief/us-life-expectancy-decline-why-arent-other-countries-suffering-same-problem.

5. E.g., Roxane Dunbar-Ortiz, *Not "A Nation of Immigrants": Settler Colonialism, White Supremacy, and a History of Erasure and Exclusion* (Boston: Beacon Press, 2021); Stuart Anderson and David Miller, "Legal Immigrants: Waiting Forever," National Foundation for American Policy, 2006, http://www.nfap.com/researchactivities/studies/NFAPStudyLegalImmigrants WaitingForever052206.pdf; Aviva Chomsky, *Undocumented: How Immigration Became Illegal* (Boston: Beacon Press, 2014).

6. E.g., "Undocumented Immigrants," New American Economy, n.d., https://www.newamericaneconomy.org/issues/undocumented-immigrants/; Jeffrey S. Passel and D'Vera Cohn, "Industries of Unauthorized Immigrant Workers," Pew Research Center, November 3, 2016, https://www.pewresearch.org/race-and-ethnicity/2016/11/03/industries-of-unauthorized-immigrant-workers/; Mary Jo Dudley, "These U.S. Industries Can't Work without Illegal Immi-

grants," CBS News Moneywatch, January 10, 2019, https://www.cbsnews.com/news/illegal
-immigrants-us-jobs-economy-farm-workers-taxes/.

7. E.g., Alan M. Kraut, *Silent Travelers: Germs, Genes, and the Immigrant Menace* (Balti-more: Johns Hopkins University Press, 1994); Howard Markel, *When Germs Travel: Six Major Epidemics That Have Invaded America since 1900 and the Fears They Have Unleashed* (New York: Pantheon, 2004); Judith Walzer Leavitt, *Typhoid Mary: Captive to the Public's Health* (Boston: Beacon Press, 1996).

8. E.g., Dan Gordon, "Life in America: Hazardous to Immigrants' Health?," UCLA News-room, December 1, 2014, https://newsroom.ucla.edu/stories/life-in-america-hazardous-to-immigrants-health. Factors negatively affecting immigrants' health, which will be discussed throughout this book, include the dangers of migration, detention and border control, immi-gration raids, fear of deportation, workplace exploitation, poverty, denial of health care, lack of insurance, discrimination, and language barriers.

9. E.g., Roberta Bivins, *Contagious Communities: Medicine, Migration, and the NHS in Post War Britain* (Oxford: Oxford University Press, 2015); Diane Sainsbury, *Welfare States and Immi-grant Rights: The Politics of Inclusion and Exclusion* (Oxford: Oxford University Press, 2012); Beatrix Hoffman, "At the Borders of the Public: Immigrant and Migrant Publics and the Right to Health," in *Publics and Their Health: Historical Problems and Perspectives*, ed. Alex Mold, Peder Clark, and Hannah J. Elizabeth (Manchester: University of Manchester Press, 2023).

10. Associated Press, "What's EMTALA, the Patient Law Central in the Latest Supreme Court Abortion Case?," Health News Florida, April 24, 2024; Beatrix Hoffman, "Emergency Rooms: The Reluctant Safety Net," in *History and Health Policy: Bringing the Past Back In*, ed. Rosemary Stevens, Charles Rosenberg, and Lawton R. Burns (New Brunswick, NJ: Rutgers Uni-versity Press, 2006).

11. E.g., Elizabeth Trovall, "Immigrants' Taxes Play an Outsize Role in the U.S. Govern-ment's Fiscal Health," Marketplace.org, April 11, 2023, https://www.marketplace.org/2023/04/11/immigrants-taxes-play-an-outsized-role-in-the-u-s-governments-fiscal-health/; Andy J. Semo-tiuk, "New Report Details Huge Contribution Immigrants Are Making to America," Forbes.com, November 15, 2023, https://www.forbes.com/sites/andyjsemotiuk/2023/11/15/new-report-details-huge-contribution-immigrants-are-making-to-america/?sh=1ed490a12824; Jeanne Batalova, "Immigrant Health-Care Workers in the United States," Migration Information Source, April 7, 2023, https://www.migrationpolicy.org/article/immigrant-health-care-workers-united-states-2021; "The Impact of Immigrants on Health Care in the United States," Immigrant Learning Center, May 6, 2022, https://www.ilctr.org/the-impact-of-immigrants-on-health-care-in-the-united-states/.

12. E.g., Pia Orrenius, "Benefits of Immigration Outweigh the Cost," *The Catalyst: A Journal of Ideas from the Bush Institute*, no. 2, Spring 2016, https://www.bushcenter.org/catalyst/north-american-century/benefits-of-immigration-outweigh-costs; Stuart Anderson, "Immigrants Make Economies More Dynamic, Increase Employment Growth," *Forbes*, February 23, 2023, https://www.forbes.com/sites/stuartanderson/2023/02/23/immigrants-make-economies-more-dynamic-increase-employment-growth/?sh=57b18708427c.

13. E.g., Albert Prago, *Strangers in Their Own Land: A History of Mexican Americans* (New York: Four Winds Press, 1973). As legal scholar Kunal Parker writes, "Designation as foreign is not a function of coming from the territorial outside. It is a political strategy that has been used inside *and* outside the country and to multiple ends." *Making Foreigners: Immigration and Citizenship Law in America, 1600–2000* (New York: Cambridge University Press, 2015), ix.

Chapter One

1. Jeffrey Ostler and Nancy Shoemaker, "Settler Colonialism in Early American History: An Introduction," *William and Mary Quarterly* 76, no. 3 (July 2019): 361–68; David Weber, *The Spanish Frontier in North America* (New Haven, CT: Yale University Press, 1992); Robert H. Jackson, "The Dynamic of Indian Demographic Collapse in the San Francisco Bay Missions, Alta California, 1776–1840," *American Indian Quarterly* 16, no. 2 (Spring 1992): 141–56.

2. Henry Harris, *California's Medical Story* (San Francisco: J. W. Stacey, 1932); Joe Rayl McBride et al., "Exchange of Medicinal Plant information in California Missions," *Journal of Ethnobiology and Ethnomedicine* 16 (2020); Pat Ireland Nixon, MD, *A Century of Medicine in San Antonio* (San Antonio, self-published, 1936), 73. See also P. I. Nixon, "Chaparro Amargosa in the Treatment of Amebic Dysentery," *Journal of the American Medical Association*, May 16, 1914, https://jamanetwork.com/journals/jama/article-abstract/455327.

3. Weber, *The Spanish Frontier in North America*, 316.

4. John Mckiernan-González, *Fevered Measures: Public Health and Race at the Texas-Mexico Border, 1848–1942* (Durham, NC: Duke University Press, 2012), 22; Mark Allan Goldberg, *Conquering Sickness: Race, Health, and Colonization in the Texas Borderlands* (Lincoln: University of Nebraska Press, 2016), 25–26. Inoculation campaigns had occurred earlier, including one led by George Washington during the Revolutionary War, but that involved live smallpox (inoculation) rather than the safer cowpox (vaccination).

5. Chester R. Burns, "Health and Medicine," Texas State Historical Association, Handbook of Texas, https://www.tshaonline.org/handbook/entries/health-and-medicine; Goldberg, *Conquering Sickness*, 22.

6. Nixon, *A Century of Medicine in San Antonio*, 16–17, 25.

7. Nixon, 28.

8. Nixon, 44–48.

9. Nixon, 73.

10. Jorge A. Hernández, "Merchants and Mercenaries: Anglo-Americans in Mexico's Northeast," *New Mexico Historical Review* 75, no. 1 (2000): 43–75, 50–52.

11. Noah Smithwick, *The Evolution of a State* (1900), quoted (without comment) in Nixon, *A Century of Medicine in San Antonio*, 42–43. This incident is also mentioned in Andrés Reséndes, *Changing National Identities at the Frontier: Texas and New Mexico, 1800–1859* (Cambridge: Cambridge University Press, 2005), 109.

12. On the age of "heroic" treatments, see, e.g., John Harley Warner, *The Therapeutic Perspective: Medical Practice, Knowledge, and Identity in America, 1820–1885* (Princeton, NJ: Princeton University Press, 2014).

13. Goldberg, *Conquering Sickness*, 141, 155, chap. 5.

14. Nixon, *A Century of Medicine in San Antonio*, 98.

15. "¿Tendremos un hospital?" (Will we have a hospital?), *El Bejareño*, June 9, 1855 (Hispanic American Newspapers database). Translation by the author.

16. Board members are listed in Nixon, *A Century of Medicine in San Antonio*, 117–18.

17. David Montejano, *Anglos and Mexicans in the Making of Texas, 1836–1986* (Austin: University of Texas Press, 1987), 29.

18. John Carranza, "Stability and Care: Establishing the Santa Rosa Infirmary in a Frontier City," *Synapsis: A Health Humanities Journal*, November 1, 2017, https://medicalhealthhumanities.com/2017/11/01/stability-and-care-establishing-the-santa-rosa-infirmary-in-a-frontier-city/.

19. E.g., Parker, *Making Foreigners*; David J. Weber, *Foreigners in their Native Land: Historical Roots of the Mexican Americans* (Albuquerque: University of New Mexico Press, 2004).

20. E.g., Goldberg, *Conquering Sickness*; McKiernan-Gonzalez, *Fevered Measures*; Natalia Molina, *How Race Is Made in America: Immigration, Citizenship, and the Historical Power of Racial Scripts* (Berkeley: University of California Press, 2014).

21. Albert Camarillo, *Chicanos in a Changing Society: From Mexican Pueblos to American Barrios in Santa Barbara and Southern California, 1848–1930* (Cambridge, MA: Harvard University Press, 1979), 66–67.

22. Mario T. García, *Desert Immigrants: The Mexicans of El Paso, 1880–1920* (New Haven, CT: Yale University Press, 1981), 136–39, 146.

23. Natalia Molina, *Fit to Be Citizens? Public Health and Race in Los Angeles, 1879–1939* (Berkeley: University of California Press, 2006), 90.

24. Guenter B. Risse, "Translating Western Modernity: The First Chinese Hospital in America," *Bulletin of the History of Medicine* 85, no. 3 (Fall 2011): 413–47, 420.

25. "County Hospital," *Daily Alta California* 33, no. 11536 (November 20, 1881): 1 (California Digital Newspaper Collection); Nayan Shah, *Contagious Divides: Epidemics and Race in San Francisco's Chinatown* (Berkeley: University of California Press, 2001), 70–71.

26. "County Hospital."

27. Erika Lee, *At America's Gates: Chinese Immigration during the Exclusion Era, 1882–1943* (Chapel Hill: University of North Carolina Press, 2003), 4.

28. Lee, 53–54.

29. Lee, 56.

30. H. M. Lai, "Island of Immortals: Chinese Immigrants and the Angel Island Immigration Station," *California History* 57, no. 1 (Spring, 1978): 95–98. See also Shah, *Contagious Divides*, chap. 7.

31. Cian T. McMahon, *The Coffin Ship: Life and Death at Sea during the Great Irish Famine* (New York: New York University Press, 2021), 4.

32. McMahon; Alan M. Kraut, "Plagues and Prejudice: Nativism's Construction of Disease in Nineteenth- and Twentieth-Century New York City," in *Hives of Sickness: Public Health and Epidemics in New York City*, ed. David Rosner (New Brunswick, NJ: Rutgers University Press, 1995), 67.

33. Kraut, *Silent Travelers*, 33.

34. John Freeman Gill, "A Quarantine Hospital So Unwelcome That New Yorkers Burned It Down," *New York Times*, May 8, 2020.

35. Hidetaka Hirota, *Expelling the Poor: Atlantic Seaboard States and the Nineteenth-Century Origins of American Immigration Policy* (New York: Oxford University Press, 2016), 92.

36. Kathryn Stephenson, "The Quarantine War: The Burning of the New York Marine Hospital in 1858," *Public Health Reports* 119, no. 1 (January–February 2004): 79–92.

37. David Oshinsky, *Bellevue: Three Centuries of Medicine and Mayhem and America's Most Storied Hospital* (New York: Doubleday, 2016), 107.

38. Charles Rosenberg, *The Care of Strangers: The Rise of America's Hospital System* (New York: Basic Books, 1987), 42; Hirota, *Expelling the Poor*, 51, 59; Oshinsky, *Bellevue*, 54–56.

39. Hirota, *Expelling the Poor*, 105.

40. Cybelle Fox, *Three Worlds of Relief: Race, Immigration, and the American Welfare State from the Progressive Era to the New Deal* (Princeton, NJ: Princeton University Press, 2012), 131–32; Hirota, *Expelling the Poor*, 201.

41. Amy Fairchild, *Science at the Borders: Immigrant Medical Inspection and the Shaping of the Modern Industrial Labor Force* (Baltimore, MD: Johns Hopkins University Press, 2003); Kraut, *Silent Travelers*, 4.

42. Howard Markel, *Quarantine! East European Jewish Immigrants and the New York City Epidemics of 1892* (Baltimore, MD: Johns Hopkins University Press, 1997), 131.

43. *Arbeiter Zeitung* quoted in Markel, 113.

44. Gail Farr Casterline, "St. Joseph's and St. Mary's: The Origins of Catholic Hospitals in Philadelphia," *Pennsylvania Magazine of History and Biography* 108, no. 3 (July 1984): 289–314; Barbra Mann Wall, *American Catholic Hospitals: A Century of Changing Markets and Missions* (New Brunswick, NJ: Rutgers University Press, 2011), 10–11.

45. Casterline, "St. Joseph's and St. Mary's," 299–300.

46. Alan M. Kraut and Deborah A. Kraut, *Covenant of Care: Newark Beth Israel and the Jewish Hospital in America* (New Brunswick, NJ: Rutgers University Press, 2007), 2–5; Edward C. Halperin, "The Rise and Fall of the American Jewish Hospital," *Academic Medicine* 87, no. 5 (May 2012): 610–14.

47. Rosenberg, *The Care of Strangers*, 112.

48. James Donnaruma to George Palmieri, April 14, 1923, Box 2, Folder 11, James V. Donnaruma Papers, Immigration History Research Center Archives, University of Minnesota (hereafter IHRC Archives).

49. Vanessa Gamble, *Making a Place for Ourselves: The Black Hospital Movement* (New York: Oxford University Press, 1995).

50. Casterline, "St. Joseph's and St. Mary's," 299–300; David Rosner, *A Once Charitable Enterprise: Hospitals and Health Care in Brooklyn and New York* (Cambridge: Cambridge University Press, 1982).

51. Risse, "Translating Western Modernity," 421–22.

52. Kenneth H. Marcus and Yong Chen, "Inside and Outside Chinatown: Chinese Elites in Exclusion Era California," *Pacific Historical Review* 80, no. 3 (August 2011): 369–400; Tamara Venit Shelton, "Curiosity or Cure? Chinese Medicine and American Orientalism in Progressive Era California and Oregon," *Oregon Historical Quarterly* 114, no. 3 (Fall 2013): 266–91.

53. Risse, "Translating Western Modernity," 421–33; Shah, *Contagious Divides*, 212.

54. Risse, "Translating Western Modernity," 433–40.

55. Shah, *Contagious Divides*, 212–13; "Chinese Hospital: History," chinesehospital-sf.org, https://chinesehospital-sf.org/history/.

56. Leonard Pitt, *The Decline of the Californios: A Social History of Spanish-Speaking Californians, 1846–1890* (Berkeley: University of California Press, 1999), 224, 265–66; Cecilia Rasmussen, "A Hospital That Made History and Preserved It," *Los Angeles Times*, October 1, 2000. The same order of nuns was sometimes called the Sisters of Charity.

57. Rasmussen, "A Hospital That Made History and Preserved It"; Pitt, *Decline of the Californios*.

58. "La 'Cruz Azul Mexicana' de este Ciudad, esta cumpliendo su Mision; La Fundacion de un Hospital para nuestra Colonia es una Obra muy Urgente," *La Prensa* (Los Angeles), October 2, 1921, 1 (Hispanic American Newspapers).

59. Casterline, "St. Joseph's and St. Mary's," 293; Rosenberg, *The Care of Strangers*, 113; Risse, "Translating Western Modernity"; National Jewish Health, "Our History," https://www.nationaljewish.org/about/history. For more on the founding of the National Jewish Hospital in Denver, see Kraut, *Silent Travelers*, 203–6.

60. Markel, *Quarantine!*, 36–37.

61. For a history of the profession, see Karen Buhler-Wilkerson, *False Dawn: The Rise and Decline of Public Health Nursing* (New Brunswick, NJ: Rutgers University Press, reprint, 2021).

62. *Report of the Henry Street Settlement, 1893–1913*, 15; *The Henry Street Settlement 1893–1918*, Box 84, Folder 5, Henry Street Collection, Social Welfare Archives, University of Minnesota; Diane Hamilton, "The Cost of Caring: The Metropolitan Life Insurance Company's Visiting Nursing Service, 1909–1953," *Bulletin of the History of Medicine* 63, no. 3 (Fall 1989): 414–34.

63. *Henry Street Nurse*, no. 2 (February 1921): 10. All issues of this journal cited are in Box 85, Henry Street Collection, Social Welfare Archives.

64. *Henry Street Nurse*, no. 2 (February 1921): 10.

65. *Henry Street Nurse* 2, no. 4 (April 1921): 9.

66. *Henry Street Nurse*, no. 2 (February 1921): 6.

67. Quote from *Trained Nurse and Hospital Review*, 1934, reprinted in Wald's memorial service. Lillian Wald Papers (Reel 1), New York Public Library.

68. "Contributor's Column," *Henry Street Nurse* 2, nos. 10–11 (June–July 1922): 9.

69. See, e.g., Marco H. D. Van Leeuwen, "Guilds and Middle-Class Welfare, 1550–1800: Provisions for Burial, Sickness, Old Age, and Widowhood," *Economic History Review* 65, no. 1 (February 2012): 61–90; "'Sou-sou': Black Immigrants Bring Savings Club Stateside," *Grio*, May 20, 2011, https://thegrio.com/2011/05/20/sou-sou-black-immigrants-bring-savings-club-stateside/.

70. José Amaro Hernández, *Mutual Aid for Survival: The Case of the Mexican American* (Malabar, FL: Krieger, 1983), 3.

71. Hernández, 16–17.

72. Julie Leininger Pycior, "*Sociedades Mutualistas*," Handbook of Texas, https://www.tsha online.org/handbook/entries/sociedades-mutualistas.

73. Hernández, *Mutual Aid for Survival*, 75–76.

74. James B. McBride, "The *Liga Protectora Latina*: A Mexican-American Benevolent Society in Arizona," *Journal of the West* 14 (October 1975): 82–90; Hernández, *Mutual Aid for Survival*, 63–65.

75. *Alianza* 23, no. 9 (September 1930), Box 127, Folder 5, Alianza Hispano Americana Papers, Hayden Library, Arizona State University (hereafter Alianza Papers).

76. Kaye Lynn Briegel, "Alianza Hispano-Americana, 1894–1965: A Mexican American Fraternal Insurance Society," PhD diss., University of Southern California, 1974.

77. "Estatutos Generales de la Alianza Hispano-Americana," May 1937, Box 116, Folder 1; Membership file of Faustina Olguin, b. Fronteras, Sonora 1889 indicating "nacionalidad Mexicana," Box 1, Folder 10, Alianza Papers.

78. Francisco E. Balderrama, *In Defense of La Raza: The Los Angeles Mexican Consulate and the Mexican Community, 1929 to 1936* (Tucson: University of Arizona Press, 1982), 39–40. Today, the consulate continues to be involved in health care for Mexican residents. See Raúl Necochea López, "Mexico's Health Diplomacy and the Ventanilla de Salud Program," *Latino Studies* 16 (2018): 482–502.

79. Robert Ernst, *Immigrant Life in New York City, 1825–1863* (New York: Columbia University Press, 1949), 56; Kraut and Kraut, *Covenant of Care*, 7; John Foster Carr, *Guide to the United States for the Jewish Immigrant: A Nearly Literal Translation of the Second Yiddish Edition* (New York: Immigrant Publication Society, 1916), 9, Newberry Library Special Collections.

80. Daniel Soyer, *Jewish Immigrant Associations and American Identity in New York, 1880–1939* (Detroit: Wayne State University Press, 1997), 1.

81. Soyer, *Jewish Immigrant Associations*, 95, 99, 143–44.

82. Gary R. Mormino and George E. Pozzetta, "The Cradle of Mutual Aid: Immigrant Co-operative Societies in Ybor City," *Tampa Bay History* 7, no. 2 (Fall/Winter 1985): 36–58, 37–47; Nancy Hewitt, *Southern Discomfort: Women's Activism in Tampa, Florida, 1880s–1920s* (Urbana and Chicago: University of Illinois Press, 2001). See also Sarah McNamara, *Ybor City: Crucible of the Latina South* (Chapel Hill: University of North Carolina Press, 2023).

83. Mormino and Pozzetta, "The Cradle of Mutual Aid"; Durward Long, "An Immigrant Co-operative Medicine Program in the South, 1887–1963," *Journal of Southern History* 31, no. 4 (November 1965): 417–34, 431; Hewitt, *Southern Discomfort*, 204.

84. Mormino and Pozzetta, "The Cradle of Mutual Aid."

85. Finding aid, Sociedad La Unión Martí-Maceo Records, University of South Florida Special Collections, https://archives.lib.usf.edu/repositories/2/resources/534.

86. Nancy Raquel Mirabal, "The Afro-Cuban Community in Ybor City and Tampa, 1886–1910," *OAH Magazine of History* 7, no. 4 (Summer, 1993): 19–22; Susan D. Greenbaum, *More than Black: Afro-Cubans in Tampa* (Gainesville: University Press of Florida, 2002), 156.

87. *El Organizador* 1 de Diciembre 1944, Box 127, Folder 4, Alianza Papers; Hernandez, *Mutual Aid for Survival*, 54.

88. Hernández, *Mutual Aid for Survival*, 137.

89. Soyer, *Jewish Immigrant Associations*, 143–44.

90. Mormino and Pozzetta, "The Cradle of Mutual Aid," 51.

91. Debbie Michaels, "Railroads, Physicians, and Hospitals," November 2017, AmericanNursingHistory.org, https://www.americannursinghistory.org/railroad-physicians-and-hospitals.

92. Mark Aldrich, "Train Wrecks to Typhoid Fever: The Development of Railroad Medicine Organizations, 1850 to World War I," *Bulletin of the History of Medicine* 75, no. 2 (Summer 2001): 254–89; J. Roy Jones, "The Old Central Pacific Hospital," Central Pacific Railroad Photographic History Museum, http://cprr.org/Museum/CPRR_Hospital.html; "The Railroad Hospital," *Sacramento Daily Union* 62, no. 40 (October 1889) (California Digital Newspaper Collection). It appears that Mexican track workers did not undergo discrimination by railroad hospitals, although more research is required to confirm this; Larry Mullaly post, "Southern Pacific Railroad Hospital in 1907" discussion, CPRR Discussion Group listserv, May 2, 2010, http://discussion.cprr.net /2010/05/dan-krieger-train-wreck-victims.html. See also Jeffrey Marcos Garcílazo, *Traqueros: Mexican Railroad Workers in the United States, 1870–1930* (Denton: University of North Texas Press, 2012); William F. Chew, *Nameless Builders of the Transcontinental Railroad: The Chinese Workers of the Central Pacific Railroad* (Bloomington, IN: Trafford Publishing, 2004).

93. Stephen J. Pitti, *The Devil in Silicon Valley: Northern California, Race, and Mexican Americans* (Princeton, NJ: Princeton University Press, 2003), 58–60, 63–64. Thanks also to Dana Yarak for sharing his research on the New Almadén mines.

94. Alan Derickson, "Naphtha Drunks, Lead Colic, and the Smelter Shakes: The Inordinate Exposure of Immigrant Workers to Occupational Health Hazards at the Turn of the Twentieth Century," *Journal of American Ethnic History* 37, no. 2 (Winter 2018): 37–61, 55.

95. Hernández, *Mutual Aid for Survival*, 41.

96. *Bisbee Daily Review*, quoted in Joseph F. Park, "The 1903 'Mexican Affair' at Clifton," *Journal of Arizona History* 18, no. 2 (Summer 1977): 19–148, 142; Linda Gordon, *The Great Arizona Orphan Abduction* (Cambridge, MA: Harvard University Press, 1999), 222.

97. Alan Derickson, *Workers' Health, Workers' Democracy: The Western Miners' Struggle, 1891–1925* (Ithaca, NY: Cornell University Press, 1988), 101–6, 120–21.

98. "Unbelievable Conditions at Durst Hop Ranch Caused the Riot Says Official Report," *Stockton Independent*, February 14, 1914 (California Digital Newspaper Collection).

99. "Oriental and Mexican Labor Unions and Strikes in California Agriculture," in *A Documentary History of Migratory Farm Labor in California*, ed. Raymond P. Barry (Oakland, CA: Federal Writers' Project, 1938), 1–3, 11.

100. "Unbelievable Conditions at Durst Hop Ranch."

101. Greg Hall, *Harvest Wobblies: The Industrial Workers of the World and Agricultural Labor in the American West* (Corvallis: Oregon State University Press, 2001), 51; Cletus E. Daniel, *Bitter Harvest: A History of California Farmworkers, 1870–1941* (Berkeley: University of California Press, 1981), 91.

102. Alice Hamilton, *Exploring the Dangerous Trades*, quoted in Derickson, "Naphtha Drunks," 43–44. See also Kraut, *Silent Travelers*, chap. 7.

103. Leo Price, "Health Program of International Ladies' Garment Workers' Union," *Monthly Labor Review* 49, no. 4 (October 1939): 811–29. The Union Health Center still exists today and still provides care for a primarily immigrant garment industry workforce.

104. Robert K. Murray, *Red Scare: A Study in National Hysteria, 1919–1920* (Minneapolis: University of Minnesota Press, 1955); Beatrix Hoffman, *The Wages of Sickness: The Politics of Health Insurance in Progressive America* (Chapel Hill: University of North Carolina Press, 2001), 158.

105. Hoffman, *The Wages of Sickness*, 117.

106. David Segal, "Why Are There Almost No Memorials to the Flu of 1918?," *New York Times*, May 14, 2020.

107. Marian Moser Jones, "The American Red Cross and Local Response to the 1918 Influenza Pandemic: A Four-City Case Study," *Public Health Reports* 125, Supp. 3 (2010): 92–104, 100. See also Alan M. Kraut, "Immigration, Ethnicity, and the Pandemic," *Public Health Reports* 125, Supp. 3 (2010): 123–33.

108. García, *Desert Immigrants*, 146; Emily K. Abel, "'Only the Best Class of Immigration': Public Health Policy toward Mexicans and Filipinos in Los Angeles, 1910–1940," *American Journal of Public Health* 94, no. 6 (June 2004): 932–39.

Chapter Two

1. See, e.g., Erika Lee, *America for Americans: A History of Xenophobia in the United States* (New York: Basic Books, 2019). Roxanne Dunbar-Ortiz also points out that the phrase "nation of immigrants" "works to erase the scourge of settler colonialism and the lives of Indigenous peoples" and also ignores enslaved Africans. Dunbar-Ortiz, *Not "A Nation of Immigrants,"* xi–xii.

2. "The Immigration Act of 1924 (The Johnson-Reed Act)," Office of the Historian, Department of State, https://history.state.gov/milestones/1921-1936/immigration-act#:~:text=The %201917%20Act%20implemented%20a,decisions%20over%20whom%20to%20exclude.

3. Lee, *America for Americans*; Roger Daniels, *Guarding the Golden Door: American Immigration Policy and Immigrants since 1882* (New York: Hill and Wang, 2005); Mae Ngai, *Impossible Subjects: Illegal Aliens and the Making of Modern America* (Princeton, NJ: Princeton University Press, 2004). Japan had voluntarily limited immigration of its subjects under the 1907 "Gentlemen's Agreement," and Filipino people were US colonial subjects and not barred from entry. Black noncitizens became eligible for naturalization in 1870.

4. Ngai, *Impossible Subjects*, 77–79; Natalia Molina, "'In a Race All Their Own': The Quest to Make Mexicans Ineligible for U.S. Citizenship," *Pacific Historical Review* 79, no. 2 (May 2010): 167–201.

5. US House of Representatives, Committee on Immigration and Naturalization, *Immigration from Countries in the Western Hemisphere*, February 21 to April 25, 1928 (Washington, DC:

US Government Printing Office, 1928), 91–93; US House of Representatives, Committee on Immigration and Naturalization, *Lack of Funds for Deportations*, January 5, 1928 (Washington, DC: US Government Printing Office, 1928), 89–90.

6. *Immigration from Countries in the Western Hemisphere*, 99–101.

7. Ngai, *Impossible Subjects*, 81. On the origins of the Border Patrol, which initially targeted Chinese, Europeans, and other groups rather than Mexicans, see Kelly Lytle Hernandez, *Migra! A History of the U.S. Border Patrol* (Berkeley: University of California Press, 2010).

8. Mckiernan-González, *Fevered Measures*, 183–89; Alexandra Minna Stern, *Eugenic Nation: Faults and Frontiers of Better Breeding in Modern America* (Berkeley: University of California Press, 2005), 61–63; "Auburn-Haired Amazon at Santa Fe Street Bridge Leads Feminine Outbreak," *El Paso Times*, January, 29, 1917, 1.

9. "Depicts Mexican Immigrants as Health Menace," *Chicago Daily Tribune*, October 19, 1928, 20; Benjamin Goldberg, MD, "Tuberculosis in Racial Types with Special Reference to Mexicans," *American Journal of Public Health* 19 (1929): 274–84, 283; Don D. Lescohier, "The Vital Problem in Mexican Immigration," *Proceedings of the National Conference of Social Work* (1927), 547–54, 553.

10. On tuberculosis among the Irish, see Michael M. Davis, *Immigrant Health and the Community* (New York: Harper & Bros., 1921), 53–57. For an incisive history of tuberculosis and race, see Samuel Kelton Roberts Jr., *Infectious Fear: Politics, Disease, and the Health Effects of Segregation* (Chapel Hill: University of North Carolina Press, 2009).

11. Goldberg, "Tuberculosis in Racial Types," 280.

12. Goldberg, 280–81.

13. Zaragosa Vargas, *Labor Rights Are Civil Rights: Mexican-American Workers in Twentieth-Century America* (Princeton, NJ: Princeton University Press, 2007), 129.

14. Emily K. Abel, "From Exclusion to Expulsion: Mexicans and Tuberculosis Control in Los Angeles, 1914–1940," *Bulletin of the History of Medicine* 77, no. 4 (Winter 2003): 823–49, 835–36.

15. Abel, 825.

16. Mary Melcher, "Times of Crisis and Joy: Pregnancy, Childbirth, and Mothering in Rural Arizona, 1910–1940," *Journal of Arizona History* 40, no. 2 (Summer 1999): 181–200, 195, 192.

17. J. Stanley Lemons, "The Sheppard-Towner Act: Progressivism in the 1920s," *Journal of American History* 55, no. 4 (March 1969): 776–86; Molly Ladd-Taylor, *Mother-Work: Women, Child Welfare, and the State, 1890–1930* (Urbana: University of Illinois Press, 1994).

18. "Report on the Midwife Survey in Texas, January 2, 1925," quoted in Molly Ladd-Taylor, "'Grannies' and 'Spinsters': Midwife Education under the Sheppard-Towner Act," *Journal of Social History* 22, no. 2 (Winter 1988): 255–75, 260.

19. Ladd-Taylor, "'Grannies' and 'Spinsters,'" 266.

20. Sandra Shackel, *Social Housekeepers: Women Shaping Public Policy in New Mexico, 1920–1940* (Albuquerque: University of New Mexico Press, 1992), 38.

21. Melcher, "Times of Crisis and Joy," 195.

22. Melcher.

23. Ladd-Taylor, "'Grannies' and 'Spinsters,'" 267–70.

24. Lemons, "The Sheppard-Towner Act," 780–81; Mrs. H. K. Schoff, *Congressional Record*, 69 Cong., 2 Sess. (January 8, 1927), 1281.

25. For example, in Newark, New Jersey, in the 1910s, "The infant mortality rate [was] lowest among the babies whose mothers are attended by midwives" rather than physicians or hospital births. Maternal deaths were also less common in midwife-assisted births. Davis, *Immigrant Health and the Community*, 213–15.

26. Excerpt, *Health News*, Albany, NY, November 28, 1927, 190, Box 57, Folder 18, Immigration and Refugee Services of America Collection, IHRC Archives.

27. On the continuation of midwifery, see, e.g., Jenny M. Luke, *Delivered by Midwives: African-American Midwifery in the Twentieth-Century South* (Oxford: University Press of Mississippi, 2018); Lena McQuade-Salzfass, "'An Indispensable Service': Midwives and Medical Officials after New Mexico Statehood," in *Precarious Prescriptions: Contested Histories of Race and Health in North America*, ed. Laurie B. Green, John Mckiernan-González, and Martin Summers (Minneapolis: University of Minnesota Press, 2014); Susan L. Smith, *Japanese American Midwives: Culture, Community, and Health Politics, 1880–1950* (Urbana: University of Illinois Press, 2005); Molina, *Fit to Be Citizens?*, 103–5.

28. Rose Anne Rennie, "Union Settlement Health Service Report, February 1934"; "Study of the Health Examinations of the Henry Street Settlement," n.d. ca 1929, both in Box 60, Folder 3, Henry Street Collection, Social Welfare Archives. On the assimilation and "whitening" of immigrant groups, see, e.g., Thomas A. Guglielmo, *White on Arrival: Italians, Race, Color, and Power in Chicago, 1890–1945* (New York: Oxford University Press, 2003).

29. "Alien Study" (1937), Box 17, Folder 7, Henry Street Collection, Social Welfare Archives.

30. "A Department of Citizenship and Naturalization at Hull House," October 1, 1935, Box 4, Folder 44; "Types of New Cases Which Now Come to the Immigrants' Protective League," April 22, 1931, Box 4, Folder 44, Immigrants' Protective League Papers, Daley Library, University of Illinois Chicago.

31. "Families Separated by Deportation," December 1932, Box 4, Folder 44, Immigrants' Protective League Papers.

32. "Families Separated by Deportation."

33. Shah, *Contagious Divides*, 213. On the 1923 *Thind* decision making South Asians ineligible for citizenship by deeming them nonwhite, and other legal decisions that kept Asians from citizenship, see, e.g., Ngai, *Impossible Subjects*, 64–76.

34. Shah, *Contagious Divides*, 212.

35. Molina, *Fit to Be Citizens?*, 75, 90. See also Abel, "'Only the Best Class of Immigration.'"

36. Goldberg, "Tuberculosis in Racial Types." Goldberg's arguments were refuted by Emil Bogen, MD, in the *American Review of Tuberculosis* in 1931. Bogen argued that TB was overdiagnosed in Mexicans and that the primary causes were environmental, not racial; Molina, *Fit to Be Citizens?*, 135.

37. "Report of the Mexican Work at the University of Chicago Settlement 1929–1930," "Mexican Work, October 1930," "Report of Mexican Case Work, 1931," all in Box 21, Mary McDowell Papers, Chicago History Museum.

38. Quoted in Gabriela F. Arredondo, *Mexican Chicago: Race, Identity, and Nation, 1916–39* (Urbana: University of Illinois Press, 2008), 95.

39. Agnes K. Hanna, "Social Services on the Mexican Border," *Proceedings of the National Conference of Social Work* (1935), 700–701.

40. Fox, *Three Worlds of Relief*, 153.

41. Goldberg, Tuberculosis in Racial Types," 284.

42. Fox, *Three Worlds of Relief*, 127.

43. Francisco E. Balderrama and Raymond Rodríguez, *Decade of Betrayal: Mexican Repatriation in the 1930s* (Albuquerque: University of New Mexico Press, 2006), 72–74; Antonio Olivo, "Ghosts of a 1931 Raid," *Los Angeles Times*, February 25, 2001.

44. Neil Betten and Raymond A. Mohl, "From Discrimination to Repatriation: Mexican Life

in Gary, Indiana, during the Great Depression," *Pacific Historical Review* 42, no. 3 (August 1973): 370–88, 373–74, 382.

45. Fox, *Three Worlds of Relief*, 134.

46. Abel, "From Exclusion to Expulsion," 844.

47. Abraham Hoffman, *Unwanted Mexican Americans in the Great Depression: Repatriation Pressures, 1929-1939* (Tucson: University of Arizona Press, 1974), 115; Balderrama and Rodríguez, *Decade of Betrayal*.

48. Abel, "'Only the Best Class of Immigration'"; Abel, "From Exclusion to Expulsion," 843–44.

49. Molina, *Fit to Be Citizens?*, 139–40.

50. Balderrama and Rodríguez, *Decade of Betrayal*, 132–33. The "carted across the line" phrase is from Carey McWilliams, "Getting Rid of the Mexican," *American Mercury* 28 (March 1933): 322–24.

51. Balderrama and Rodríguez, *Decade of Betrayal*, 140–41; Betten and Mohl, "From Discrimination to Repatriation," 386.

52. Abel, "From Exclusion to Expulsion," 847.

53. Balderrama and Rodríguez, *Decade of Betrayal*, 247, 308.

54. Fox, *Three Worlds of Relief*, 163, 183; one million figure, Balderrama and Rodríguez, *Decade of Betrayal*.

55. For examples, see Balderrama and Rodríguez, *Decade of Betrayal*.

56. Fox, *Three Worlds of Relief*, 148.

57. Comite de Beneficencia Mexicana, "Mr. Chairman, Ladies and Gentlemen," 1931; untitled typescript, n.d., both in Box 20, Folder 6, Ron Lopez Papers, UCLA Chicano Studies Research Center; Balderrama, *In Defense of La Raza*, 26, 42. On the founding of the Comite de Beneficencia, see Balderrama, 37–46.

58. Balderrama, *In Defense of La Raza*, 24–28, 31–32.

59. Amelia Sears and Joseph Moss, quoted in Fox, *Three Worlds of Relief*, 137–38.

60. Fox, *Three Worlds of Relief*, 140, 143.

61. "Mexican Work, October 1930," "Mexican Case Work, November 1931," Box 21, Folder "Mexican Work (Reports)," McDowell Papers.

62. Molina, *Fit to Be Citizens?*, 121, 125, 127.

63. Mexican Work Reports, March 1932, November 1, 1932, Box 21, Folder "Mexican Work (Reports)," McDowell Papers; Fox, *Three Worlds of Relief*, 139; "10,000 Chicagoans Join 'Hunger March,'" *New York Times*, November 1, 1932, 3.

64. Fox, *Three Worlds of Relief*, 151.

65. The Spanish-American Society was founded in Tucson in the 1890s and apparently provided medical care; one of its officers was the "Supreme Physician." James Henry McClintock, *Arizona: The Youngest State* (Chicago: S. J. Clarke Publishing Company, 1916), 847.

66. Michael Grey, *New Deal Medicine: The Rural Health Programs of the Farm Security Administration* (Baltimore, MD: Johns Hopkins University Press, 1999), 27; Verónica Martínez-Matsuda, *Migrant Citizenship: Race, Rights, and Reform in the U.S. Farm Labor Camp Program* (Philadelphia: University of Pennsylvania Press, 2020), 152.

67. Anita E. Faverman, MD, "A Study of the Health of 1,000 Children of Migratory Agricultural Laborers in California," July 1936–June 1937, 16, 22–24, Box 15, Folder 51, Paul Taylor Papers, Bancroft Library, University of California, Berkeley.

68. Joe Smith and Clifford F. Baughman, "Survey of Kern County Migratory Labor Pro-

gram," July 1, 1938, Box 15, Folder 54, Paul Taylor Papers. These studies mentioned but did not systematically record racial/ethnic categories.

69. Faverman, "A Study of the Health of 1,000 Children of Migratory Agricultural Laborers in California," 31–36.

70. Bertha S. Underhill, "A Study of 132 Families in California Cotton Camps with Reference to Availability of Medical Care," 1937, 3, 23–31, Box 15, Folder 52, Paul Taylor Papers. On the migrant stream, see, e.g., John Weber, *From South Texas to the Nation: The Exploitation of Mexican Labor in the Twentieth Century* (Chapel Hill: University of North Carolina Press, 2015).

71. Martínez-Matsuda, *Migrant Citizenship*, 156, 153.

72. Grey, *New Deal Medicine*, 82–83.

73. Martínez-Matsuda, *Migrant Citizenship*, 156.

74. Verónica Martínez-Matsuda, "'A Transformation for Migrants': Mexican Farmworkers and Federal Health Reform during the New Deal Era," in *Precarious Prescriptions: Contested Histories of Race and Health in North America*, ed. Laurie B. Green, John McKiernan-Gonzalez, and Martin Summers (Minneapolis: University of Minnesota Press, 2014); Martínez-Matsuda, *Migrant Citizenship*, 147–48.

75. Faverman, "A Study of the Health of 1,000 Children of Migratory Agricultural Laborers in California," 5–6, 9.

76. Brandt Ayers, "Living Different under U.S. Control," *Raleigh Times*, July 3–7, 1961, reprinted in *Health Clinics for Migratory Farmworkers: Hearing before a Subcommittee of the Committee on Interstate and Foreign Commerce, House of Representatives*, 87th Cong., February 15, 1962 (Washington, DC: US Government Printing Office, 1962), 77.

77. Fox, *Three Worlds of Relief*, 252. See also Mary Poole, *The Segregated Origins of Social Security: African Americans and the Welfare State* (Chapel Hill: University of North Carolina Press, 2006).

78. Martínez-Matsuda, *Migrant Citizenship*, 252.

79. Lee A. Stone, County Health Officer, Madera County, "Axioms for the Employer of Labor," n.d., Box 15, Folder 54, Paul Taylor Papers.

80. Daniel, *Bitter Harvest*; Charles Wollenberg, "Race and Class in Rural California: The El Monte Berry Strike of 1933," *California Historical Quarterly* 51, no. 2 (Summer 1972): 155–64; Frank P. Barajas, "Resistance, Radicalism, and Repression on the Oxnard Plain: The Social Context of the Betabelero Strike of 1933," *Western Historical Quarterly*, no. 1 (Spring, 2004): 28–51; Ramón D. Chacon, "Labor Unrest and Industrialized Agriculture in California: The Case of the 1933 San Joaquin Valley Cotton Strike," *Social Science Quarterly* 65, no. 2 (June 1984): 336–53; Vicki Ruiz, *From Out of the Shadows: Mexican Women in Twentieth-Century America* (New York: Oxford University Press, 1998), chap. 4.

81. Ruiz, *From Out of the Shadows*, 93.

82. Vicki Ruiz, *Cannery Women, Cannery Lives: Mexican Women, Unionization, and the California Food Processing Industry, 1930–1950* (Albuquerque: University of New Mexico Press, 1987), 49–51; Vargas, *Labor Rights Are Civil Rights*, 1–3; Zaragosa Vargas, "Tejana Radical: Emma Tenayuca and the San Antonio Labor Movement during the Great Depression," *Pacific Historical Review* 66, no. 4 (November 1997): 553–80, 570–71.

83. George Sanchez, *Becoming Mexican American: Ethnicity, Culture, and Identity in Chicano Los Angeles, 1900–1945* (New York: Oxford University Press, 1993), 234–35.

84. "Immigration and Assimilation—Symposium," *Proceedings of the National Conference on Social Work* (1927), 585–86.

85. On poll taxes and their impact on Mexican American voting, see, e.g., Brian Behnken,

Fighting Their Own Battles: Mexican Americans, African Americans, and the Struggle for Civil Rights in Texas (Chapel Hill: University of North Carolina Press, 2011). On anti-Mexican school segregation, see, e.g., Sanchez, *Becoming Mexican American.*

Chapter Three

1. Bracero History Archive, https://braceroarchive.org/about; Pam Belluck, "Mexican Laborers in U.S. during War Sue for Back Pay," *New York Times,* April 29, 2001.

2. Natalia Molina, "Borders, Laborers, and Racialized Medicalization: Mexican Immigration and US Public Health Practices in the 20th Century," *American Journal of Public Health* 101, no. 6 (June 2011): 1024–31; Henry P. Anderson, "The Bracero Program in California with particular Reference to Health Status, Attitudes, and Practices," School of Public Health, University of California, Berkeley, 1961; Deborah Cohen, *Braceros: Migrant Citizens and Transnational Subjects in the Postwar United States and Mexico* (Chapel Hill: University of North Carolina Press, 2011), 106. Quotation from Cohen, *Braceros,* 98–99.

3. Mary E. Mendoza, "La Tierra Pica/The Soil Bites: Hazardous Environments and the Degeneration of Bracero Health, 1942–64," in *Disability Studies and the Environmental Humanities: Toward an Eco-Crip Theory,* ed. Sarah Jaquette Ray and J. C. Sibara (Lincoln: University of Nebraska Press, June 2017), 482–93. Numerous additional examples are in Anderson, "The Bracero Program in California"; Lori A. Flores, "A Town Full of Dead Mexicans: The Salinas Valley Bracero Tragedy of 1963, the End of the Bracero Program, and the Evolution of California's Chicano Movement," *Western Historical Quarterly* 44, no. 2 (Summer 2013): 124–43.

4. Grace L. Wiest, *Health Insurance for the Bracero: A Study of Its Development and Implementation under Public Law 78* (Grand Forks: University of North Dakota Press, 1968); Anderson, "The Bracero Program in California."

5. Jesus Hernandez Medrano interview, Manuel Leal Altamirano interview, Bracero History Archive, braceroarchive.org, translation by Daniel Tamayo; Ernesto Galarza, *Strangers in Our Fields* (US Section, Joint United States–Mexico Trade Union Committee, Washington, DC, 1956,), 57–58.

6. Galarza, *Strangers in Our Fields,* 57.

7. Galarza, 58.

8. Galarza, 58.

9. "U.S. Dept. of Labor Prevents Domestic Farmworkers from Working," October 15, 1963, Box 1, Folder 6, Ben Yellen Papers, University of California, San Diego Special Collections (digitized); "How the Meek Inherit the Earth," June 1, 1959, Box 1, Folder 2, Ben Yellen Papers.

10. *Farm Labor: Hearings before the Subcommittee on Equipment, Supplies, and Manpower of the Committee on Agriculture,* House of Representatives, June 9, 10, 11, and 12 and July 2, 1958, 507. Gomez's statement was presented as part of the National Agricultural Workers' Union (AFL-CIO) testimony opposing the bracero program.

11. "How the Meek Inherit the Earth"; "U.S. Dept. of Labor Prevents Domestic Farmworkers from Working."

12. Chantel Rodriguez, "Challenging the Labor Contract: Mexican Guest Workers, US Good Neighbors, and the Fight to Expand Health Rights during the Railroad Bracero Program of World War II," paper presented at the Borderlands and Latino/a Studies Seminar, Newberry Library, December 7, 2018. For additional discussion of bracero complaints and activism, see, e.g., Mireya Loza, *Defiant Braceros: How Migrant Workers Fought for Racial, Sexual, and Political Freedom* (Chapel Hill: University of North Carolina Press, 2016); Ngai, *Impossible Subjects,* 165–68.

13. "Bracero Complaints to Be Considered," *Valley Morning Star* (Harlingen, TX), June 2, 1950, 5. See also "Bracero Complaints Mount in Arkansas," *Tyler Morning Telegraph* (Tyler, TX), December 9, 1949, 2; "300 Braceros Continue Protests over Conditions in Isleton Area," *Sacramento Bee*, September 22, 1966, 44; "Braceros' Complaints Found Justified," *Valley Morning Star*, November 18, 1951, 13 (newspapers.com).

14. Wiest, *Health Insurance for the Bracero*, 16, 20.

15. Henry Anderson, *Fields of Bondage*, quoted in Truman E. Moore, *The Slaves We Rent* (New York: Random House, 1965), 90–91.

16. "U.S. Dept. of Labor Prevents Domestic Farmworkers from Working"; "Cause of Action, *Yellen vs. Imperial Valley Farmers Assoc. et al.*," November 12, 1959, Box 5, Folder 6, Ben Yellen Papers. Worker's name redacted by the author.

17. Wiest, *Health Insurance for the Bracero*, 49. On opposition to the bracero program, see, e.g., Galarza, *Strangers in the Fields*; Kitty Calavita, *Inside the State: The Bracero Program, Immigration, and the I.N.S.* (New Orleans: Quid Pro Books, 1992); Kenneth C. Burt, *The Search for a Civic Voice: California Latino Politics* (Claremont, CA: Regina Books, 2007).

18. Wiest, *Health Insurance for the Bracero*, 42–50.

19. "Farm Labor to Be from Out of State Sources," *Redlands Daily Facts*, January 17, 1964, 5 (newspapers.com).

20. Martínez-Matsuda, *Migrant Citizenship*, 212–16.

21. Louis Fiset, "Medical Care in Camp," *Densho Encyclopedia* https://encyclopedia.densho.org/Medical_care_in_camp/; Gwenn M. Jensen, "System Failure: Health-Care Deficiencies in the World War II Japanese American Detention Centers," *Bulletin of the History of Medicine* 73, no. 4 (Winter 1999): 602–28, 604–6, 609. In Arizona, the dust even carried an endemic fungal disease, coccidioidomycosis.

22. Jensen, "System Failure," 609–11, 613–17, 619–23.

23. Jensen, 606–9, 623–25.

24. Jensen, 608, 625; "Heart Mountain," *Densho Encyclopedia*, https://encyclopedia.densho.org/Heart_Mountain/.

25. Smith, *Japanese American Midwives*, 160–61.

26. Gerald B. Breitigam, "Welcomed Mexican Invasion," *New York Times*, June 20, 1920, 6.

27. Ngai, *Impossible Subjects*, 168–71.

28. Quoted in Calavita, *Inside the State*, 50.

29. W. G. Kneeland, "Farmers Hire Illegal Workers," *Arizona Republic*, July 30, 1953, 28; Ngai, *Impossible Subjects*, 173.

30. Juan Ramon García, *Operation Wetback: The Mass Deportation of Mexican Undocumented Workers in 1954* (Westport, CT, and London: Greenwood Press, 1980), 157–58; Lytle Hernandez, *Migra!*, 179.

31. García, *Operation Wetback*, 216, 224–25.

32. Eladio B. Bobadilla, "'One People without Borders': The Lost Roots of the Immigrants' Rights Movement, 1954–2006," diss., Duke University, 2019, 58.

33. García, *Operation Wetback*, 201, 220–21; "4 Wetbacks Drowned: 36 Leap into Sea— Crowding on Vessel Is Charged," *New York Times*, August 27, 1956, 40; "Port Chief Suspended: Involved in Deportation Ship Incident in Tampico," *New York Times*, September 2, 1956, S9.

34. "Case #6," "Case #13," Typewritten reports, n.d. ca. 1954, Box 15, Folder 4, Edward Roybal Papers, Special Collections, University of California, Los Angeles.

35. García, *Operation Wetback*, 198, 201–2.

36. Garcia, 230–31.

37. David Gutiérrez, *Walls and Mirrors: Mexican Americans, Mexican Immigrants, and the Politics of Ethnicity* (Berkeley: University of California Press, 1995), 81.

38. Gutiérrez; Behnken, *Fighting Their Own Battles.*

39. Henry A. J. Ramos, *American G.I. Forum: In Pursuit of the American Dream* (Houston, TX: Arté Publico Press, 1998), 4, 8.

40. Ramos, 3–4; Hector García, "Letters to the People," September 24, 1948, Box 45, Folder 10, Hector P. García Papers, Texas A&M University. Their fight for a VA hospital never succeeded; Steve Taylor, "Valley Veterans to Consider Class Action Lawsuit," *Rio Grande Guardian*, March 8, 2015, https://riograndeguardian.com/valley-veterans-to-consider-class-action-lawsuit/.

41. Hector García, "Letters to the People."

42. Invitation letter signed by J. A. Garcia (LULAC), June 24, 1948, Box 161, Folder 20; Hector P. García to County of Nueces, February 9, 1949, Box 161, Folder 20, Hector García Papers.

43. Carmel Zarate, "To Whom It May Concern," 1953, Box 160, Hector García Papers.

44. Ed Idar Jr. to "The Mayor," July 2, 1953, Box 161, Folder 19, Hector García Papers; Behnken, *Fighting Their Own Battles*, 62.

45. Behnken, *Fighting Their Own Battles.*

46. Fred L. Koestler, "Operation Wetback," Texas Historical Association, Handbook of Texas, https://www.tshaonline.org/handbook/entries/operation-wetback.

47. Behnken, *Fighting Their Own Battles*, 33–34.

48. Gutiérrez, *Walls and Mirrors*, 159, 166. See also Michael D. Aguirre, "Identities, Quandaries, and Emotions: Labor in the Imperial-Mexicali Borderlands," *Southern California Quarterly* 102, no. 3 (Fall 2020): 222–49, 230–31.

49. Gutiérrez, *Walls and Mirrors*, 168–71.

50. Edith M. Hettema and Ruth Ranson, "Nursing in a Medical Care Program for Farm Workers," *Public Health Nursing* 39 (August 1947): 398–402, 398.

51. Public Health Service Monthly Report, October 1960, 4, Carton 21, Folder 13, National Council on Agricultural Life and Labor Records, Bancroft Library.

52. *Fair Labor Standards Act Amendments of 1949, Hearings before the Subcommittee of the Committee on Labor and Public Welfare, United States Senate*, April 11–14 and 18–22, 1949 (Washington, DC: US Government Printing Office, 1949).

53. "Migrant Labor Health Legislation," December 17, 1947, Carton 2, Folder 17, National Council on Agricultural Life and Labor Records, Bancroft Library.

54. Robert S. Robinson, "Taking the Fair Deal to the Fields: Truman's Commission on Migratory Labor, Public Law 78, and the Bracero Program, 1950–1952," *Agricultural History* 84, no. 3 (Summer 2010): 381–402, 393.

55. *Migratory Labor in American Agriculture*, 153.

56. Lyman Jones, "We Live Off Their Sweat," unidentified clipping (likely *Texas Observer*, 1957), Box 201, Folder 8, Hector García Papers.

57. *Health Clinics for Migratory Farm Workers*, 72, 76.

58. Tom Gavin, "Senators Kill Plan to Study Migrant Camps," *Rocky Mountain News*, February 8, 1956, Typed copy of article, Box 201, Folder 8, Hector García Papers.

59. Amy M. Hay, "Migrant Health," Handbook of Texas, https://www.tshaonline.org/handbook/entries/migrant-health.

60. Brandt Ayers, "Army of Despair Begins Its Annual Odyssey," "A Stark, Personal Migrant's Drama," *Raleigh Times*, July 3–7, 1961, reprinted in *Health Clinics for Migratory Farm Workers*, 73, 74.

61. Donald H. Grubbs, "The Story of Florida's Migrant Farm Workers," *Florida Historical*

Quarterly 40, no. 2 (October 1961): 103–22; "Employment Covered under the Social Security Program, 1935–84," *Social Security Bulletin* 48, no. 4 (April 1985).

62. Grubbs, "The Story of Florida's Migrant Farm Workers," 117 (his phrase is "torn from").

63. Public Health Service Monthly Report, October 1960, 4, Carton 21, Folder 13, National Council on Agricultural Life and Labor Records, Bancroft Library.

64. *CBS Reports: Harvest of Shame*, first broadcast November 25, 1960, https://www.youtube .com/watch?v=yJTVF_dya7E.

65. Grubbs, "The Story of Florida's Migrant Farm Workers," 121; *Harvest of Shame* reviewed in *Time*, March 31, 1961, https://web.archive.org/web/20131029204422/http://www2.vcdh.virginia .edu/HIUS316/mbase/docs/harvest.html.

66. *Health Clinics for Migratory Farmworkers*, Statement of William Fitts Ryan, 48–49; Testimony of C. L. Brumback, 53; Kenneth A. Roberts and Donald Harting, 22.

67. *Health Clinics for Migratory Farmworkers*, Testimony of Boisfeuillet Jones of National Institutes of Health, 22; Testimony of Donald Harting, 31; Statement of Harrison Williams, 79.

68. *Health Clinics for Migratory Farmworkers*, 80, 13.

69. *Health Clinics for Migratory Farmworkers*, Testimony of Donald Harting, 46; Harrison, 79.

70. *Health Clinics for Migratory Farmworkers*, Testimony of the American Public Health Association, 64; Fay Bennett, 81.

71. *Health Clinics for Migratory Farmworkers*, Statement of the Friends Committee on National Legislation Regarding Farm Labor, 80. On the Puerto Rican farm labor program, see Ismael García-Colón, *Colonial Migrants at the Heart of Empire: Puerto Rican Workers on US Farms* (Berkeley: University of California Press, 2020).

72. Louise S. Ward, "Migrant Health Policy: History, Analysis, and Challenge," *Policy, Politics, & Nursing Practice* 4, no. 1 (February 2003): 45–52, 48.

73. John F. Kennedy, "Special Message to the Congress on Improving the Nation's Health," February 7, 1963.

74. Helen L. Johnston, *Health for the Nation's Harvesters: A History of the Migrant Health Program in Its Economic and Social Setting* (Farmington Hills, MI: National Migrant Worker Council, Inc., 1985), 151.

75. Florida State Board of Health, Annual Progress Report, Migrant Health Grant MG-18B R (65), 1, Florida Christian Migrant Ministry Records, Walter Reuther Library, Wayne State University.

76. Florida State Board of Health, Annual Progress Report, Migrant Health Grant, 9.

77. Florida State Board of Health, Annual Progress Report, Migrant Health Grant, 8.

78. Florida State Board of Health, Annual Progress Report, Migrant Health Grant, 2.

79. National Center for Farmworker Health, "History of America's Agricultural Workers and the Migrant Health Movement," http://www.ncfh.org/history.html.

80. *Migrant Health Services: Hearings before the Subcommittee on Health of the Committee on Labor and Public Welfare, United States Senate, Ninety-first Congress, First Session, on S. 2660, to Extend and Otherwise Amend Certain Expiring Provisions of the Public Health Service Act for Migrant Health Services, October 21 and 22, 1969* (Washington, DC: US Government Printing Office, 1969), 1–2, 6, 9, 10.

81. Nicole Rodriguez-Robbins, "Honoring the Migrant Health Program and the Workers It Serves," RCHN Community Health Foundation, https://www.rchnfoundation.org/?p=613; "Special Populations: Migrant Health Centers," *Chronicles: The Community Health Center Story*, https://www.chcchronicles.org/stories/special-populations-migrant-health-centers.

82. Florida State Board of Health, Annual Progress Report, 7–8.

83. Johnston, *Health for the Nation's Harvesters*, 168–69.

84. Johnston, 168. Johnston doesn't provide a citation or a year for this change, but the Migrant Health Act language in the early 1980s (when she was writing) did not include the word "domestic." Johnston, Appendix VII: Public Health Service Act, Title III, Part D, Migrant Health, 43.

85. Cybelle Fox, "Unauthorized Welfare: The Origins of Immigrant Status Restrictions in American Social Policy," *Journal of American History* 102, no. 4 (March 2016): 1051–74.

86. Edwin Maldonado, "Contract Labor and the Origins of Puerto Rican Communities in the United States," *International Migration Review* 13, no. 1 (Spring 1979): 103–21; Maria L. Quintana, *Contracting Freedom: Race, Empire, and U.S. Guestworker Programs* (Philadelphia: University of Pennsylvania Press, 2022), chap. 5.

87. García-Colón, *Colonial Migrants at the Heart of Empire* (Berkeley: University of California Press, 2020); Quintana, *Contracting Freedom*, 234; Ismael García-Colón, "'We Like Mexican Laborers Better': U.S. Immigration and Citizenship Policies in Puerto Rican Farm Labor Migration," *Centro Voices*, Summer 2017, https://centropr-archive.hunter.cuny.edu /centrovoices/chronicles/"we-mexican-laborers-better"-us-immigration-and-citizenship -policies-puerto.

88. Edgardo Meléndez, *Sponsored Migration: The State and Puerto Rican Postwar Migration to the United States* (Columbus: Ohio State University Press, 2017); Lilia Fernández, *Brown in the Windy City: Mexicans and Puerto Ricans in Postwar Chicago* (Chicago: University of Chicago Press, 2012); Laura Briggs, *Reproducing Empire: Race, Sex, Science, and U.S. Imperialism in Puerto Rico* (Berkeley: University of California Press, 2002).

89. Case Histories, Box 18, Folder 5 and Folder 6, Henry Street Collection.

90. "Puerto Rican Community Study," 1954, Box 19, Folder 1, Henry Street Collection.

91. Guglielmo, *White on Arrival*; Eric L. Goldstein, *The Price of Whiteness: Jews, Race, and American Identity* (Princeton, NJ: Princeton University Press, 2008).

92. "Puerto Rican Community Study," 1954, Box 19, Folder 1, Henry Street Collection.

93. "Health Study," 1962, Folder 3, Box 19, Henry Street Collection. These reports occasionally used initials but more often include the patients' names; I have used initials for all cases.

94. "Health Study," 1962, Folder 3; Handwritten report, Folder 6, both in Box 19, Henry Street Collection.

95. "Health Study," 1962, Folder 3, Box 19, Henry Street Collection.

96. Handwritten reports, Folder 6, Box 19, Henry Street Collection.

97. Hongdeng Gao, "Community Struggles for a New Gouverneur: Tackling the Deeper Roots of the City's Inadequate Hospital Care," Gotham Center for New York History, January 5, 2021, https://www.gothamcenter.org/blog/community-struggles-for-a-new-gouverneur.

98. Helen Hall, William J. Calise, Dora Tannenbaum, and Dr. Sidney Rosenfelt to Robert F. Wagner, June 28, 1956, Box 77, Folder 1, Henry Street Collection.

99. Gao, "Community Struggles for a New Gouverneur."

100. Edward Roybal, speech to Western Branch of the American Public Health Association, San Diego, CA, June 26, 1961, Box 13, Folder 3, Roybal Papers.

Chapter Four

1. Jacques E. Levy, *Cesar Chavez: Autobiography of La Causa* (1975; reprint, Minneapolis: University of Minnesota Press, 2007), book 4, chap. 2. On the CSO's limited efforts to include

farmworkers, see Lori Flores, *Grounds for Dreaming: Mexican Americans, Mexican Immigrants, and the California Farmworker Movement* (New Haven, CT: Yale University Press, 2016), 129–34.

2. On permanent and temporary visas, see Calavita, *Inside the State*.

3. "The National Farm Workers Association . . . ," n.d., Box 3, Folder 1, Marion Moses M.D. Papers, Reuther Library; "Farm Workers Health Clinic," *El Malcriado*, June 7, 1967, 10; Marion Moses, "Viva La Causa!," *American Journal of Nursing* 73, no. 5 (May 1973): 842–48, 844, United Farm Workers Administration Files, Reuther Library. Some material in this chapter first appeared in Beatrix Hoffman, "'¡Viva la Clinica!': The United Farm Workers' Fight for Medical Care," *Bulletin of the History of Medicine* 93, no. 4 (2019): 518–49, Copyright © 2019, The Johns Hopkins University Press.

4. "Clinic Program 7/22/69," Box 103, Folder 33, UFW Administration Files, Reuther Library.

5. "Farm Workers Health Clinic," *El Malcriado*, June 7, 1967, 10; Interview with Caleb Foote, Farmer Consumer Reporter, December 1971–January 1972, clipping in Box 2, folder 9, Anne Loftis Papers, Stanford University Special Collections.

6. "Farm Workers Health Clinic," *El Malcriado*, June 7, 1967, 10; "Farm Workers Health Clinic-Clinica Medica Campesina," n.d., Box 21, Folder 7, UFW Administration Files.

7. "Jim Drake shows Robert Kennedy a UFW Clinic trailer" (photo, n.d.), Farm Worker Movement Online Gallery, Farmworkers Movement Documentation Project (hereafter FMDP), University of California, San Diego Library, https://libraries.ucsd.edu/farmworkermovement/.

8. "Farm Workers Union Will Build a Clinic in Delano," *El Malcriado*, January 15, 1971, 9–13.

9. "UFW Chronology," https://ufw.org/research/history/ufw-chronology/.

10. "Terronez Clinic," Box 21, Folder 12, UFW Administration Files; National Farm Worker Health Group, "RTMC Program," July 14, 1972, Box 36, Folder 25, United Farm Workers Information and Research Files, Reuther Library; Peter Rudd, MD, "The United Farm Workers Clinic in Delano, Calif.: A Study of the Rural Poor," *Public Health Reports* 90, no. 4 (July–August 1975): 331–39.

11. "Clinic Opens in Delano," Box 6, Folder 16, Douglas Adair United Farm Workers Collection, California State Polytechnic University, Pomona Special Collections.

12. Levy, *Autobiography of La Causa*, 178; LeRoy Chatfield, "Forty Acres Delano: United Farm Workers," n.d., FMDP; Cesar Chavez and Peggy McGivern, "Rodrigo Terronez Memorial Clinic," n.d., Box 3, Folder 1, Marion Moses Papers; "Terronez Clinic"; "Clinic Opens in Delano."

13. Rudd, "United Farm Workers Clinic," 332, 337.

14. Dan Murphy, Essay, FMDP.

15. Report on Terronez Clinic April 3, 1970, Box 36, Folder 20, UFW Information and Research Files; Rudd, "United Farm Workers Clinic," 337.

16. Rudd, "United Farm Workers Clinic," 332.

17. Abby Flores Rivera, July 5, 2004, Listserv Archive, FMDP.

18. Sheldon Rosen, MD, to Cesar Chavez, March 13, 1970, Box 103, Folder 32, UFW Administration Files.

19. Joyce A. Fettner to "Dear _____," November 12, 1971, Box 10, Folder 2, UFW-Arizona State Office Collection, Reuther Library.

20. "Farm Workers Union Will Build a Clinic in Delano."

21. Kathy Lynch Murguia, September 30, 2004 (2), Listsev Archive, FMDP.

22. Dan Murphy, Essay, FMDP; Julie Greenfield, December 31, 2004, Listserv Archive, FMDP.

23. Cesar Chavez, speech to National Farm Worker Health Group, n.d., Box 36, Folder 36, UFW Information and Research Files. Capitalization in original. The same wording appears in Philip Traynor, "What Makes a Farm Workers Union Clinic," UFW Administration Files.

24. "Terronez Clinic"; "RTMC Program"; Kate Colwell July 4, 2004, Listserv Archive, FMDP.

25. "Farm Workers Union Will Build a Clinic in Delano."

26. "Clinic in Delano," *El Malcriado*, December 15, 1972.

27. "Terronez Clinic," Folder 12, Box 21, UFW Administration Files.

28. On the Calexico clinic, see Khati Hendry, "UFW Memories," Essay, FMDP. Eventually there would also be UFW clinics in Mexicali, Mexico; in Coachella, California; and in Tijuana and Florida. "Commentary by Leroy Chatfield," FMDP.

29. "The Robert F. Kennedy Farm Workers Medical Plan," Box 6, Folder 6, Douglass Adair United Farm Workers Collection. For more on the RFK Plan, see Hoffman, "'¡Viva la Clinica!'"

30. Kennedy Planning Conference, July 18–21, 1978, Box 102, Folder 11, UFW Administration Files; Frank Bardacke, *Trampling Out the Vintage: Cesar Chavez and the Two Souls of the United Farm Workers* (London and New York: Verso, 2011), 669–71; Miriam Pawel, *The Union of Their Dreams: Power, Hope, and Struggle in Cesar Chavez's Farm Worker Movement* (New York: Bloomsbury, 2009), 296–313; numerous discussions, Listserv Archive, FMPD.

31. Margaret Murphy July 4, 2004, Listserv Archive, FMDP.

32. A California Rural Manpower Report estimated that about 120,000 undocumented workers did some farm labor in California in 1974. Frank Bardacke notes, "If that figure is correct, then in the year that the Campaign Against Illegals became the UFW's number one priority, more than half of the people working in the California fields were undocumented." Bardacke, *Trampling Out the Vintage*, 490. For a discussion of the role of Mexican national workers in the Salinas lettuce strike, see Lori Flores, *Grounds for Dreaming*, chap. 7.

33. Miriam Pawel, *The Crusades of Cesar Chavez: A Biography* (New York: Bloomsbury, 2014), 293–94.

34. Quoted in Bardacke, *Trampling Out the Vintage*, 488.

35. Liza Hirsch to Boycott Cities, July 6, 1974, Box 105, Folder 60, UFW Administration Files.

36. Cesar E. Chavez, "Press Statement," July 1, 1974, Box 38, Folder 7, UFW Information and Research. Thanks to Kristen Chinery of Reuther Archives for locating this document.

37. "Visit to the County Health Department by Bill Plum and Diane Sklarr, 6/24/74," Box 39, Folder 12, UFW Information and Research Files.

38. Paul A. Pumphrey to Cesar Chavez, June 17, 1974; New Orleans Support Committee to UFW, August 15, 1974; Eight Farmworker Supporters, Kalamazoo, Michigan, to Cesar Chavez, August 25, 1974; and many more letters, all in Box 39, Folder 6, UFW Information and Research Department Files.

39. The decision still causes anguish and bewilderment among former volunteers. See numerous discussions on the Listserv Archive, 2004, FMDP.

40. R. W. Chamberlain, MD, and J. F. Radebaugh, MD, "Delivery of Primary Health Care—Union Style: A Critical Review of the Robert F. Kennedy Plan for the United Farm Workers of America," *New England Journal of Medicine* 294, no. 12 (March 18, 1976): 641–45; Dan Murphy Essay, FMPD; Ken Tittle resignation letter to Cesar Chavez and Pearl McGivney, February 7, 1975, Box 103, Folder 45, UFW Administration Files.

41. Dan Murphy Essay, FMPD. Murphy was not the only UFW physician to complain of top-down control; see John Radebaugh, MD, *House Calls with John* (Portsmouth, NH: Peter E. Randall, 2006), 53.

42. Sapir Essay, FMDP; Bardacke, *Trampling Out the Vintage*, 581.

43. Dan Spelce, May 16, 2004, Listserv Archive, FMDP.

44. Legislation to further protect farmworkers' union rights was passed in California in 2022.

45. Dan Spelce, May 16, 2004, Listserv Archive, FMDP; Randy Shaw, *Beyond the Fields: Cesar Chavez, the UFW, and the Struggle for Justice in the 21st Century* (Berkeley: University of California Press, 2008).

46. Khati Hendry, July 5, 2004, Listserv Archive, FMDP.

47. Hendry, July 5, 2004.

48. Bonnie Lefkowitz, *Community Health Centers: A Movement and the People Who Made It Happen* (New Brunswick, NJ: Rutgers University Press, 2007), 3–4.

49. Lefkowitz, 6–8.

50. Lefkowitz, 10, 12; Alice Sardell, *The U.S. Experiment in Social Medicine: The Community Health Center, Program, 1965–1986* (Pittsburgh: University of Pittsburgh Press, 1988), 218.

51. Box 6, Muscatine Migrant Committee Records, Iowa Women's Archives.

52. Ray Esparza, "Community Based and Controlled Migrant Health Service," Report of the Southwest States Chicano Consumer Conference on Health, January 1972, San Antonio, 16; Interview with Tomás Villanueva, Seattle Labor Rights and History Project, June 4, 2016, https://www.yakimaherald.com/activist-and-organizer-tom-s-villanueva-describes-the-founding-of-the-yakima-valley-farmworkers-clinic/article_d7261246-2a8d-11e6-a499-977ab4d21232.html. According to Villanueva, Ray Esparza was a farmworker who had served as a medic in Vietnam.

53. Esparza, "Community Based and Controlled Migrant Health Service," 16–17.

54. Application for Funding, Campaign for Human Development, "Proposal—La Casa de Buena Salud," 1974, Box 19, Folder 27, Frank I. Sanchez Papers, University of New Mexico Center for Southwest Research.

55. Virginia Espino, "Equal Medical Care for All: Chicana and Chicano Health Activism in Late 1960s Los Angeles," Conference Abstract, American Historical Association Annual Meeting, January 2000, https://www.researchgate.net/publication/267541017_Equal_Medical_Care_for_All_Chicana_and_Chicano_Health_Activism_in_Late_1960s_Los_Angeles; Frank Aguilera, "The Birth of the East Los Angeles Health Task Force," Report of the Southwest States Chicano Consumer Conference on Health.

56. Herbert K. Abrams, MD, Interview, Medicine and Health Care Delivery in Southern Arizona, Arizona Historical Society Oral History Project, Arizona Historical Society, 15–21.

57. Abrams Interview, 8.

58. Interview with Tomás Villanueva. From their website, it's unclear whether the clinic today includes any farmworkers on its board. https://www.yvfwc.com/about/board-members/

59. Casa de Amistad Community Center Newsletter, September, 1970, Box 5, Folder 15; Complaint, Yellen et al. vs. Casa de Amistad et al., September 28, 1970, Box 5, Folder 15, Yellen Papers.

60. Vernon E. Wilson, MD (HEW) to Ben Yellen, September 25, 1970, Box 4, Folder 9, Yellen Papers.

61. Complaint, Yellen et al.

62. "Workshop Notes: Migrant Health Workshop," Report of the Southwest States Chicano Consumer Conference on Health, 67. On the history of the Chicano Movement, see, e.g., Mario T. García, *The Chicano Generation: Testimonios of the Movement* (Berkeley: University of California Press, 2015).

63. "Workshop Notes: Migrant Health Workshop," Report of the Southwest States Chicano Consumer Conference on Health, 67.

64. "Workshop Notes: Migrant Health Workshop," Report of the Southwest States Chicano Consumer Conference on Health, 67.

65. Report of the Southwest States Chicano Consumer Conference on Health, 137.

66. Report of the Southwest States Chicano Consumer Conference on Health, 71, 136.

67. Erasmo Andrade, "Planning and Development of Health Services," Report of the Southwest States Chicano Consumer Conference on Health, 35.

68. Report of the Southwest States Chicano Consumer Conference on Health, 146, 150.

69. Report of the Southwest States Chicano Consumer Conference on Health, 119–55.

70. Howard Phillips to James Cavanaugh, March 21, 1973, Box 17, Folder 17, James Vizzard Papers, Stanford University Special Collections.

71. Report of the Southwest States Chicano Consumer Conference on Health, 73.

72. "National Chicano Health Association," Box 2, Folder 38, Enriqueta Chavez Papers, San Diego State University. On medical student militance in the 1960s, see Naomi Rogers, "Radical Visions of American Medicine: Politics and Activism in the History of Medicine," *Bulletin of the History of Medicine* 96, no. 4 (Winter 2022): 545–611.

73. Joe Dimas, "Health Agency: N.C.H.O. Starts," *Model Cities News*, April 6, 1972, Box 20, Folder 20, Frank I. Sanchez Papers.

74. "Statement," Health Manpower Conference, March 10–11 [1972], Chicago, Box 20, Folder 20, Frank I. Sanchez Papers.

75. "National Chicano Health Organization," Box 42, Folder 14, Frank I. Sanchez Papers.

76. "Prepare for Medical School," n.d., Box 21, Folder 7, Frank I. Sanchez Papers.

77. "Wanted: Chicano and Chicana Nurses," n.d. ca. 1972, Box 1, Folder 1, Gloria Arellanes Papers, California State University, Los Angeles Special Collections. NCHO later became La Raza Medical Association and then the Latino Medical Students Association.

78. East Los Angeles Health Task Force Newsletter, June 1971, Ricardo Cruz/Catolicos por la Raza Papers, University of California, Santa Barbara Special Collections; American G.I. Forum, "Memorial Hospital Emergency Room," November 23, 1977, Box 46, Folder 3, Hector García Papers.

79. "Let's Fight for Gouverneur!," ca. June 1969, Box 77, Folder 1, Henry Street Collection.

80. "Let's Fight for Gouverneur!"

81. Dorothy and Thomas Hoobler, *From Street Fair to Medical Home: Charles B. Wang Community Health Center/Chinatown Health Clinic* (New York: Charles B. Wang Community Health Center, 2011), 14.

82. Hoobler and Hoobler, 22–23.

83. Gao, "Community Struggles for a New Gouverneur"; Hoobler and Hoobler, *From Street Fair to Medical Home*, 24–25; Rudy Johnson, "Gouverneur Hospital to Open in '72, Protesters Told," *New York Times*, November 17, 1971, 51.

84. Hoobler and Hoobler, *From Street Fair to Medical Home*, 27–29.

85. Hoobler and Hoobler, 39, 41, 45.

86. "Betances Health Center: History," https://www.betances.org/history; Hoobler and Hoobler, *From Street Fair to Medical Home*, 43–47.

87. Merlin Chowkwanyun, *All Health Politics Is Local: Community Battles for Medical Care and Environmental Health* (Chapel Hill: University of North Carolina Press, 2022), 41–44; Johanna Fernández, *The Young Lords: A Radical History* (Chapel Hill: University of North Carolina Press, 2020), 280–82.

88. Fernández, *The Young Lords*, chaps. 3 and 5.

89. Fernández, 291–92.

90. Alondra Nelson, *Body and Soul: The Black Panther Party and the Fight against Medical Discrimination* (Minneapolis: University of Minnesota, 2011), 49.

91. Fernández, *The Young Lords*, 291.

92. Fernández, 271–73.

93. Eveline Chao, "How Asian-American Radicals Brought 'Yellow Power' to Chinatown," *Gothamist*, October 19, 2016, https://gothamist.com/news/how-asian-american-radicals-brought -yellow-power-to-chinatown. I am grateful to the Corky Lee Estate for permission to reprint two of the amazing photos he took of these events.

94. Philip B. Gonzales, "Struggle for Survival: The Hispanic Land Grants of New Mexico, 1848–2001," *Agricultural History* 77, no. 2 (Spring, 2003): 293–324; David Correia, "'Rousers of the Rabble' in the New Mexico Land Grant War: *La Alianza Federal de Mercedes* and the Violence of the State," *Antipode* 40, no. 4 (2008): 561–83.

95. *25 Years of La Clinica's History*, 1994, La Cooperación del Pueblo de Tierra Amarilla Collection, UNM Center for Southwest Research; Maria Varela, "Volunteer Health Service," Report of the Southwest States Chicano Consumer Conference on Health, 54.

96. La cooperacion del pueblo, "Dear Friend," September 1975, La Cooperación del Pueblo de Tierra Amarilla Collection.

97. Varela, "Volunteer Health Service," Report of the Southwest States Chicano Consumer Conference on Health, 53–54.

98. La cooperacion del pueblo, "Dear Friend," September 1975, La Cooperación del Pueblo de Tierra Amarilla Collection; Varela, "Volunteer Health Service," 57–61.

99. Typescript, Box 1, Folder 1, Gloria Arellanes Papers; George Thurlow, "Chicano Student Activist Builds a Health Empire," *Coastlines*, Spring 2019, https://www.alumni.ucsb.edu /coastlines/spring-2019/chicano-activists-builds-health-empire.

100. Carolina Sanchez, "Bobby Garcia Memorial Clinic," *El Grito del Norte*, October 2, 1971, 12; "Chicanos Holding Dorm Allowed to Start School," *Albuquerque Journal*, August 28, 1973, 26; "Mobile Medical Clinic Aids Strikers," *Albuquerque Journal*, March 4, 1973, 76.

101. Betita Martinez, "Health Is a Human Right," *El Grito del Norte*, May 1, 1973, 10.

102. Varela, "Volunteer Health Service," 53–54.

103. Correia, "'Rousers of the Rabble'"; "La cooperacion del pueblo" newsletter, n.d. ca 1975; "Dear Friend," October 1976, La Cooperación del Pueblo de Tierra Amarilla Collection.

104. David Correia, "Return of the Albuquerque Death Squads," *Counterpunch*, November 23, 2011, https://www.counterpunch.org/2011/11/23/the-return-of-the-albuquerque-death -squads/.

105. Felipe Hinojosa, "¡*Medicina Sí Muerte No!* Race, Public Health, and the 'Long War on Poverty' in Mathis, Texas, 1948–1971," *Western Historical Quarterly* 44, no. 4 (Winter 2013): 437–58.

106. Fernández, *Brown in the Windy City*, 198–99; Jessica Jerome, "Much More than a Clinic: Chicago's Free Health Centers, 1968–1972," *Medical Anthropology* 38, no. 6 (2019): 537–50.

107. Dionne Espinoza, "'Revolutionary Sisters': Women's Solidarity and Collective Identification among Chicana Brown Berets in East Los Angeles, 1967–1970," *Aztlán* 26, no. 1 (Spring 2001): 17–58; "Special Points of Courtesy," Box 1, Folder 9, Arellanes Papers; Arellanes testimonio in Garcia, *The Chicano Generation*, 204.

108. Elena R. Gutiérrez, *Fertile Matters: The Politics of Mexican-Origin Women's Reproduction* (Austin: University of Texas Press, 2008). At least one Chicana feminist organization, the Chicana Welfare Rights Organization, partnered for a time with the "pro-life" movement. See News Release, December 7, 1974, Box 18, Folder 36, Alicia Escalante Papers, University of California, Santa Barbara Special Collections.

109. Jennifer Nelson, "'Abortions under Community Control': Feminism, Nationalism, and the Politics of Reproduction among New York City's Young Lords," *Journal of Women's History* 13, no. 1 (Spring 2001): 157–80.

110. On the history of forced sterilization in the US, see, e.g., Gutierrez, *Fertile Matters*; Wendy Kline, *Building a Better Race: Gender, Sexuality, and Eugenics from the Turn of the Century to the Baby Boom* (Berkeley: University of California Press, 2005); Natalie Lira, *Laboratory of Deficiency: Sterilization and Confinement in California, 1900–1950s* (Oakland: University of California Press, 2022).

111. Antonia Hernández interview, "La Biblioteca and Latina Sterilizations in *Madrigal v. Quilligan*," Library of Congress podcast, October 5, 2021; Box 16, Folder 2, Ricardo Cruz Papers; City News Service, "LA County Seeks Reparations," *Los Angeles Daily News*, July 13, 2021. See also https://irle.ucla.edu/portfolio-item/virginia-espino/ and the excellent documentary "No Mas Bebes," http://www.nomasbebesmovie.com.

112. Gutiérrez, *Fertile Matters*, 44.

113. Gutiérrez, 49.

114. Gutiérrez, 103; Antonia Hernández interview.

115. See e.g. Sam Kalen, "Durational Residency Requirements and the Equal Protection Clause," *Journal of Urban and Contemporary Law* 25 (January 1983): 329–59.

116. Interview, Augusto Ortíz, MD, May 26, 1994, Medicine and Health Care Delivery in Southern Arizona, Arizona Historical Society Oral History Project.

117. *Memorial Hosp. v. Maricopa County*, 415 U.S. 250 (1974); *Shapiro, Commissioner of Welfare of Connecticut v. Thompson*, 394 U.S. 618 (1969).

118. Interview, Augusto Ortíz.

119. The Hastings Center, "Undocumented Immigrants in the United States: U.S. Health Policy and Access to Care," n.d., https://undocumented.thehastingscenter.org/issuebrief/health-policy-and-access-to-care/.

120. "Gloria Arellanes" oral history in Garcia, *The Chicano Generation*, 204; "La Clínica Familiar del Barrio" poster, Box 1, Folder 9, Arellanes Papers.

121. "Mini-Conference, Health, Mental Health and Alcohol Workshop," June 5, 1980, Chicano Federation of San Diego County, Inc., Subject files, Box 20, Folder 5, Herman Baca Papers, Special Collections and Archives, University of California, San Diego.

122. Gutiérrez, *Walls and Mirrors*, 183–99; "National Chicano/Latino Conference on Immigration and Public Policy, October 28–30, San Antonio, Texas," 1977, José Angel Gutiérrez Papers, Box 74, Benson Library, University of Texas at Austin.

Chapter Five

1. Maddalena Marinari, *Unwanted: Italian and Jewish Mobilization against Restrictive Immigration Laws, 1882–1965* (Chapel Hill: University of North Carolina Press, 2020); David M. Reimers, *Still the Golden Door: The Third World Comes to America* (New York: Columbia University Press, 1985).

2. In Mexico, "The percentage of income available to the poorer half of society fell from 19 percent in 1950 to 16 percent in 1957. It dropped again to 15 percent in 1963 and 13 percent in 1975. The wealthiest 20 percent of Mexican society, however, claimed a near steady 60 percent of the available income." Hernandez, *Migra!*, 214.

3. Ngai, *Impossible Subjects*, 280–81; Fox, "Unauthorized Welfare," 1059; Congressional estimate, *Illegal Aliens; A Review of Hearings Conducted during the 92d Congress* (Serial No. 13, pts. 1–5) by Subcommittee No. 1 of the Committee on the Judiciary, House of Representatives, 93rd Congress, First Session—February 1973, 3. Undocumented immigrants were not counted or estimated in the US census until 1986. Robert Warren and Jeffrey S. Passel estimate 1,116,000

undocumented immigrants resided in the US in 1974; "A Count of the Uncountable: Estimates of Undocumented Aliens Counted in the 1980 United States Census," *Demography*, August 1987. Media reports, e.g., Reuters, "10 Million Illegal Immigrants Told," *Des Moines Register*, January 10, 1972, 2; Chavez, *The Latino Threat*, 26–28.

4. Lee, *America for Americans*, 255.

5. American Medical Association, *Ronald Reagan Speaks Out against Socialized Medicine* (L.P. recording, 1961); Sharon M. Keiger, "Reagan's 'New Federalism' and the 1971 California Medi-Cal Reforms," *Urban and Social Change Review* 16, no. 2 (1983): 3–8.

6. Rosie C. Bermudez, "Chicana Militant Dignity Work: Building Coalition and Solidarity in the Los Angeles Welfare Rights Movement," *Southern California Quarterly* 102, no. 4 (Winter 2020): 420–55. Escalante's physician was Herbert Karlow, who cofounded health centers for the poor in New York and Los Angeles with his partner Pauline Furth. For additional discussion of Escalante's work, see Jenna M. Loyd, *Health Rights Are Civil Rights: Peace and Justice Activism in Los Angeles, 1963–1978* (Minneapolis: University of Minnesota Press, 2014).

7. Keiger, "Reagan's 'New Federalism'"; Fox, "Unauthorized Welfare," 1064. For a detailed discussion of California's adoption of welfare restrictions, and a similar effort in New York State, see Cybelle Fox, "'The Line Must Be Drawn Somewhere': The Rise of Legal Status Restrictions in State Welfare Policy in the 1970s," *Studies in American Political Development* 33, no. 2 (2019).

8. California State Social Welfare Board, "Position Statement: Issue: Aliens in California," June 1972, Box H23, Reagan Gubernatorial Papers, Ronald Reagan Presidential Library. Thanks to Jessica Adler for this citation.

9. Handwritten notes (likely for speeches), n.d., Folder 18, Box 21, Escalante Papers.

10. Handwritten notes, Escalante Papers.

11. M. Kevin Leary, "Welfare Cutbacks Protested," *Oakland Tribune*, March 18, 1971, 13.

12. Fox, "Unauthorized Welfare," 1052–53. The welfare rights cases were *Shapiro v. Thompson* (1968), which ended state residency requirements for public assistance based on the right to travel, and *Graham v. Richardson* (1971), which banned states from denying welfare to legal immigrants.

13. Study quoted in "Plight of Undocumented Aliens in America," December 23, 1976, Baca Papers.

14. Mike Goodman, "Epidemics a Barrio Specter," *Los Angeles Times*, September 16, 1973, 35.

15. Philip R. Lee and Barry Ensminger, "Reagan Health Policy? Look at California," *New York Times*, May 29, 1981, 27.

16. Jesus (surname not indicated) to Edmund D. Edelman, March 23, 1976, Box 313, Edmund D. Edelman Papers, Huntington Library. Some material in this chapter also appears in Beatrix Hoffman, "Immigrant Sanctuary or Danger: Health Care and Hospitals in the United States," *Migration and Society* 4, no. 1 (June 2021): 62–75; and Beatrix Hoffman, "The Politics of Immigration Meets the Politics of Health Care," in *The Edinburgh Companion to the Politics of American Health*, ed. Martin Haliwell and Sophie A. Jones (Edinburgh: Edinburgh University Press, 2022).

17. Jesus to Edelman.

18. L. A. Weatherill to "Each Supervisor," December 6, 1976, Box 313, Edelman Papers. He did not mention the name of the organization.

19. Ronald A. Zumbrun to Baxter Ward, October 29, 1976, Box 33, Folder 1, Centro de Acción Social Autónomo Papers, Stanford University Special Collections.

20. John M. Fredenburg to John H. Larson, Los Angeles County Counsel, April 12, 1977, Box 6, Folder 7, Baca Papers.

21. Jean Merl, "Battle on Alien Health Care Revived," *Los Angeles Times*, March 16, 1981, 32. Hufford also announced that undocumented people were not eligible for county services except for emergency care and communicable diseases. Jean McDowell to Inter-Religious Committee on Human Needs, March 22, 1977, Greater Los Angeles Community Action Agency file, Baca Papers. Individuals and groups organizing in opposition to Hufford included the Catholic auxiliary bishop, United Neighborhood Organization, the Los Angeles Democratic Central Committee, ACLU, Legal Aid Foundation of Los Angeles, One Stop Immigration Center, THE (To Help Everyone) Clinic for Women, East Los Angeles Health Task Force, Community Health Foundation of East Los Angeles, and the National Health Law Program. "Denial of Health Services to Undocumented Persons—Taxation without Representation," Greater Los Angeles Community Action Agency file, Baca Papers. The Mexican American Legal Defense and Education Fund also filed a suit against the Board of Supervisors on Fourteenth Amendment grounds. Judy Hammond, "Board May Face Suit over Health Care for Aliens," clipping in Box 129, Folder 9, Mexican American Legal Defense and Educational Fund Records (hereafter MALDEF Records), Stanford University Special Collections.

22. Coalition for Health and Justice for All Taxpayers, "Contact Your Legislators . . . ," February 21, 1979, Greater Los Angeles Community Action Agency file, Baca Papers; Gail Diane Cox, "Supervisors Quietly Drop Alien Health Rule," *Los Angeles Daily Journal*, April 10, 1985, 1, clipping in Box 313, Edelman Papers.

23. Jean Merl, "L.A. Board Lawyers Get 2nd Health Suit," *Los Angeles Times*, March 26, 1981, 6; Myrna Oliver, "Court Bars Alien Health Care Curb," *Los Angeles Times*, May 30, 1981, 15.

24. Cox, "Supervisors Quietly Drop Alien Health Rule."

25. "Discussion Paper, Undocumented Aliens and Health Services," August 25, 1986, Box 313, Edelman Papers. Schabarum finally left office when his district was redrawn to be majority Latino.

26. *Medical Treatment of Illegal Aliens: Hearing before the Subcommittee on Health and the Environment of the Committee on Interstate and Foreign Commerce*, House of Representatives, June 9, 1977 (Washington, DC: Government Printing Office, 1977), 2. Hereafter, *Medical Treatment of Illegal Aliens*.

27. *Medical Treatment of Illegal Aliens*, 10–11.

28. *Medical Treatment of Illegal Aliens*, 21–22.

29. *Medical Treatment of Illegal Aliens*, 23.

30. *Medical Treatment of Illegal Aliens*, 15, 28.

31. Nancy Plaxico to Indigent Medical Care Commission, December 27, 1979, Box 17, Folder 8, Samuel Hayakawa Papers, San Diego State University.

32. *Medical Treatment of Illegal Aliens*, 29–30.

33. According to a 1979 HHS study, "hospitals do not have systematic methods for determining the alienage status of their patients. As a result, none of the hospitals had exact figures on the amount of money lost due to the treatment of undocumented persons." Grace Flores, "Unpaid Medical Costs and Undocumented Aliens" (summary), HHS Evaluation Documentation Center, *Compendium of HHS Evaluations and Relevant Other Studies*, 1985.

34. Lew Scarr, "Doctor Absolved of Wrongdoing for Refusing to Authorize Transfer," *San Diego Union*, June 2, 1979; "SD Hospital Gets a Warning," *Escondido Times-Advocate*, September 21, 1979, 25.

35. Gina Lubrano, "Hospital Bias Alleged, U.S. Probe Sought," *San Diego Union*, n.d., clipping in Box 17, Folder 8, Hayakawa Papers; "SD Hospital Gets a Warning." The organizations were the National Association for Equal Educational Opportunities, La Raza Lawyers Asso-

ciation of San Diego, Metropolitan Area Advisory Committee, the Chicano Federation of San Diego, and the San Diego Affirmative Action Coalition.

36. Jan Cook, "Hospital's Race Query Faulted," unidentified clipping in Box 17, Folder 8, Hayakawa Papers; Herman Baca to Mario Obledo, April 24, 1979, Box 21, Folder 20, Baca Papers. On Baca's activism in this case, see Joe Applegate, "Some People in This Town Don't Like Herman Baca," *San Diego Reader*, June 21, 1979, https://www.sandiegoreader.com/news/1979/jun/21/cover-some-people-in-this-town-dont-like-herman-b/.

37. "County Alien Care Suit Rejected," *San Diego Tribune*, December 11, 1979, B-4.

38. E.g., Edith Jones to Samuel Hayakawa, "Cost to San Diego County Hospitals for Illegal Alien Inpatient Care," March 10, 1980, Box 17, Folder 8, Hayakawa Papers.

39. "Remarks to Press Conference on Illegal Aliens," May 12, 1986, "Golding, San Diego Mayor Susan—False Statistics," Box 23, Folder 5, Baca Papers.

40. Press release, Committee on Chicano Rights, May 14, 1986, "Golding, San Diego Mayor Susan—False Statistics," Box 23, Folder 5, Baca Papers.

41. Press Release, Committee on Chicano Rights.

42. Heidi L. Holmblad, "Board Agrees to Study Impact of Aliens," *Escondido Times-Advocate*, June 15, 1986, 21; H. G. Reza, "Golding Wants U.S. to Pick Up Alien Tab," *Los Angeles Times*, May 13, 1986, 42, 44.

43. Susan Golding form letter, June 17, 1986, "Golding, San Diego Mayor Susan—False Statistics," Box 23, Folder 5, Baca Papers.

44. Holmblad, "Board Agrees to Study Impact of Aliens"; "Remarks to Press Conference on Illegal Aliens," May 12, 1986, "Golding, San Diego Mayor Susan—False Statistics," Box 23, Folder 5, Baca Papers.

45. Golding form letter.

46. Golding form letter.

47. Handwritten notes, "Golding, San Diego Mayor Susan—False Statistics," Baca Papers (spelling corrected).

48. Bardacke, *Trampling Out the Vintage*, chap. 24. See chap. 4 for additional discussion of UFW's policy toward the undocumented.

49. Guadalupe L. Sánchez and Jesús Romo, "Organizing Mexican Farm Workers on Both Sides of the Border," Working Papers in US-Mexican Studies 27, 1981, Program in US-Mexico Studies, University of California, San Diego, 4.

50. Ana Raquel Minian, *Undocumented Lives: The Untold Story of Mexican Migration* (Cambridge, MA: Harvard University Press, 2018), 161–62.

51. "Maricopa County Organizing Project Records: Historical Note," Online Archive of Arizona; Minian, *Undocumented Lives*, 164–65.

52. Sánchez and Romo, "Organizing Mexican Undocumented Farm Workers," 8.

53. Gabe Valdez to Lupe Sánchez, June 1, 1987, Box 95, Folder 21, Maricopa County Organizing Project Records, Hayden Library, Arizona State University (hereafter MCOP Records).

54. Don Harris, "Farm Union Enters New Season," *Arizona Republic*, February 20, 1984. For examples of some of their successful projects, see Minian, *Undocumented Lives*, 165.

55. Minian, *Undocumented Lives*, 161.

56. Guadalupe Sánchez to Cesar Chavez, April 24, 1979, FMDP; Sánchez and Romo, "Organizing Mexican Undocumented Farm Workers," 12. Numerous documents collected in the Farmworkers Movement Documentation Project indicate that the UFW attempted to disrupt the AFWU's efforts: http://library.ucsd.edu/dc/object/bb7373369s/_1.pdf.

57. "Our Story," http://adelantehealthcare.com/about-adelante-healthcare/our-story/; "El Mirage Anxiously Awaits Planned Opening of Clinic," *Arizona Republic*, January 23, 1980, 93.

58. "Agreement for Services," n.d., Box 16, Folder 55, MCOP Records.

59. Mass mailing, n.d., Box 16, Folder 50, MCOP Records.

60. Mass mailing, translation by the author.

61. *Arizona Republic*, December 5, 1984, clipping in Box 16, Folder 56, MCOP Records.

62. Minian, *Undocumented Lives*, 166.

63. "The First International Conference in Defense of the Full Rights of Undocumented Workers," Mexico City, April 28, 29, and 30, 1980, Box 61, Folder 1, MCOP Records. The rights enumerated include legal permanent residence, civil rights, family reunification, and the right to unionize, as well as housing and health services.

64. Minian, *Undocumented Lives*, 176–79; Michael A. Olivas, *No Undocumented Child Left Behind: Plyler v. Doe and the Education of Undocumented Schoolchildren* (New York: New York University Press, 2012); Sarah R. Coleman, *The Walls Within: The Politics of Immigration in Modern America* (Princeton, NJ: Princeton University Press, 2021), chap. 2.

65. Olivas, *No Undocumented Child Left Behind*, 60, 36.

66. https://casetext.com/case/lewis-v-thompson-2.

67. Consolidated Omnibus Budget Reconciliation Act of 1986, Section 9406(a).

68. Consolidated Omnibus Budget Reconciliation Act of 1986, Section 9121.

69. Although it is likely that they had permission to commute to work in the US (i.e. were "green card commuters"), I have not been able to determine the Guerreros' documentation status.

70. Transcript, *Guerrero v. Copper Queen*, Office of the County Clerk, Cochise County, Bisbee, Arizona.

71. *Guerrero v. Copper Queen Hospital*, https://law.justia.com/cases/arizona/supreme-court /1975/11958-pr-0.html.

72. *Guerrero v. Copper Queen Hospital*. Hays was a "noted conservative," https://en.wikipedia .org/wiki/Jack_D._H._Hays, so his decision was likely not related to a desire to expand the rights of noncitizens.

73. Consolidated Omnibus Budget Reconciliation Act of 1986, Section 9121.

74. "Brief of 104 Health Law Professors as *Amici Curiae* in Support of Petitioners," January 13, 2012, https://www.kellogghansen.com/assets/htmldocuments/Professors%20amicus %20brief%20in%20ACA%20case.pdf, 13.

75. Beatrix Hoffman, "Emergency Rooms: The Reluctant Safety Net," in *History and Health Policy: Bringing the Past Back In*, ed. Rosemary Stevens, Charles Rosenberg, and Lawton R. Burns (New Brunswick, NJ: Rutgers University Press, 2006).

76. See chapter 7 for further discussion of emergency room utilization.

77. Coleman, *The Walls Within*, 44.

78. Coleman, chap. 4.

79. Coleman, 91.

80. IRCA, Title II, "Temporary Disqualification of Newly Legalized Aliens from Receiving Certain Public Welfare Assistance."

81. "Dos and Don'ts" pamphlet, Coalition for Humane Immigration Rights of Los Angeles, Box 68, Folder 17, Grace Montanez Davis Papers; US Department of Justice, "Medical Examination of Aliens Seeking Adjustment of Status," February 14, 1987, Box 45, Folder 20, Hector García Papers.

82. "New Challenges for the Newly Legalized" Conference, August 23, 1988, 12–13, Box 47, Folder 2, American Friends Service Committee—US-Mexico Border Program Records, University of California, San Diego Special Collections and Archives (hereafter AFSC Papers).

83. Minian, *Undocumented Lives*, 201–2.

84. Immigration and Naturalization Service, "Estimates of the Unauthorized Immigrant Population Residing in the United States: 1990 to 2000," January 31, 2003, https://www.dhs.gov /sites/default/files/publications/Unauthorized%20Immigrant%20Population%20Estimates %20in%20the%20US%201990%20to%202000%20Exec%20Summ.pdf. On how IRCA unintentionally ended circular migration patterns, see Douglas S. Massey, Jorge Durand, and Nolan J. Malone, *Beyond Smoke and Mirrors: Mexican Immigration in an Era of Economic Integration* (New York: Russell Sage Foundation, 2003), and Minian, *Undocumented Lives*, chap. 8.

85. Daniel Martinez HoSang, *Racial Propositions: Ballot Initiatives and the Making of Postwar California* (Berkeley: University of California Press, 2010), 163–65.

86. HoSang, 164.

87. Proposition 187, chap. 1.3.

88. HoSang, *Racial Propositions*, 179–82; Taxpayers against 187, "Vote No," Box 679, Gloria Molina Papers, Huntington Library.

89. "Vote No."

90. "Vote No": Editorial, *San Francisco Chronicle*, July 28, 1994, Box 679, Molina Papers; MALDEF, "Preliminary Section-By-Section Analysis of the S.O.S. Initiative," June 30, 1994, Box 43, Folder 3, AFSC Papers.

91. "Vote No"; Peter Schrag, "SOS to Put Californians in Service of Big Brother," *Sacramento Bee*, July 14, 1994, 28.

92. HoSang, *Racial Propositions*, 184–85.

93. Isaac Guzman, "Students at UCLA Protest Prop. 187," *Los Angeles Times*, October 7, 1994, 384; "Protest: Students Oppose Prop. 187," *Los Angeles Times*, November 3, 1994, 25; Matt Spetalnik, "Huge L.A. march against Prop. 187," *San Francisco Examiner*, October 17, 1994, 4.

94. Amy Pyle and Greg Hernandez, "10,000 Students Protest Prop. 187," *Los Angeles Times*, November 3, 1994, 97; Jane Ballinger, "Students Protest Prop. 187," *Tulare Advance-Register*, November 4, 1994, 1.

95. "7,000 Attend Protest Denouncing Proposition 187," *Los Angeles Times*, October 31, 1994, 96.

96. HoSang, *Racial Propositions*, 197.

97. MALDEF Los Angeles, "Update on Litigation Challenging Proposition 187," March 24, 1995.

98. "187 Update," November 23, 1994, Box 1, Folder 27; Bill Tamayo to Concerned Organizations, November 17, 1994, Box 1, Folder 27, Eduardo Hernandez-Chavez Papers, University of New Mexico Center for Southwest Research; Department of Public Health, City and County of San Francisco, "Common Questions Regarding Proposition 187," Box 679, Folder 2, Molina Papers.

99. Lee Romney, Jeff Brazil, and Martin Miller, "Child Cited as Prop. 187 Casualty Had Leukemia," *Los Angeles Times*, Orange County ed., November 24, 1994, A24.

100. Romney et al., "Child Cited as Prop. 187 Casualty Had Leukemia," A43.

101. Romney et al., A40.

102. Walter L. Gray to Carrie Sutkin, November 15, 1994, Box 679, Folder 2, Molina Papers.

103. Nancy Otto to All Forum Members (National Immigration Forum), February 17, 1995;

Nancy Otto to Forum Members, December 5, 1994, both in Box 1, Folder 31, Hernandez-Chavez Papers. Expletive redacted in original.

104. HoSang, *Racial Propositions*, 200; Alex Nowrasteh, "Proposition 187 Turned California Blue," Cato Institute, July 20, 2016, https://www.cato.org/blog/proposition-187-turned-california-blue.

105. "Immigrant Rights Are Human Rights!," Box 1, Folder 34, Hernandez-Chavez Papers.

106. "Nuevo Mexicanos en Contra de la Propuesta 187" pamphlet, n.d., Box 1, Folder 27, Hernandez-Chavez Papers.

107. Coleman, *The Walls Within*, 126–27.

Chapter Six

1. Richard Breitman and Alan Kraut, *American Refugee Policy and European Jewry, 1933–1943* (Bloomington: Indiana University Press, 1988); "Refugee Timeline," https://www.uscis.gov/about-us/our-history/history-office-and-library/featured-stories-from-the-uscis-history-office-and-library/refugee-timeline. Three hundred and fifty thousand were admitted under the Displaced Persons Act. The 1952 Immigration and Nationality Act, also known as McCarren-Walter, reaffirmed nationality quotas and included no specific provisions for refugees.

2. "A Brief History of U.S. Refugee Resettlement from World War Two to the Obama Administration," *International Crisis Group* (2018), 4–6; "Refugee Timeline."

3. Refugee Relief Act of 1953. US Statutes at Large, Public Law 203, Ch. 336, 400–407. The public charge provision continued a policy known as the "Corporate Affidavit Program" started by Harry Truman in 1946 that allowed voluntary agencies to serve as guarantors, permitting entry for refugees who otherwise would have been subject to public charge exclusions. Norman L. Zucker, "Refugee Resettlement in the United States: The Role of Voluntary Organizations," *Michigan Journal of International Law* 3, no. 1 (1982): 155–77.

4. Public Law 87-510, "An Act to enable the United States to participate in the assistance rendered to certain migrants and refugees," June 28, 1962, 76 Stat., 121–24.

5. National Park Service, "Freedom Tower," nps.gov. In 1960 Eisenhower had established a Cuban Refugee Center in Miami, run by voluntary organizations. Zucker, "Refugee Resettlement in the United States," 157.

6. The Cuban Adjustment Act of 1966. Cuban refugees had unlimited access to public assistance programs, without waiting periods or time limits; US Office of Refugee Resettlement, "Refugees and General Assistance: A Short-Term Evaluation of the Effects of the Changes in Federal Refugee Assistance Policy on State and Local Governments and on Refugees." Washington, DC, 1983, 4.

7. Public Law 94-23, Ninety-Fourth Congress, "An Act to Enable the United States to Render Assistance to, or in Behalf of, Certain Migrants and Refugees," May 23, 1975, 89 Stat., 87–88.

8. "A Brief History of U.S. Refugee Resettlement," 6.

9. Public Law 96-212, March 17, 1980, 94 Stat., 102–18; "Refugee Program Policy Issues on Cash and Medical Assistance," n.d., Box 27, Folder 14, Comisión Feminil Mexicana Nacional Collection, University of California, Santa Barbara Special Collections.

10. "Testimony of William French Smith, Attorney General, before the Senate Subcommittee on Immigration and Refugee Policy and the House Subcommittee on Immigration, Refugees, and International Law," July 30, 1981, 17, Baca Papers.

11. "Testimony of William French Smith," 17–18.

12. Statement of Robert A. Peterson, General Accounting Office, to the Subcommittee on Immigration and Refugee Policy, Senate Committee on the Judiciary, on "Resettlement and Medical Problems of Indochinese Refugees in the United States," September 13, 1982.

13. Rubén G. Rumbaut, Leo R. Chavez, Robert J. Moser, Sheila M. Pickwell, and Samuel M. Wishick, "The Politics of Migrant Health Care: A Comparative Study of Mexican Immigrants and Indochinese Refugees," *Research in the Sociology of Health Care* 7 (1988): 143–202, 162. For a fascinating study of Cambodian refugee health and medicine, see Aihwa Ong, *Buddha Is Hiding: Refugees, Citizenship, the New America* (Berkeley: University of California Press, 2003).

14. Rumbaut et al., "The Politics of Migrant Health Care," 176.

15. Rumbaut et al., 176.

16. House of Representatives, Ninety-Fourth Congress, "Enable United States to Render Assistance to Migrants and Refugees," 1 (1975), 3. By the end of the century, an additional five hundred thousand Indochinese refugees were resettled in the US.

17. Carl Rowan and David Mazie, "New Bill Offers Solution to Immigration Nightmare," *Wichita Eagle-Beacon*, December 19, 1982, 3; F. James Sensenbrenner Jr., "The Immigration Problem," *Modesto Bee*, August 5, 1981, 11. Under the 1980 Refugee Act, the number of persons who may be admitted to the United States as refugees each year is set by the president, in consultation with Congress.

18. Rowan and Mazie, "New Bill Offers Solution."

19. E.g. Devyn Benson and Danielle Clealand, "Re-Narrating Mariel: Black Cubans, Racial Exclusion, and Building Community in Miami," *Anthurium: A Caribbean Studies Journal* (December 14, 2021), https://anthurium.miami.edu/articles/10.33596/anth.462/.

20. Felix Masud-Piloto, *From Welcomed Exiles to Illegal Immigrants: Cuban Migration to the U.S., 1959–1995* (Lanham, MD: Rowman and Littlefield, 1996), 84.

21. Masud-Piloto, 86–87.

22. The INS continued to detain Cubans with criminal convictions. See Mark Dow, *American Gulag: Inside U.S. Immigration Prisons* (Berkeley: University of California Press, 2004).

23. See, e.g., William M. LeoGrande, *Our Own Backyard: The United States in Central America, 1977–1992* (Chapel Hill: University of North Carolina Press, 1998); María Cristina García, *Seeking Refuge: Central American Migration to Mexico, the United States, and Canada* (Berkeley: University of California Press, 2006), chap. 1.

24. García, *Seeking Refuge*, 31–32; Ann Crittenden, *Sanctuary: A Story of American Conscience and Law in Collision* (New York: Weidenfelt and Nicholson, 1988), xvi–xvii.

25. Norma Stoltz Chinchilla, Nora Hamilton, and James Loucky, "The Sanctuary Movement and Central American Activism in Los Angeles," *Latin American Perspectives* 36, no. 6 (November 2009): 101–26.

26. Lefkowitz, *Community Health Centers*, 127.

27. Leonard Cizewski with assistance from Barbara Burdulis, Jacquelyn Tomberlan, and Cheryl Robinson, "A Short Guide to Refugee Health Care," *Links: Central American Health Rights Network* 2 (n.d.): 8. Part 2, Box 1, Folder 4, Chicago Religious Task Force on Central America Records, Wisconsin Historical Society.

28. "The Many Responses to Refugee Health Needs," *Links: Central American Health Rights Network* 2 (n.d.): 10. Part 2, Box 1, Folder 4, Chicago Religious Task Force on Central America Records; "Handbook of Health Care Services for Low-Income Spanish-Speaking Clients," 1987, Box 68, Folder 22, Grace Montañez Davis Papers, Chicano Studies Research Center, UCLA. See also Mario García, *Father Luis Olivares, a Biography: Faith Politics and the Origins of the Sanctuary Movement in Los Angeles* (Chapel Hill: University of North Carolina Press, 2018).

29. Health-related solidarity groups included the Nicaragua Medical Aid Project and the Central American Health Rights Network. Brittany McWilliams, "Treating the Revolution: Health Care and Solidarity in Nicaragua and El Salvador in the 1980s," MA thesis, University of Massachusetts Amherst, 2020. See also Michael Terry with Laura Turiano, "Brigadistas and Revolutionaries: Health and Social Justice in El Salvador," in *Comrades in Health: U.S. Health Internationalists, Abroad and at Home*, ed. Anne-Emanuelle Birn and Theodore H. Brown (New Brunswick, NJ: Rutgers University Press, 2013).

30. García, *Seeking Refuge*, 112–13. In US policy, refugees are given that designation before arrival; asylum seekers seek recognition of their claims individually, after arrival.

31. García, 111–12.

32. Yuriko Doku and Oscar A. Chacón, "TPS Extension: A New Hope for Salvadorans," University of Nebraska Office of Latino/Latin American Studies, March 2019, https://www.unomaha.edu/college-of-arts-and-sciences/ollas/research/tps-blog.php.

33. American Immigration Council, "Temporary Protected Status: An Overview," https://www.americanimmigrationcouncil.org/research/temporary-protected-status-overview.

34. "A Timeline on HIV and AIDS," HIV.gov, https://www.hiv.gov/hiv-basics/overview/history/hiv-and-aids-timeline#year-1987. See also Jennifer Brier, *Infectious Ideas: US Political Responses to the AIDS Crisis* (Chapel Hill: University of North Carolina Press, 2009), especially chap. 3.

35. Rona Morrow, "AIDS and Immigration: The United States Attempts to Deport a Disease," *University of Miami Inter-American Law Review* 20, no. 1 (Fall 1988): 131–73.

36. Morrow, 147.

37. "Dear Activists," Box 4, Folder 7, ACT UP/Los Angeles Records, ONE Gay and Lesbian Archives, University of Southern California.

38. Sandy Dwyer, "Protest at INS" (unidentified clipping), Box 4, Folder 7, ACT UP/Los Angeles Records.

39. Benita Roth, *The Life and Death of ACT UP/LA* (New York: Cambridge University Press, 2017), 101; Sarah Schulman, *Let the Record Show: A Political History of ACT UP New York, 1987–1993* (New York: Farrar, Straus and Giroux, 2021).

40. "La Resistencia Protest at Mardi Gras Motel INS Detention Center," March 19, 1988, Box 4, Folder 15; "Shut Down the INS National Phone Zap," Box 6, Folder 19 April 5, 1990, ACT UP/Los Angeles Records.

41. "Shut Down the INS National Phone Zap."

42. "Case Examples of Persons Assisted by HIV Task Force Members That Demonstrate Nature and Consequence of Civil Surgeon Counseling," Box 6, Folder 22, San Francisco Department of Public Health AIDS Office Records, San Francisco Public Library.

43. Kenneth W. Kizer to Richard Norton, January 9, 1989, Box 6, Folder 22, San Francisco Department of Public Health AIDS Office Records; Karma R. Chávez, *The Borders of AIDS* (Seattle: University of Washington Press, 2021), 70. As of July 1990, the INS "has denied thirty-seven out of fifty-nine waiver applications." Bettina M. Fernandez, "HIV Exclusion of Immigrants under the Immigration Reform & Control Act of 1986," *La Raza Law Journal* 5 (1992): 65–107, 68.

44. "United States HIV Immigration and Travel Policy," ACT UP NY Historical Archive, https://actupny.org/actions/Immigration.html; Associated Press, "Tomas Fabregas; AIDS Crusader, 36," *New York Times*, September 26, 1994, Section D, 9.

45. "Closing the Gaps," June 1991, Box 8, Folder 10, ACT UP/Los Angeles Records.

46. Dr. David Butler-Jones, ACT UP NY Historical Archive, https://actupny.org/actions

/Immigration.html. On the adoption of a human rights approach to pandemic control, see Elizabeth Fee and Manon Perry, "Jonathan Mann, HIV/AIDS, and Human Rights," *Journal of Public Health Policy* 29, no. 1 (Apr., 2008): 54–71.

47. On the history of US racism toward Haitians, see, e.g., Malissia Lenox, "Refugees, Racism, and Reparations: A Critique of the United States' Haitian Immigration Policy," *Stanford Law Review* 45, no. 3 (February 1993): 687–724.

48. Carl Lindskoog's *Detain and Punish: Haitian Refugees and the Rise of the World's Largest Immigration System* (Gainesville: University of Florida Press, 2018), brilliantly discusses the history of refugee detention in the US.

49. *Caribbean Refugee Crisis: Cubans and Haitians. Hearing before the Committee on the Judiciary, United States Senate*, May 12, 1980, 53–59.

50. Lindskoog, *Detain and Punish*, 51–62.

51. AP, "Haitians removed from AIDS risk list," *New York Times*, April 10, 1985; https://www.nytimes.com/1990/04/21/nyregion/fda-policy-to-limit-blood-is-protested.html.

52. A. Naomi Paik, *Rightlessness: Testimony and Redress in U.S. Prison Camps since World War II* (Chapel Hill: University of North Carolina Press, 2016), 97.

53. Paik, 105–6; "ACT UP Turns to HIV-Positive Haitian Detainees," Guantánamo Public Memory Project, https://gitmomemory.org/timeline/resisting-and-protesting-guantanamo/act-up-turns-to-hiv-positive-haitian-detainees/. See Paik's remarkable book for a detailed discussion of the refugees' experiences at Guantánamo.

54. Lindskoog, *Detain and Punish*, 2; Smita Ghosh, "How Migrant Detention Became American Policy," *Washington Post*, July 19, 2019.

55. Jessica Ordaz, *The Shadow of El Centro* (Chapel Hill: University of North Carolina Press, 2021), 62–64; Katrina Shull, *Detention Empire: Reagan's War on Immigrants and the Seeds of Resistance* (Chapel Hill: University of North Carolina Press, 2002), 176–77. On the history of detention, see also Ana Raquel Minian, *In the Shadow of Liberty: The Invisible History of Immigrant Detention in the United States* (New York: Viking, 2024).

56. Minutes of Centro de Asuntos Migratorios Board of Directors Meeting, April 28, 1982, Box 45, Folder 10, AFSC Records. The AFSC's long-standing US-Mexico Border Program also had a project, the Centro de Asuntos Migratorios, that reported on abusive treatment of migrants, including cases of migrants who were denied medical attention while detained by border officials. See the Centro files in AFSC Records, University of California, San Diego, and Michael Huspek, Roberto Martinez, and Leticia Jimenez, "Violations of Human and Civil Rights on the U.S.-Mexico Border, 1995 to 1997: A Report," *Social Justice* 25, no. 2 (Summer 1998): 110–30. See also Legal Aid Society of San Diego, Inc., "Petition for Congressional Investigation," Box 31, Folder 2, Baca Papers.

57. Ordaz, *Shadow of El Centro*, 64–65; *Links* newsletter, n.d., in Part 2, Box 1, Folder 4, Chicago Religious Task Force on Central America Records.

58. "Hunger Strike Declared at Center," *Tulare Advance-Register*, May 28, 1985, 2. For a full discussion of the 1985 hunger strike, see Ordaz, *Shadow of El Centro*, chap. 5.

59. AFSC, "Human Rights at the Mexico-US Border," March 1990, Box 7, Chicago Religious Task Force on Central America Records. The report did not specify the names of the detention centers.

60. Transcript of the Special Hearing on Human Rights and Civil Rights Abuses in the US-Mexico Border Region, n.d., 29, Box 17, Folder 23, AFSC Records.

61. Lindskoog, *Detain and Punish*, 116–31.

62. William J. Clinton, "Remarks on the Immigration Policy Initiative and an Exchange

with Reporters," February 7, 1995, American Presidency Project; Kristina Davis, "Operation Gatekeeper at 25: Look Back at the Turning Point That Transformed the Border," *Los Angeles Times*, September 30, 2019. In August of 2000, right before the end of his term, Clinton did issue an executive order favorable to immigrant health, Executive Order 13166, which requires all recipients of federal funding, including hospitals, to provide individuals with limited English proficiency "meaningful" access to language services.

63. William J. Clinton, "Address before a Joint Session of Congress on the State of the Union," January 24, 1995, American Presidency Project.

64. Michael E. Fix, Randy Capps, and Neeraj Kaushal, "Immigrants and Welfare: Overview," Russel Sage Foundation, 1; Coleman, *The Walls Within*, 116–18.

65. Fix et al., "Immigrants and Welfare," 1; Coleman, *The Walls Within*, 116–18.

66. Coleman, *The Walls Within*, 116–18, 135.

67. Willie L. Brown to Dianne Feinstein, n.d., Box 21, Folder 18, Frank I. Sanchez Papers.

68. National Latina Health Organization, "National Welfare Reform: An Analysis of its Impact on Latinas," September 1995, Box 38, Folder 16, Grace Molina de Pick Papers, San Diego State University Special Collections; "Welfare Reform: Evolving Impact," *Latino Health News* 6, no. 1 (January 1997), Box 8, Folder 27, MELA (Madre del Este de Los Angeles) Collection, California State University, Northridge Special Collections and Archives.

69. Lisa Sun-Hee Park, *Entitled to Nothing: The Struggle for Immigrant Health Care in the Age of Welfare Reform* (New York: New York University Press), 92–93; Lynn Fujiwara, *Mothers without Citizenship: Asian Immigrant Families and the Consequences of Welfare Reform* (Minneapolis: University of Minnesota Press, 2008), xv–xvi.

70. Bruce Goldstein and Shelley Davis, "Farmworkers and Public Benefits in the Era of Welfare Reform," *In Defense of the Alien* 20 (1997): 64; Carol Morello, "Aid Cutoff Driving Immigrants to Suicide," *Philadelphia Inquirer*, May 25, 1997, 1, 14.

71. "Ruling Deals Blow to Illegal Immigrants on Prop. 187," *Tribune* (San Luis Obispo), November 4, 1996, 26. The judge was Mariana R. Pfaelzer.

72. "Texas Public Hospitals May Not Provide Preventive Care to Undocumented Immigrants, State AG Determines," *Kaiser Daily Health Policy Report*, July 13, 2001; "Interpretations Vary on Health Care," *Odessa American*, September 8, 2001, 5B. Levin quotations: Kristalee Guerra, "The Policy and Politics of Illegal Immigrant Health Care in Texas," *Houston Journal of Health Law and Policy* 3 (2002): 113–50, 136. Levin went on to become a conservative talk radio host and Fox News commentator.

73. Kristalee Guerra, "The Policy and Politics of Illegal Immigrant Health Care in Texas," *Houston Journal of Health Law and Policy* 3 (2002): 113–50, 135; Marisa Treviño, "Immigrants Are Human Beings Too," *El Paso Times*, August 26, 2001, 9A; Pam Easton (Associated Press), "Health Care for Illegal Immigrants Debated," *Abilene Reporter-News*, September 2, 2001, 3AA; Jim Yardley, "Immigrants' Medical Care Is Focus of Texas Dispute," *New York Times*, August 12, 2001, 18.

74. "Texas Senate Approves Measure That Would Allow Preventive Care for Undocumented Immigrants," *Kaiser Daily Health Policy Report*, May 7, 2003. On media and rights group' reactions to Cornyn's AG opinion, see Guerra, "The Policy and Politics of Illegal Immigrant Health Care in Texas."

75. Easton, "Health Care for Illegal Immigrants Debated."

76. *Lewis v. Thompson*, 252 F.3d 567 (2d Cir. 2001).

77. "Undocumented Immigrants in the United States: Access to Prenatal Care," Hastings Center Issue Brief, September 12, 2014, https://undocumented.thehastingscenter.org/issuebrief /undocumented-immigrants-in-the-united-states-access-to-prenatal-care/.

78. Linda S. Smith, "Health of American Newcomers," *Journal of Community Health Nursing* 18, no. 1 (Spring 2001): 53–68, 58. Abortion rights advocates also feared that the "unborn child option" would define the fetus as a person. Vicki Kemper, "White House Issues Regulation that Defines Fetuses as Children," *Los Angeles Times*, September 28, 2022, A23.

79. Gabrielle Lessard and Leighton Ku, "Gaps in Coverage for Children in Immigrant Families," *Future of Children* 13, no. 1 (Spring 2003): 100–115, 108; Jacqueline Hagan, Nestor Rodriguez, Randy Capps, and Nika Kabiri, "The Effects of Recent Welfare and Immigration Reforms on Immigrants' Access to Health Care," *International Migration Review* 37, no. 2 (2003): 444–63, 447. Attempts to include legal immigrant children fully in SCHIP were defeated in the reauthorizations of 2007 and 2009.

80. Lessard and Ku, "Gaps in Coverage for Children in Immigrant Families," 108.

81. Hagan et al., "The Effects of Recent Welfare and Immigration Reforms on Immigrants' Access to Health Care."

82. Smith, "Health of American Newcomers"; Lucas Guttentag and Lee Gelernt, "Health Care Reform and the Rights of Immigrants," *In Defense of the Alien* 17 (1994): 42–49.

83. Coleman, *The Walls Within*, 64.

84. Christian Zlolniski, "Labor Control and Resistance of Mexican Immigrant Janitors in Silicon Valley," *Human Organization* 62, no. 1 (Spring 2003): 39–49, 42.

85. "Janitors Stage Vigil," *Los Angeles Times*, March 31, 1988, part 2, 10.

86. Ruth Milkman, *L.A. Story: Immigrant Workers and the Future of the U.S. Labor Movement* (New York: Russell Sage Foundation, 2006), 147, 127–30, 159. See also Hector Delgádo, *New Immigrants, Old Unions: Organizing Undocumented Workers in Los Angeles* (Philadelphia: Temple University Press, 1994).

87. Robert Pear, "34.7 Million Lack Health Insurance, Studies Say," *New York Times*, December 19, 1991, B17.

88. Bob Baker, "Largest Non-Union Janitorial Service Agrees to Labor Pact," *Los Angeles Times*, February 27, 1991, B6; Cynthia J. Cranford, "Networks of Exploitation: Immigrant Labor and the Restructuring of the Los Angeles Janitorial Industry," *Social Problems* 52, no. 3 (August 2005): 379–97, 394.

89. Edna Bonacich, "Organizing Immigrant Workers in the Los Angeles Apparel Industry," *Journal of World-Systems Research* 4 (1998): 10–19, 12.

90. Kenneth B. Noble, "Thai Workers Are Set Free in California," *New York Times*, August 4, 1995, A1.

91. Barbara J. Burgel, Nanette Lashuay, Leslie Israel, and Robert Harrison, "Garment Workers in California: Health Outcomes of the Asian Immigrant Women Workers Clinic," *AAOHN Journal* 52, no. 11 (2004): 465–75; Jennifer Jihye Chun, George Lipsitz, and Young Chin, "Immigrant Women Workers at the Center of Social Change: Asian Immigrant Women Advocates," in *Immigrant Women Workers in the Neoliberal Age*, ed. Nilda Flores-González, Anna Romina Guevarra, Maura Toro-Morn, and Grace Chang (Urbana: University of Illinois Press, 2013). On the "worker center" movement, which emerged as an adjunct and alternative to union organizing, see, e.g., Kent Wong, "A New Labor Movement for a New Working Class: Unions, Worker Centers, and Immigrants," *Berkeley Journal of Employment and Labor Law* 36, no. 1 (2015): 205–13.

92. Glenn Omatsu, "Immigrant Workers Take the Lead: A Militant Humility Transforms L.A. Koreatown," in *Immigrant Rights in the Shadows of Citizenship*, ed. Rachel Ida Buff, (New York: New York University Press, 2008); "About Miguel Contreras," Miguel Contreras Foundation, https://miguelcontrerasfoundation.org/about/miguel-contreras/. See also, e.g., Eileen Boris

and Jennifer Klein, *Caring for America: Home Health Workers in the Shadow of the Welfare State* (New York: Oxford University Press, 2012).

93. Leonardo Salvaggio, "World Trade Center: An Interview with Former Windows on the World Cook Sekou Siby," *Undicisettembre*, April 29, 2002, https://undicisettembre.blogspot.com /2022/04/world-trade-center-interview-with-sekou.html.

94. Evan Osnos (*Chicago Tribune*), "Added Pain for 'Undocumented,'" *Rochester Democrat and Chronicle*, October 14, 2001, 16A.

95. Osnos.

96. Jocelyn Solis and Liliana Rivera-Sanchez, "Recovering the Forgotten: The Effects of September 11th on Undocumented Latin American Victims and Families," *Canadian Journal of Latin American and Caribbean Studies/Revue canadienne des études latino-américaines et cara-ïbes* 29, no. 57/58 (2004): 93–115, 101, 103.

97. "Windows of Hope Family Relief Fund: A Five-Year Report on the Accomplishments of the Fund," 2006, https://www.windowsofhope2001.org/wp-content/uploads/2017/01/5-year -report.pdf.

98. "Disaster Relief Medicaid Evaluation Project," Prepared for the Office of Medicaid Management, New York State Department of Health by Cornell University, School of Industrial Relations, December 2005; Solis and Rivera-Sanchez, "Recovering the Forgotten," 113.

Chapter Seven

1. Christina Headrick and Vicki Chang, "Some Link Citizenship, Transplants," *News and Observer* (Raleigh, NC), March 4, 2004, A1; Beatrix Hoffman, "Sympathy and Exclusion: Access to Health Care for Undocumented Immigrants in the United States," in *A Death Retold: Jesica Santillan, the Bungled Transplant, and Paradoxes of Medical Citizenship in the United States*, ed. Keith Wailoo, Julie Livingston, and Peter Garbaccia (Chapel Hill: University of North Carolina Press, 2006).

2. Wailoo, Livingston, and Garbaccia, *A Death Retold*; Headrick and Chang, "Some Link Citizenship, Transplants," A1, A6; Michelle Malkin, "America: Medical Welcome Mat to the World," VDare.com, February 20, 2003, https://vdare.com/articles/america-medical-welcome -mat-to-the-world.

3. "Illegal Immigrant Hoping for Liver Transplant," Cleveland19 News, July 19, 2002, https:// www.cleveland19.com/story/863793/illegal-immigrant-hoping-for-liver-transplant/; Headrick and Chang, "Some Link Citizenship, Transplants."

4. Headrick and Chang, "Some Link Citizenship, Transplants"; Hoffman, "Sympathy and Exclusion," 245.

5. Malkin, "America: Medical Welcome Mat to the World."

6. The number of US hospitals peaked in the 1970s at 7,174 and by 2013 had declined to 5,686; "5 Statistics about Hospital Capacity over Time," *Becker's Hospital Review*, March 17, 2015, https://www.beckershospitalreview.com/patient-flow/5-statistics-about-hospital-capacity-over -time.html. Reasons that hospitals closed include low patient numbers, declining reimbursements, mergers and consolidations, and the overall shift from inpatient to outpatient services during this time period. For further analyses of the factors behind hospital closures, see, e.g., Department of Health and Human Services, Office of the Inspector General, "Trends in Urban Hospital Closure, 1990–2000," May 2003, https://www.govinfo.gov/content/pkg/GOVPUB-HE -PURL-gpo72133/pdf/GOVPUB-HE-PURL-gpo72133.pdf; Nicholas C. Petris Center on Health

Care Markets and Consumer Welfare, "California's Closed Hospitals, 1995–2000," January 2001, revised April 2001, https://petris.org/wp-content/uploads/2013/02/ClosedHospitals.pdf.

7. Arizona College of Emergency Physicians, "The Critical State of Emergency Care in Arizona," December 6, 2000, Debi Wells Papers, Series 3, Subseries 8, Box 6, Folder "ER 'Crisis,'" Arizona State Archives. Some material from this section also appeared in Beatrix Hoffman, "The Politics of Immigration Meets the Politics of Health Care" in *The Edinburgh Companion to the Politics of American Health*, ed. Martin Haliwell and Sophie A. Jones (Edinburgh: Edinburgh University Press, 2022).

8. Jeff Biggers, *State Out of the Union: Arizona and the Final Showdown over the American Dream* (New York: Nation Books, 2012).

9. Arizona Hospital and Healthcare Association, n.d., "The Perfect Storm: Hospitals Brace for Winter Crisis," Box 6, Folder "ER 'Crisis,'" Wells Papers.

10. Todd B. Taylor, MD, "Amendment to Restore Imperiled Safety Net Care," Box 6, Folder "ER 'Crisis,'" Wells Papers; Michael K. Gusmano and Frank J. Thompson, "Safety Net Hospitals at the Crossroads: Whither Medicaid DHS?," in *The Health Care Safety Net in a Post-Reform World*, ed. Mark A. Hall and Sara Rosenbaum (New Brunswick, NJ: Rutgers University Press, 2012).

11. "Flow of 2000 Medicaid Disproportionate Share Funds," Wells Papers. No statistics on the amount of DSH funds that went to undocumented immigrants' care were available for any state; Congressional Research Service, "Federal Funding for Unauthorized Aliens' Emergency Medical Expenses," October 18, 2004, CRS Report for Congress, RL31630, 7.

12. "Federal Funding for Unauthorized Aliens' Emergency Medical Expenses," 8. In a separate maneuver, a House committee established a single payment solely for four counties in southern Arizona (10).

13. Dana Rohrabacher, "Providing Health Care for Illegal Aliens" (Statement), January 21, 2004, https://votesmart.org/public-statement/40778/providing-health-care-for-illegal-aliens#.X29VCS2z3OR; Hoffman, "Sympathy and Exclusion," 249.

14. "Statement of Congresswoman Linda Sánchez on the Undocumented Alien Emergency Medical Assistance Amendments of 2004, H.R. 3722," May 17, 2004, https://lindasanchez.house.gov/media-center/press-releases/statement-congresswoman-linda-s-nchez-undocumented-alien-emergency; Sheila Jackson-Lee, "Undocumented Alien Emergency Medical Assistance Amendments of 2004," May 17, 2004, https://votesmart.org/public-statement/37912/undocumented-alien-emergency-medical-assistance-amendments-of-2004#.X2eBMy2z3OQ.

15. Ken Alltucker, "Hospitals' Funding for Unpaid Bills to End," *Arizona Republic*, September 21, 2008.

16. US Government Accountability Office, Report to Congressional Requesters, "Undocumented Aliens: Questions Persist about Their Impact on Hospitals' Uncompensated Care Costs," GAO-04-472, May 2004.

17. Oliver W. Jones, MD, "Health Care for California's Undocumented Mexican Immigrants," Division of Medical Genetics, vol. 1, no. 1, University of California, San Diego, n.d. ca. 1980; Lyndon B. Johnson School of Public Affairs, "The Use of Public Services by Undocumented Aliens in Texas: A Study of State Costs and Revenues," Policy Research Project Report No. 60, University of Texas at Austin, 1984, 87, 159.

18. Leo R. Chavez, "Unauthorised Immigrants and Access to Health Services: A Game of Pass the Buck," *Migration Today* 11, no. 1 (1983): 14–19; Leo R. Chavez, *Shadowed Lives: Undocumented Immigrants in American Society* (Forth Worth, TX: Harcourt Brace, 1992), 75.

19. Leo R. Chavez, Estevan T. Flores, and Marta Lopez-Garza, "Undocumented Latin

American Immigrants and U.S. Health Services: An Approach to a Political Economy of Utilization," *Medical Anthropology Quarterly*, new series, 6, no. 1 (March 1992): 6–26, quotation from abstract.

20. Steven P. Wallace, Jacqueline Torres, Tabashir Sadegh-Nobari, Nadereh Pourat, E. Richard Brown, "Unauthorised Immigrants and Health Care Reform," Final Report to the Commonwealth Fund, August 31, 2012, 21.

21. W. Tarraf, W. Vega, and H. M. Gonzales, "Emergency Department Services Use among Immigrant and Non-immigrant Groups in the United States," *Journal of Immigrant and Minority Health* 16, no. 4 (August 2014): 595–606; Alberto Coutasse, Andrea L. Lorden, Vishal Nemarugommula, and Karan Singh, "Uncompensated Care Cost: A Pilot Study Using Hospitals in a Texas County," *Hospital Topics* 82, no. 2 (February 2009): 3–11, 5.

22. Deborah Sontag, "Deported, by U.S. Hospitals: Immigrants, Spurned on Rehabilitation, Are Forced Out," *New York Times*, August 3, 2008, 1. Some material in this section also appeared in Beatrix Hoffman, "At the Borders of the Public: Immigrant and Migrant Publics and the Right to Health" in *Publics and Their Health: Historical Problems and Perspectives*, ed. Alex Mold, Peder Clark, and Hannah J. Elizabeth (Manchester: University of Manchester Press, 2023).

23. Sontag, "Deported, by U.S. Hospitals," 18; Lori A. Nessel, "Disposable Workers: Applying a Human Rights Framework to Analyze Duties Owed to Seriously Injured or Ill Migrants," *Indiana Journal of Global Legal Studies* 19, no. 1 (January 2012): 61–103.

24. Sontag, "Deported, by U.S. Hospitals," 18. For a claim that DSH funds are insufficient, see James W. Jones, Laurence B. McCullough, and Bruce W. Richman, "My Brother's Keeper: Uncompensated Care for Illegal Immigrants," *Journal of Vascular Surgery* 44, no. 3 (September 1, 2006): 679–82.

25. Seton Hall Law School and New York Lawyers for the Public Interest, "Discharge, Deportation, and Dangerous Journeys: A Study on the Practice of Medical Repatriation," December 2012, https://www.immigrationresearch.org/system/files/Seton_Hall_Discharge_Deportation_and_Dangerous_Journeys.pdf.

26. Associated Press, "Report: U.S. Hospitals Deported Hundreds of Immigrants," CBS News, April 23, 2013, https://www.cbsnews.com/news/report-us-hospitals-deported-hundreds-of-immigrants/.

27. Abby Kaighin, "Nowhere to Go," *Austin American-Statesman*, April 11, 1982, 1.

28. "Case of: Candida Cassas and Paradise Valley Hospital," Subject Files, Baca Papers.

29. "Formerly Comatose Honduran Woman to Stay in U.S.," *Arizona Republic*, May 21, 2008, B7. I was not able to determine the outcome of the San Diego case.

30. Judith Graham, Becky Schlikerman, and Abel Uribe, "Seriously Injured, Abruptly Deported," *Chicago Tribune*, February 7, 2011, 1; "Discharge, Deportation, and Dangerous Journeys."

31. "Seriously Injured, Abruptly Deported"; "Quadriplegic Immigrant Dies after Chicago-Area Hospital Returned Him to Mexico," *Chicago Tribune*, January 4, 2012, 5.

32. Kevin Sack, "Hospital Falters as Refuge for Illegal Immigrants," *New York Times*, November 20, 2009.

33. Kevin Sack, "Atlanta Judge Rules Dialysis Unit Can Be Closed," *New York Times*, September 25, 2009.

34. For other examples of US cases reported to the Inter-American Commission, see Margaret Huang, "'Going Global': Appeals to International and Regional Human Rights Bodies," in *Bringing Human Rights Home: A History of Human Rights in the United States*, ed. Cynthia Soohoo, Catherine Albisa, and Martha F. Davis, abridged ed. (Philadelphia: University of Pennsylvania Press, 2009), 244.

35. "Lawyers for Grady Memorial Dialysis Patients Seek International Stage," *Atlanta Journal-Constitution*, January 11, 2010, https://www.healthleadersmedia.com/finance/lawyers -grady-memorial-dialysis-patients-seek-international-stage; Inter-American Commission on Human Rights, "PM 385-09-31 Undocumented Immigrants Residing in Atlanta, Georgia, United States," https://www.oas.org/en/IACHR/decisions/precautionary.asp?Year=2010.

36. "Human Rights Group Looks at Dialysis Clinic Closure," *Atlanta Journal-Constitution*, January 21, 2010, https://www.ajc.com/news/local/human-rights-group-looks-grady-dialysis -clinic-closure/H40s3rRr7wspXWaAG5F3yM/.

37. Misty Williams, "Grady, Dialysis Provider Strike Three-Year Deal," *Atlanta Journal-Constitution*, September 9, 2011, https://www.ajc.com/news/local/grady-dialysis-provider-strike -year-deal/bUPxvxWl6AtvGrIhu2ISjP/.

38. Jonathan Springston, "Grady Extends Dialysis amidst Human Rights Inquiry," *Atlanta Progressive News*, January 20, 2010, https://atlantaprogressivenews.com/2010/01/10/grady -extends-dialysis-deadline-amidst-human-rights-inquiry/; Free Migration Project, *Fatal Flights: Medical Deportation in the U.S.*, 2021, 5; Kevin Sack, "For Sick Illegal Immigrants, No Relief Back Home," *New York Times*, December 31, 2009.

39. Free Migration Project, *Fatal Flights*, iii.

40. Free Migration Project, 3.

41. For a critical discussion of this literature, see Stacey A. Teruya and Shahrzad Bazargan-Hejazi, "The Immigrant and Hispanic Paradoxes: A Systematic Review of Their Predictions and Effects," *Hispanic Journal of Behavioral Science* 35, no. 4 (September 5, 2015): 486–509.

42. Shawn Malia Kanaiaupuni, "Child Well-Being and the Intergenerational Effects of Undocumented Immigrant Status," Institute for Research on Poverty, Discussion Paper no. 1210-00, June 2000. For important anthropological research on the intersection of undocumented status, low-wage work, and health, see Seth Holmes, *Fresh Fruit, Broken Bodies: Migrant Farmworkers in the United States* (Berkeley: University of California Press, 2013); and Sarah Bronwen Horton, *They Leave Their Kidneys in the Fields: Illness, Injury, and Illegality among U.S. Farmworkers* (Berkeley: University of California Press, 2016).

43. Leo R. Chavez, *Anchor Babies and the Challenge of Birthright Citizenship*, Kindle ed. (Stanford: Stanford University Press, 2017), location 1138.

44. Sol Pía Juárez, Helena Honkaniemi, Andrea C. Dunlavy, Robert W. Aldridge, Mauricio L. Barreto, Srinivasa Vittal Katikireddi, and Mikael Rostila, "Effects of Non-Health-Targeted Policies on Migrant Health: A Systematic Review and Meta-Analysis," *Lancet Global Health* 7, no. 4 (April 1, 2019). See also Collin W. Mueller and Bryce J. Bartlett, "U.S. Immigration Policy Regimes and Physical Disability Trajectories among Mexico-U.S. Immigrants," *Journals of Gerontology Series B: Psychological Sciences and Social Sciences* 74, no. 4 (April 2019): 725–34, showing correlation between the health of aging immigrant populations and the policy regimes they live under.

45. Luis H. Zayas, *Forgotten Citizens: Deportation, Children, and the Making of American Exiles and Orphans* (New York: Oxford University Press, 2015), 88–99.

46. William D. Lopez, *Separated: Family and Community in the Aftermath of an Immigration Raid* (Baltimore, MD: Johns Hopkins University Press, 2019), 23.

47. Lopez, 77–80. See also Nolan Kline, *Pathogenic Policing: Immigration Enforcement and Health in the U.S. South* (New Brunswick, NJ: Rutgers University Press, 2019); Karen Hacker, Jocelyn Chu, Carolyn Leung, Robert Marra, Alex Pirie, Mohamed Brahimi, Margaret English, Joshua Beckman, Dolores Acevedo-Garcia, and Robert P. Marlin, "The Impact of Immigration

and Customs Enforcement on Immigrant Health: Perceptions of Immigrants in Everett, Massachusetts, USA," *Social Science and Medicine* 73, no. 4 (August 2011): 586–94.

48. Nicole L. Novak, Arline T. Geronimus, and Aresha M. Martinez-Cardoso, "Change in Birth Outcomes among Infants Born to Latina Mothers after a Major Immigration Raid," *International Journal of Epidemiology* 46, no. 3 (June 1, 2017): 839–49; Marci Ybarra, Angela Garcia, and Youngjin Stephanie Hong, "Deportation Threat and Infant Birth Weight: Evidence from California," Abstract, Society for Social Work and Research, January 14, 2022, https://sswr.confex .com/sswr/2022/webprogram/Paper46501.html.

49. "Affidavit of Guadalupe Alonzo," June 22, 1979, Box 31, Folder 2, Petition for Congressional Investigation, Subject Files, Baca Papers.

50. Legal Aid Society of San Diego, Inc., "Petition for Congressional Investigation," Box 31, Folder 2, Baca Papers. I have not been able to determine whether the government responded to the petition.

51. Statement of Bruce Wheeler, Tucson City Council, *Border Violence: Hearing before the Subcommittee on International Law, Immigration, and Refugees of the Committee on the Judiciary, House of Representatives*, September 29, 1993, 93–98.

52. *Border Violence*, 45.

53. *Border Violence*, 84, 125, 131.

54. *Border Violence*, 135–36.

55. *Border Violence*.

56. Mid-Valley Community Centers, Resolution, March 6, 1989, Box 422, Folder 6, MALDEF Records.

57. *McAllen Monitor*, December 2, 1990, 2–3, clipping in Box 422, Folder 6, MALDEF Records.

58. *McAllen Monitor*, December 2, 1990, 2–3, clipping in Box 422, Folder 6, MALDEF Records.

59. Mid-Valley Community Centers, Resolution; Peggy Fikac, "Indigent Care Crisis Looms, Hospitals Say," *McAllen Monitor*, November 22, 1991, 1.

60. Texas Rural Legal Aid to Davis A. Sanders, July 26, 1991, Box 422, Folder 5, MALDEF Records. The US Civil Rights Commission accepted the complaint for investigation, but I have not been able to find a resolution.

61. *McAllen Monitor*, December 2, 1990, 2–3, clipping in Box 422, Folder 6, MALDEF Records.

62. Fikac, "Indigent Care Crisis Looms," 14A.

63. No More Deaths, "Human Rights Abuses of Migrants in Short-Term Custody on the Arizona/Sonora Border," 2008, Box 2, Folder 6, San Francisco Pride at Work Records, San Francisco State University Archives; "About No More Deaths," https://nomoredeaths.org/about-no -more-deaths/.

64. Adam Goodman, *The Deportation Machine* (Princeton, NJ: Princeton University Press, 2021), 176.

65. No More Deaths, "Human Rights Abuses of Migrants in Short-Term Custody"; *No More Deaths/No Más Muertes Volunteer Resource Book*, Summer 2009, Box 2, Folder 6, San Francisco Pride at Work Records.

66. Timothy Egan, "Border Desert Proves Deadly for Mexicans," *New York Times*, May 23, 2004, N1; No More Deaths, "Human Rights Abuses of Migrants"; "About No More Deaths."

67. Susan James, "Health Care Eludes Families in the Shadows," *New York Times*, May 7, 2006, N1.

68. Quoted in Leo R. Chavez, *The Latino Threat: Constructing Immigrants, Citizens, and the Nation* (Stanford, CA: Stanford University Press, 2008), 137–38.

69. Oscar Avila and Antonio Oliva, "A Show of Strength: Thousands March in the Loop for Immigrant Rights," *Chicago Tribune*, March 11, 2006, 1.1.

70. Kim Voss and Irene Bloemraad, *Rallying for Immigrant Rights: The Fight for Inclusion in 21st Century America* (Berkeley: University of California Press, 2011), 15–16. See also Amalia Pallares and Nilda Flores-González, eds., *¡Marcha! Latino Chicago and the Immigrant Rights Movement* (Urbana: University of Illinois Press, 2010).

71. "Reform: Sensenbrenner Stands Firm," *Kenosha News*, June 23, 2006, A4.

72. Voss and Bloemraad, *Rallying for Immigrant Rights*, 16.

73. E.g., Amy Sherman, "Obama Has Mixed Record on Immigration Worksite Enforcement," Politifact, January 6, 2016, https://www.politifact.com/truth-o-meter/promises/obameter /promise/287/crack-down-on-employers-who-hire-undocumented-immi/; "Remarks by the President at Univision Town Hall with Jorge Ramos and Maria Elena Salinas," September 20, 2012, https://obamawhitehouse.archives.gov/the-press-office/2012/09/20/remarks-president -univision-town-hall-jorge-ramos-and-maria-elena-salina; "President Barack Obama's Inaugural Address," https://obamawhitehouse.archives.gov/blog/2009/01/21/president-barack-obamas -inaugural-address.

74. On the debates over Obamacare and the role of the Tea Party, see, e.g., Richard Kirsch, *Fighting for Our Health: The Epic Battle to Make Health Care a Right in the United States* (Albany, NY: Rockefeller Institute Press, 2022).

75. Charlene Galarneau, "Still Missing: Undocumented Immigrants in Health Care Reform," *Journal of Health Care for the Poor and Underserved* 22, no. 2 (2011): 424.

76. Kirsch, *Fighting for Our Health*, Kindle location 4304.

77. Peter Wallsten, "Obama's Shift on Immigrants Stokes Dissent," *Chicago Tribune*, September 16, 2009, 1.13.

78. Kevin Sack, "Issue of Illegal Immigrants," *New York Times*, November 12, 2009.

79. A congressional oversight committee found that a 2005 law requiring proof of citizenship for all Medicaid applicants "had resulted in a decline in . . . recipients" in half of the states surveyed, "and most of those affected were believed to be eligible citizens." James Oliphant, David G. Savage, and Theresa Watanabe, "Health Care Debate Turns to Citizenship," *Chicago Tribune*, September 14, 2009, sec. 1, 4.

80. Kline, *Pathogenic Policing*, chap. 6. Kline points out that the ACA's phasing out of Disproportionate Share Hospital payments would also hurt uninsured immigrants since hospitals would lose a source of reimbursement for their care.

81. Caroline L. Behr, Peter Hull, John Hsu, Joseph P. Newhouse, and Vicki Fung, "Geographic Access to Federally Qualified Health Centers before and after the Affordable Care Act," *BMC Health Services Research* 22 (March 23, 2022): 385.

82. Wallace et al., "Unauthorized Immigrants and Health Care Reform," 21.

83. March video, https://www.youtube.com/watch?v=2TjWf6HC3Ow, Speech excerpts; "Out of the Shadows and into the Streets," March 16, 2010, SocialistWorker.org, https://socialistworker .org/2010/03/16/out-of-the-shadows.

84. Richard Fausset, "Young Migrants Protest Uncertain Fate," *Los Angeles Times*, April 10, 2011, A18.

85. Griselda Nivarez, "Obama Urged to Give DACA Recipients Access to Affordable Health Care," *La Opinión*, October 14, 2014.

86. Osea Giuntella and Jakub Lonsky, "The Effects of DACA on Health Insurance, Access to Care, and Health Outcomes," Discussion Paper Series, IZA Institute of Labor Economics, April 2018.

87. Pratheepan Gulasekaram and S. Karthik Ramakrishnan, *The New Immigration Federalism* (New York: Cambridge University Press, 2015); Human Rights Watch, "No Way to Live: Alabama's Immigration Law," December 14, 2011, https://www.hrw.org/report/2011/12/14/no-way -live/alabamas-immigrant-law.

88. Cesar L. Escalante and Tianyuan Luo, "Stringent Immigration Enforcement and the Mental Health and Health-Risk Behaviors of Hispanic Adolescent Students," Working Paper, Center for Growth and Opportunity at Utah State University, January 2020; Kari White, Valerie A. Yeager, Nir Menachemi, and Isabel C. Scarinci, "Impact of Alabama's Immigration Law on Access to Health Care among Latina Immigrants and Children: Implications for National Reform," *American Journal of Public Health* 104, no. 3 (March 2013): 397–405, also citing additional studies.

89. Medha D. Makhlouf, "Laboratories of Exclusion: Medicaid, Federalism and Immigrants," *New York University Law Review* 95 (2020): 1680–1777, 1710–13.

90. Democratic Party dominance is Makhlouf's observation. For an example of a local legislator committed to immigrant rights, see Patrick McGreevey, "Sen. Ricardo Lara, Point Man in the Push for Immigrant Rights," *Los Angeles Times*, July 27, 2013, latimes.com. For more on local campaigns, see Beatrix Hoffman, "Activism for Undocumented Immigrants' Health Coverage: A Tale of Two States," in *Resistance, Activism, and Social Movements in Health and Health Care*, ed. Ryan Essex, Rita Issa, and James Smith (New York: Oxford University Press, forthcoming).

91. Helen B. Marrow, "The Power of Local Autonomy: Expanding Health Care to Unauthorized Immigrants in San Francisco," *Ethnic and Racial Studies* 35, no. 1 (January 2012): 72–87, 79; A. Elizabeth Iten, Elizabeth A. Jacobs, Maureen Lahiff, and Alicia Fernández, "Undocumented Immigrant Status and Diabetes Care among Mexican Immigrants in Two Immigration 'Sanctuary' Areas," *Journal of Immigrant and Minority Health* 16 (2014): 229–38.

92. See., e.g., Catherine Ceniza Choy, *Empire of Care: Nursing and Migration in Filipino American History* (Durham, NC: Duke University Press, 2002); Eram Alam, "Cold War Crises: Foreign Medical Graduates Respond to US Doctor Shortages, 1965–1975," *Social History of Medicine* 33, no. 1 (2018): 132–51; E. E. Glaessel-Brown, "Use of Immigration Policy to Manage Nursing Shortages," *Image: The Journal of Nursing Scholarship* 30, no. 4 (1999): 323–27.

93. New Latthivongskorn biography: Mark Tuschman, "Immigrants Are Us," https://www .immigrantsareus.org/immigrant-bios/new_latthivongskorn/.

94. https://www.phdreamers.org; Gabrielle Redford, "DACA Students Risk Everything to Become Doctors," aamc.org, September 17, 2019, https://www.aamc.org/news-insights/daca -students-risk-everything-become-doctors; National Conference of State Legislatures, "Professional and Occupational Licenses for Immigrants," January 17, 2017, https://www.ncsl.org /immigration/professional-and-occupational-licenses-for-immigrants.

95. Muzaffar Chishti, Sarah Pierce, and Jessica Bolter, "The Obama Record on Deportations: Deporter in Chief or Not?," *Migration Information Source*, January 25, 2017, https:// www.migrationpolicy.org/article/obama-record-deportations-deporter-chief-or-not#:~:text= Barack%20Obama%20was%20famously%20labeled,being%20soft%20on%20unauthorized%20 immigrants.

96. Alden Woods, "A Phoenix Health Clinic Offers Hope for People with No Insurance, No Access to Care," *Arizona Republic*, June 21, 2017, https://www.azcentral.com/story/news /local/phoenix-best-reads/2017/06/21/phoenix-allies-community-health-free-clinic/315473001/. Phoenix Allies for Community Health was founded by anti-SB1070 activists in 2010. *Salud Sin Papeles: Health Undocumented* is a 2020 documentary film about the clinic; https://vimeo.com /ondemand/healthundocumentedfilm.

97. Joseph Nwadiuko, Jashalynn German, Kavita Chapla, Frances Wang, Maya Venkata-rama, Dhananjay Vaidya, and Sarah Polk, "Changes in Health Care Use among Undocumented Patients, 2014–2018," *JAMA Network Open* 4, no. 3 (2021).

98. Nicole Rodriguez, "Key Detail Changes in Saga of 10-Year-Old Girl Detained by Im-migration Officials after Surgery," *Newsweek*, November 17, 2017; "Among Other Outrages, Im-migration Agents Arrest Newborn's Parents at Texas Hospital," America's Voice Press Release, September 21, 2017, https://americasvoice.org/press_releases/among-outrages-immigration -agents-arrest-newborns-parents-texas-hospital/; Tom Dart, "Salvadoran Asylum Seeker with Brain Tumor Seized from Texas Hospital," *Guardian*, February 24, 2017.

99. Officials had actually started implementing the zero tolerance policy in the El Paso bor-der sector in mid-2017. Separations also continued after the Trump policy was officially ended on June 20. A smaller number of family separations also occurred under the Obama administra-tion. Southern Poverty Law Center, "Family Separation: A Timeline," March 23, 2022, https:// www.splcenter.org/news/2022/03/23/family-separation-timeline.

100. Dr. M. Carballo to Dr. O. W. Christenson, April 25, 1979, M5-372-4 Co-ordination with UN on the protection of social and human rights of migrant workers, Jacket No. 2, World Health Organization Archives, Geneva, Switzerland; "Report of the DHS Advisory Committee on Family Residential Centers," September 30, 2016; Nick Cumming-Bruce, "U.N. Rights Head 'Shocked' by Treatment of Migrant Children at U.S. Border," *New York Times*, July 8, 2019; Hajar Habbach, Kathryn Hampton, and Ranit Mishori, "'You Will Never See Your Child Again: The Persistent Psychological Effects of Family Separation," February 25, 2020, https://phr.org/our -work/resources/you-will-never-see-your-child-again-the-persistent-psychological-effects-of -family-separation/.

101. Wendy E. Parmet, "The Trump Administration's New Public Charge Rule: Implications for Health Care and Public Health," *Health Affairs*, August 13, 2019; Janet M. Calvo, "Trump Order Mandating Deportation for Health Service Use: Not Legally Sufficient," *American Journal of Public Health* 107, no. 8 (August 2017): 1240–41; Leslie Berestein Rojas, "Thousands of LA Immigrant Families Are No Longer Enrolled in Public Benefits. A Pending Trump Rule Could Be Why," *LAist*, August 2, 2019, https://laist.com/news/thousands-of-la-immigrant-families-are -no-longer-enrolled-in-public-benefits-a-pending-trump-rule-co. The final rule was not issued until August 2019.

102. Michael Ollove, "New Trump Rule on Medical Interpreters Could Leave Immigrants Behind," *Stateline* (Pew Memorial Trust), August 29, 2019, https://www.pewtrusts.org/en /research-and-analysis/blogs/stateline/2019/08/29/new-trump-rule-on-medical-interpreters -could-leave-immigrants-behind. The right to interpreter services in hospitals is based in several federal laws and regulations: Title VI of the 1964 Civil Rights Act banning discrimination on the basis of national origin; Bill Clinton's 2000 Executive Order mandating "meaningful access" to federally funded services for persons with limited English proficiency; and several sections (1001, 1331, and 1557) of the 2009 Affordable Care Act. "A Quick Primer on Affordable Care Act Language Service Requirements," Language Scientific, 2024, https://www.languagescientific.com /a-quick-primer-on-affordable-care-act-language-service-requirements/.

103. "By the President of the United States of America, A Proclamation," Office of the Press Secretary, October 4, 2019, https://www.politico.com/f/?id=0000016d-9904-dbde-a17d -9dc451db0001. Since Trump also attempted to rescind the Affordable Care Act, his concern to protect health care benefits for US citizens was rhetorical only.

104. Sarah Jones, "Stephen Miller Sure Seems Like a White Nationalist," *New York Magazine*, November 12, 2019, https://nymag.com/intelligencer/2019/11/stephen-miller-may-be-even-more

-racist-than-previously-known.html; Southern Poverty Law Center, "Stephen Miller's Affinity for White Nationalist Revealed in Leaked Emails," November 12, 2019, https://www.splcenter .org/hatewatch/2019/11/12/stephen-millers-affinity-white-nationalism-revealed-leaked-emails ?gclid=CjwKCAiAuK3vBRBOEiwA1IMhusH_Uip87MxEQv2IJYmeZ8qtxXOWWvjP24MlcTUk KaU3CW9YcJeqNBoC57YQAvD_BwE.

105. Jessica Guynn, "Facebook Fundraiser to Help Immigrant Children Tops $20 Million with Global Donations," *USA Today*, June 24, 2018; Ranit Mishori, "Why I Wore My White Doctor's Coat to Protest Family Separation and Detention," *USA Today*, July 18, 2018. See also Matthias Gaffni, "Doctors, Nurses Protest ICE, Trump Immigration Policies," *San Francisco Chronicle*, August 26, 2019; Bonnie Castillo, "Nurses March on ICE, Child Internment Camps to Say 'Zero Tolerance' Immigration Policy Is a Public Health Crisis," National Nurses United Blog, June 25, 2018, https://www.nationalnursesunited.org/blog/nurses-march-ice-child-internment-camps -say-zero-tolerance-immigration-policy-public-health-crisis.

106. Jeff Gammage, "Immigrant Avoids Deportation, Goes to Long-Term Care," *Philadelphia Daily News*, August 31, 2020, A12; Lisa Schenker, "Cook County to Start Program to Help Uninsured Get Health Care," *Chicago Tribune*, September 14, 2016; Community Catalyst, "Illinois Case Study: A State Campaign to Expand Health Coverage to Noncitizen Older Adults," April 2022, https://www.communitycatalyst.org/resources/publications/document/Illinois-Case -Study.pdf; Bobby Allyn, "California Is 1st State to Offer Health Benefits to Adult Undocumented Immigrants," NPR, July 10, 2019, https://www.npr.org/2019/07/10/740147546/california-first -state-to-offer-health-benefits-to-adult-undocumented-immigrants; Hoffman, "Activism for Undocumented Immigrants' Health Coverage."

107. Alexander Bolton, "All Candidates Raise Hands on Giving Health Care to Undocumented Immigrants," *Hill*, June 27, 2019, https://thehill.com/homenews/campaign/450797-all -candidates-raise-hands-on-giving-health-care-to-undocumented-immigrants/.

Epilogue

1. Examples: Kimberley M. Horner, Elizabeth Wrigley-Field, and Jonathon P. Leider, "A First Look: Disparities in COVID-19 Mortality among U.S. and Foreign-Born Minnesota Residents," *Population Research Policy Review* 41, no. 2 (2022): 465–78; Esther Yoon-Ji Kang, Natalie Moore, and María Inés Zamudio, "50 Lives in 4 ZIP Codes," WBEZ Chicago, August 17, 2020, https:// www.wbez.org/stories/a-perfect-storm-50-lives-and-4-zip-codes-tell-chicagos-story-of-covid -19-inequality/50b822ae-523e-47fa-a823-3c6a1c3ee12f; Lan N. Doan, Stella K. Chong, Supriya Misra, Simona C. Kwon, and Stella S. Yi, "Immigrant Communities and Covid-19: Strengthening the Public Health Response," *American Journal of Public Health* 111, S3 (October 2021): S169–S232. Because of unreliable or nonexistent (due to the end of the public health emergency) data, I do not attempt to provide a definitive number or percentage of immigrant deaths or infections due to COVID.

2. Rebecca Solnit, "'The Way We Get through This Is Together': The Rise of Mutual Aid under Coronavirus," *Guardian*, May 14, 2020; Chinese Progressive Association, "Mutual Aid in the Time of Covid-19," https://cpasf.org/updates/mutual-aid/; Lizzie Tribone, "Mutual Aid, for and by Undocumented Immigrants," *American Prospect*, https://prospect.org/coronavirus/mutual-aid -for-and-by-undocumented-immigrants/. Cash funds ran out quickly due to the very high demand. Some states and localities also offered small grants to residents regardless of citizenship.

3. Maira Khwaja, Trina Reynolds-Tyler, Dominique James, and Hannah Nyhart, "Our Year of Mutual Aid," *New York Times*, March 11, 2021.

4. Food Chain Workers Alliance, "We Are Not Disposable: Food Workers Organizing on the Covid Frontlines," February 2023, https://foodchainworkers.org/wp-content/uploads/2021/02 /Food-Workers-Organizing-on-the-COVID-Frontlines-FINAL.pdf; Marta Martinez, "In Their Own Words: 5 Latina Immigrant Housekeepers on How the Pandemic Has Impacted Their Lives," *Washington Post*, October 6, 2021, https://www.washingtonpost.com/gender-identity /in-their-own-words-5-latina-immigrant-housekeepers-on-how-the-pandemic-has-impacted -their-lives/.

5. Taylor Telford, "Covid Cases and Deaths Grossly Underestimated among Meatpackers, House Investigation Finds," *Washington Post*, October 27, 2021.

6. Laurel Ramsley, "Tyson Foods Fires 7 Plant Managers over Betting Ring on Workers Getting COVID-19," NPR.org, December 16, 2020; Matt Sebastian, "Feds Hit JBS Plant with $15,000 Fine for Failing to Protect Greeley Plant Workers from Covid-19," *Denver Post*, January 11, 2020; Araceli Cruz, "Lawsuit: Tyson Managers Took Bets on How Many Employees Would Get Covid," Americano News, November 19, 2020, https://theamericanonews.com/2020/11/19/tyson -covid/.

7. Shefali Milczarek-Desai, "Opening the Pandemic Portal to Re-Imagine Paid Sick Leave for Immigrant Workers," Arizona Legal Studies Discussion Paper no. 22-04, February 2022; Jennifer Tolbert, "What Issues Will Uninsured People Face with Testing and Treatment for COVID-19?," KFF.org, March 16, 2020, https://www.kff.org/coronavirus-covid-19/fact-sheet/what-issues-will -uninsured-people-face-with-testing-and-treatment-for-covid-19/.

8. Jane Spencer (*Guardian*) and Christina Jewett, "12 Months of Trauma: More than 3,600 US Health Care Workers Died in Covid's First Year," Kaiser Health News, April 8, 2021, https:// khn.org/news/article/us-health-workers-deaths-covid-lost-on-the-frontline/; https://www .asianjournal.com/usa/dateline-usa/report-83-filipino-registered-nurses-in-the-us-have-died-of -covid-19/; National Nurses United, "Nurses Condemn Biden Administration for Ripping Away Protections from Health Care Workers, Patients," December 28, 2021, https://www.national nursesunited.org/press/nurses-condemn-biden-administration-for-ripping-away-protections -for-health-care-workers.

9. Caitlin Dickerson and Michael D. Shear, "Before Covid-19, Trump Aide Sought to Use Disease to Close Borders," *New York Times*, May 3, 2020; "Covid 'Hate Crimes' against Asian Americans on Rise," BBC News, May 21, 2021; Jasmine Aguilera, "Biden Is Expelling Migrants on COVID-19 Grounds, but Health Experts Say That's All Wrong," *Time*, October 12, 2021.

10. By July of 2020, "11 countries have confirmed that deportees returned home with Covid-19." Emily Kassie and Barbara Marconi, "'It Was Like a Time Bomb': How ICE Helped Spread the Coronavirus," *New York Times*, July 10, 2020; Renuka Rayasam, "Shelter Sickness: Migrants See Health Problems Linger and Worsen While Waiting at the Border," CBS News, August 15, 2022.

11. "1,300 Medical Professionals from 49 U.S. States and Territories Call on CDC to End 'Junk Science' Border Expulsion Policy," Press Release, Physicians for Human Rights, October 28, 2021, https://phr.org/our-work/resources/u-s-medical-professionals-demand-cdc-end -title-42/; Kirk Siegler, "There Are Protests along the US-Mexico Border after Judge Blocks Ending Title 42," NPR News/Morning Edition, May 25, 2022, https://www.npr.org/2022/05/25 /1101141269/there-are-protests-along-the-u-s-mexico-border-after-judge-blocks-ending-title-4; Haitian Bridge Alliance, UndocuBlack Network, and Quixote Center, *The Invisible Wall: Title 42 and Its Impact on Haitian Migrants* (2021).

12. Brett Samuels, "Trump Says That Undocumented Immigrants Can Get Tested for Coronavirus without Fear of Deportation," *Hill*, March 22, 2020, https://thehill.com/homenews /administration/488940-trump-says-undocumented-immigrants-can-get-tested-for-coronavirus/.

13. "DHS Statement on Equal Access to Covid-19 Vaccines and Vaccine Distribution Sites," February 1, 2021, https://www.dhs.gov/news/2021/02/01/dhs-statement-equal-access-covid-19 -vaccines-and-vaccine-distribution-sites.

14. Rima Abelkader, Sara Mhaidli, and Carmen Sesin, "'A Death Sentence': Activists Call on Florida Governor to Prioritize Vaccines for Farmworkers," NBC News, February 11, 2021, https://www.nbcnews.com/news/latino/death-sentence-activists-call-florida-governor-prioritize -vaccines-farmworkers-n1257204.

15. Dulce Gonzalez, Michael Karpman, and Hamutal Bernstein, "COVID-19 Attitudes among Adults in Immigrant Families in California," Urban Institute, April 2021, https://www .urban.org/sites/default/files/publication/103973/covid-19-vaccine-attitudes-among-adults-in -immigrant-families-in-california_0_0.pdf; Liz Hamel, Samantha Artiga, Alaunda Safarpour, Mellisha Stokes, and Mollyann Brodie, "COVID-19 Vaccine Access, Information, and Experiences among Hispanic Adults in the U.S.," KFF COVID-19 Vaccine Monitor, May 13, 2021, https://www.kff.org/coronavirus-covid-19/poll-finding/kff-covid-19-vaccine-monitor-access -information-experiences-hispanic-adults/.

16. Katelynn Laws, "Community Organizers Are Helping Immigrants Navigate COVID Misinformation," *Yes Magazine*, December 15, 2021, https://www.yesmagazine.org/social-justice /2021/12/15/covid-misinformation-immigrants-community-organizers; Mauricio Peña, "After 17 Months of Battling Coronavirus, Hard-Hit Gage Park Gets Vaccination Site: 'It's a Game-Changer,'" Block Club Chicago, February 17, 2021, https://blockclubchicago.org/2021/02/17 /after-11-months-of-battling-coronavirus-hard-hit-gage-park-gets-vaccination-site-its-a-game -changer/; "Covid-19 Vaccine Doses by Zip Code—At Least One Dose," Chicago Data Portal, https://data.cityofchicago.org/Health-Human-Services/COVID-19-Vaccine-Doses-by-ZIP-Code -At-Least-One-Do/c28u-q29v; Laura Rodríguez Presa, "As COVID-19 Vaccines Arrive in Chicago's Hard-Hit Latino Communities, Hope Is Revived but Outreach to Spanish-Speakers and Skeptics Still Needed," *Chicago Tribune*, March 4, 2021.

17. Beatrix Hoffman and Dana Yarak, "La Primera Línea: Latina/o Frontline Health Workers during COVID-19's First Wave," *U.S. Latino and Latina Oral History Journal* 5 (2021): 10–32; "Meet the U.S. Scientist Who Invented the N95 Mask Filter," US Embassy in Georgia, August 12, 2020, https://ge.usembassy.gov/meet-the-u-s-scientist-who-invented-the-n95-mask-filter/; "The Impact of Immigrants on Health Care in the United States," Immigrant Learning Center, May 6, 2022, https://www.ilctr.org/the-impact-of-immigrants-on-health-care-in-the-united-states/.

18. "Immigrant Essential Workers Are Crucial to America's COVID-19 Recovery," FWD .us, December 16, 2020, https://www.fwd.us/news/immigrant-essential-workers/; https://www .americanprogress.org/article/immigrants-essential-workers-covid-19/ .

19. Senator Dick Durbin Floor Speech, December 20, 2022, https://www.facebook.com /watch/live/?extid=CL-UNK-UNK-UNK-IOS_GK0T-GK1C&mibextid=2Rb1fB&ref=watch _permalink&v=833094887955273. A photo of Flores is in chapter 7.

20. Devon Link, "Fact Check: House Bill Would Only Temporarily Protect Essential Workers in U.S. Legally," *USA Today*, May 19, 2020, https://www.usatoday.com/story/news /factcheck/2020/05/19/fact-check-bill-temporarily-protects-essential-undocumented-workers /5203282002/.

21. Sofya Aptekar and Miriam Ticktin, "Must Immigrants Sacrifice Themselves to COVID-19 for Basic Rights?," OpenDemocracy, February 6, 2021, https://www.opendemocracy.net/en /must-immigrants-sacrifice-themselves-covid-19-basic-rights/.

22. Beatrix Hoffman, "Expendable Workers and the Statecraft of Mass Death," keynote address, Pandemics and the State Conference, University College London, July 5, 2022.

23. Although it has not been covered in this book, another example of how borders shape health care access is medical tourism: for example, when US citizens travel to Mexico for cheaper medical and dental care and prescription drugs or to Canada for cheaper prescription drugs.

24. The Care Collective (Andreas Chatzidakis, Jamie Hakim, Jo Litter, and Catherine Rottenberg), *The Care Manifesto* (London: Verso Books, 2020), 5 (spelling Americanized). I continue to learn from activists and thinkers who are developing powerful analyses of borders and care. E.g., Harsha Walia, "There Is No 'Migrant Crisis,'" *Boston Review*, November 16, 2022; Beatrice Adler-Bolton and Artie Vierkant, *Health Communism* (London: Verso Books, 2022); Premilla Nadasen, *Care: The Highest Stage of Capitalism* (Chicago: Haymarket Books, 2023); Eithne Luibhéid and Karma R. Chávez, *Queer and Trans Migrations: Dynamics of Illegalization, Detention, and Deportation* (Urbana and Chicago: University of Illinois Press, 2020); Silky Shah, *Unbuild Walls: Why Immigrant Justice Needs Abolition* (Chicago: Haymarket, 2024)

25. E.g., "What It Means That We Shut Down Homestead Detention Center," American Friends Service Committee, November 1, 2019, https://afsc.org/news/what-it-means-we-shut-down-homestead-detention-center; Jeff Gammage, "Berks Immigrant Detention Center to Close," *Philadelphia Inquirer*, November 30, 2022; Carlos Ballesteros, "Illinois Just Ended ICE Detention," Injustice Watch, February 16, 2022, https://www.injusticewatch.org/news/immigration/2022/illinois-ice-detention-ended/.

Index

Page numbers in italics refer to figures.